Delmar's Dental Assisting Exam Review

MELISSA THIBODEAUX, CDA, RDA, BS
San Joaquin Valley College, Inc.

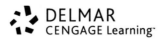
DELMAR
CENGAGE Learning™

Australia • Brazil • Japan • Korea • Mexico • Singapore • Spain • United Kingdom • United States

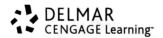

Delmar's Dental Assisting Exam Review
Melissa Thibodeaux

For product information and technology assistance, contact us at
Cengage Learning Customer & Sales Support, 1-800-354-9706
For permission to use material from this text or product,
submit all requests online at **www.cengage.com/permissions**
Further permissions questions can be emailed to
permissionrequest@cengage.com

Library of Congress Control Number: 98-55682

ISBN-13: 978-0-8273-9071-3

ISBN-10: 0-8273-9071-8

Delmar
Executive Woods
5 Maxwell Drive
Clifton Park, NY 12065
USA

Cengage Learning is a leading provider of customized learning solutions with office locations around the globe, including Singapore, the United Kingdom, Australia, Mexico, Brazil, and Japan. Locate your local office at **international.cengage.com/region**

Cengage Learning products are represented in Canada by Nelson Education, Ltd.

For your lifelong learning solutions, visit **www.cengage.com/delmar**

Visit our corporate website at **www.cengage.com**

Notice to the Reader
Publisher does not warrant or guarantee any of the products described herein or perform any independent analysis in connection with any of the product information contained herein. Publisher does not assume, and expressly disclaims, any obligation to obtain and include information other than that provided to it by the manufacturer. The reader is expressly warned to consider and adopt all safety precautions that might be indicated by the activities described herein and to avoid all potential hazards. By following the instructions contained herein, the reader willingly assumes all risks in connection with such instructions. The publisher makes no representations or warranties of any kind, including but not limited to, the warranties of fitness for particular purpose or merchantability, nor are any such representations implied with respect to the material set forth herein, and the publisher takes no responsibility with respect to such material. The publisher shall not be liable for any special, consequential, or exemplary damages resulting, in whole or part, from the readers' use of, or reliance upon, this material.

Printed in the United States of America
9 10 11 12 13   14 13 12 11 10

ED306

DEDICATION

This text is dedicated to all of the dental assistants who are committed to total patient care—and to Ron and Jordan, without whose support this manual would not have been possible.

Contents

Preface

The purpose of this manual is to assist you in preparing for the Dental Assisting National Board Examination or other dental assisting exams that you may encounter in your dental assisting career. Whether you are a dental assisting student preparing to take the Dental Assisting National Board of Examination or a seasoned assistant interested in expanding your credentials, this manual will be an invaluable tool for studying and reviewing basic dental assisting information. This review manual is arranged in an outline format to enable you to easily review dental assisting material that will appear on the Dental Assisting National Board Examination. The beginning of the chapter outlines the material that will be covered, and the end-of-chapter questions are available to assist you in reviewing. Whatever method you choose to study for the Dental Assisting National Board Examination, the most important concept to keep in mind is that reviewing should be a way to refresh already-learned concepts.

Acknowledgments

It takes many people working together, doing their own specialized tasks, to create a quality textbook. This project is a perfect example of the skills, timing, and individual effort that are involved in creating a quality product. The following people were instrumental in making this a success:

To Linda DeMasi, Project Manager, your experience and knowledge when it comes to the demands of producing a manuscript are flawless. Thank you for making this such a great experience.

To the professional staff at Delmar, for taking me from the beginning to the end and providing every resource to keep our objectives on task.

I would like to thank the following reviewers who made the commitment to look over the manuscript and gave me some great advice and professional guidance.

Lori Burch, RDA
   Corinthian College
   Reseda, California

Robin Caplan, CDA, EFDA, DRT
   Medix School
   Owings Mills, Maryland

Ellen Dietz, CDA, AAS, BS
   Mesa, Arizona

Darlene Hunziker, CDA, RDA
   Eton Technical Institute
   Everett, Washington

Fred Rich
   Gwinett School of Dental Assisting
   Liburn, Georgia

To Jeff Gordon, my fellow coworker and friend, for opening the door to being published.

And, finally, to Ron Campbell, for his ability to give quick reference information about anatomy and physics. His skills as "Mr. Mom" when it came to Jordan allowed me to spend many hours at the computer working on this project. You are my best friend and you are appreciated.

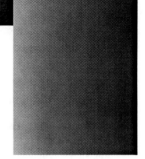

Study Techniques

When it comes to taking a test, we all get a little anxious. We wouldn't be human if we didn't. There is no substitute for knowledge. To pass a test successfully, you must simply know the material you are being tested on. However, there are some strategies that you can follow to help increase the probability of passing with a higher score.

MULTIPLE-CHOICE QUESTIONS

The Certified Dental Assistant Examination (CDA) may contain questions known as A-type and K-type questions.

A-Type Questions
(one best answer)

A-type questions are multiple-choice questions that consist of a stem and four or five lettered response options: three or four distractors and "one best answer." It is helpful to remember the following tips when answering these types of questions:

1. Read the question thoroughly before answering.
2. Try not to read into the question. It is better to just read it and take it the way it is written. By the same token, do not omit any information.
3. Before reviewing the options, try to answer the question in your head.
4. If you cannot determine the answer on your own or the answer is not one of the options available, try to eliminate the answers you know are not correct.
5. Always go with your first choice. Never go back and change an answer unless you know with certainty that it is incorrect. Chances are your initial response is the most accurate.
6. When completing questions that are sentences, eliminate the grammatically incorrect options.

7. Do not choose an option that is partially true or partially false.
8. Questions regarding patient care that imply all is well, a lack of professionalism, or deny patient feelings are usually distractors and should be avoided.
9. Pay close attention to words that are capitalized, italicized, underlined, or in bold type.
10. Never leave anything blank. Blanks are automatically wrong answers. When all else fails, just guess. There is a one in four or five chance that you will be right.

If you are totally perplexed by a question, mark it and come back to it. Chances are you will read other questions containing similar material that could jog your memory.

Other approaches may include the following:

1. Choose one of two options that are similar except for a word or two.
2. Choose one of two options that sound or look familiar.
3. Choose the answer that is most complex or wordy.

If you are still bewildered, guess! There is no penalty for guessing. But if you do, be sure to guess the same letter each time because this, too, will increase the probability of a right answer.

K-Type Questions (complex multiple choice)

K-type questions are the most complex of the multiple-choice questions. These questions contain more than one right answer in the choices and are a favorite on this type of exam. They contain a stem and four numbered words or phrases, as shown in the following example:

The oral cavity contains which of the following?

1. Tongue
2. Hard palate
3. Dentition
4. Sinuses

A. if only 1, 2, and 3 are correct.
B. if only 1 and 3 are correct.
C. if only 1 and 4 are correct.
D. if all are correct.

The correct answer is A.

The best way to tackle this type of question is to look at all of the answers. Mark with your pencil the answers that you know with certainty are not correct. Then using these numbers, look at the options and circle the corresponding answers containing those numbers. By process of elimination, you should be able to get the correct combination.

True-False Questions

True-false questions should be answered carefully. Remember, if any part of the question as stated is false, the whole question should be regarded as false and marked appropriately. Also, if the words "always," "never," "all," and "none" are used, this will generally make the statement false.

Fill in the Blank

To correctly complete a sentence or phrase, a question is asked and it is up to you to choose the correct word or phrase to fill in the blank. These are sometimes the toughest questions because they require complete knowledge of the subject. As with essay questions, you must know the material completely to successfully answer the question correctly.

Identifying

You may be asked to identify certain items on the CDA such as radiographs, instruments, or oral hygiene aids. These questions are strictly clinical in nature and should not be a problem for the experienced dental assistant. However, before the exam, go through your textbooks and the office if possible and refamiliarize yourself with your clinical surroundings.

Negative Format

Negative format questions are designed to force the candidate to choose the one answer that does not fit. The choices that are available are correct except for one. It's just the reverse of choosing one best answer.

Matching

You may be asked to match certain terms or concepts with their definitions. These questions are routine and usually grouped by subjects. For example, all questions will be about one subject such as radiographs or infection control protocols.

Attitude

Attitude is probably the number one area that gets us in trouble. It doesn't matter whether you pass this exam on the first try. What matters is that you have studied and put forth the effort to sit for it. Failing is not a measure of self-worth—it means only that receiving your CDA is postponed. If you do not pass, you know what needs to be done next time. It will help you to define what areas you need to study more. You will be better prepared the second time around because you know what to expect from the exam. Keeping a positive attitude will make the difference. Talk to yourself. Tell yourself you are ready mentally and that you have the knowledge to successfully pass this exam. You know the material. You work around it every day, and taking this exam will only validate this fact. If, on the other hand, you have not been in the field on a steady basis and have not really studied, go ahead and take the exam and do the very best you can. If for some reason you don't pass the exam, don't make excuses about why you didn't study or that you weren't given enough time to take the test. This will only make the situation worse and could lead to feelings of low self-esteem. Instead, take control of the situation and remind yourself that you will be better prepared next time. Keep telling yourself that you are a competent dental assistant and that this exam is worth taking and passing.

TIPS TO REMEMBER
BEFORE TAKING THE EXAM

1. Get plenty of rest the night before.
2. Eat before taking the exam. Even if it's a light meal, you will need something in your stomach to get you through the four hours it will take to complete the exam.
3. Relax. Take a deep breath and remind yourself that you know the material.
4. Bring at least two sharpened pencils and possibly a small pencil sharpener.
5. Bring a valid form of identification and any registration material that was sent to you. You must present this before taking the exam.
6. Wear something comfortable.
7. Set your alarm at least 30 minutes ahead of time so that you can get to the testing facility a few minutes early.
8. If it is possible, drive by the test site the day before the test if you are not familiar with the location.
9. Don't pick the night before to cram for the test.

USING THIS REVIEW MANUAL

This study guide provides you with a comprehensive outline format and questions at the end of each chapter for your review. It is best to review the chapter, and then using a separate sheet of paper, answer the questions at the end of the chapter. After correcting the review questions, go over the questions that were missed. In a couple of days, go back to the questions and test yourself again. If you find that you continue to miss the same questions, look for an approved textbook to brush up on that particular area. Do not rely on the review manual as your sole source of reference when taking this national exam. The Dental Assisting National Board uses many sources when compiling examination questions. Use other materials to refresh your memory on certain aspects of dental assisting. Refer to the appendices of this book for approved sources for study.

CHAPTER 2

Basic Oral Anatomy

CHAPTER OVERVIEW

This chapter outlines structures of the oral cavity, cranial and facial bones, head and neck musculature, nerve innervation, and tooth morphology and histology.

KEY TERMS

alveolar process

attachment apparatus

cranial bones

cranial nerves

deciduous teeth

facial bones

frenum

frontal sinuses

gag reflex

hard palate

lining mucosa

masticatory mucosa

maxillary sinuses

soft palate

I. INTRODUCTION

A. Dental anatomy is defined as the scientific study of the structures and functions of the oral cavity and maxillofacial components.

B. The dentition or two dental arches make up one *set* of teeth.
   1. Two dental arches
      a. Maxilla—upper arch.
      b. Mandible—lower arch.
   2. Deciduous teeth, also known as primary teeth, are the first set of dentition that begins to emerge into the mouth between the sixth and eighth month of life. There are 20 teeth in the human primary dentition. By the age of 2½ to 3 years, all deciduous teeth have erupted and at about 6 years, the permanent teeth start to erupt. Primary dentition has no premolars or third molars. Following is a listing of the growth development pattern for deciduous teeth:
      a. Mandibular central incisors: 6 months.
      b. Mandibular lateral incisors: 7 months.
      c. Maxillary central incisors: 7½ months.
      d. Maxillary lateral incisors: 8 months.
      e. Mandibular first molars: 12–16 months.
      f. Maxillary first molars: 14 months.
      g. Mandibular cuspids: 16 months.
      h. Maxillary cuspids: 18 months.
      i. Mandibular second molars: 20 months.
      j. Maxillary second molars: 24 months.

3. Permanent dentition takes the place of lost deciduous teeth. There are 32 teeth in the permanent human dentition. Following is a listing of the growth development pattern for permanent teeth:
   a. Mandibular first molars: 6–7 years.
   b. Maxillary first molars: 6–7 years.
   c. Mandibular central incisors: 6–7 years.
   d. Mandibular lateral incisors: 7–8 years.
   e. Maxillary central incisors: 7–8 years.
   f. Maxillary lateral incisors: 8–9 years.
   g. Mandibular cuspids: 9–10 years.
   h. Maxillary first premolars: 10–11 years.
   i. Mandibular first premolars: 10–12 years.
   j. Maxillary second premolars: 11–12 years.
   k. Mandibular second premolars: 11–12 years.
   l. Maxillary cuspids: 11–12 years.
   m. Mandibular second molars: 11–13 years.
   n. Maxillary second molars: 12–13 years.
   o. Third molars: 17–21 years.

II. STRUCTURES OF THE ORAL CAVITY

A. The oral cavity is the inner portion of the mouth that contains the dentition and the hard and soft tissues. The oral cavity includes the palate, or roof of the mouth; the alveolar ridges; the tongue and its musculature; and the opening of the lips and throat, or oropharynx.

B. Oral mucosa and gingival tissue
   1. Masticatory mucosa covers the areas subject to stress such as gingival tissue and the hard palate.
   2. Specialized mucosa covers the area that has the specific function of taste on the dorsum of the tongue.
   3. Lining mucosa covers all other areas of the oral cavity such as the inner surfaces of the lips and cheeks and the floor and roof of the mouth.
   4. Attached gingiva extends from the free gingival groove, which demarcates it from the free or marginal gingivae, to the mucogingival junction, which separates it from the alveolar mucosa. This tissue is firm and dense and tightly bound down to the underlining periosteum, tooth, and bone.
   5. Free gingiva is the unattached coronal portion of the gingiva that encircles the tooth to form the gingival sulcus.

C. Structures inside the oral cavity
   1. Palate is the concave surface that is known as the roof of the mouth.
      a. Hard palate: The bony anterior two-thirds of the palate that is covered with mucosa.
      b. Soft palate: The posterior third of the palate, made up of muscular fibers covered with mucosa.
      c. Rugae: The irregular ridges that cover the anterior portion of the hard palate.
      d. Uvula: The pendent fleshy mass that is suspended in the back of the throat.
      e. Frenum: A fold of mucous membrane attaching the cheeks, lips, and tongue to the floor of the mouth.
         (1) Buccal frenum: The fold of tissue attaching the cheek to the alveolar ridge near the second premolar.
         (2) Labial frenum: The fold of tissue attaching the lip to the alveolar ridge near the midline.
         (3) Lingual frenum: The fold of tissue attaching the tongue to the floor of the mouth.
      f. Tongue: The muscular organ that is the main articulatory element in the production of speech and accounts for the clarity and fluidity of speech. The tongue also contains taste buds and is responsible for preparing food for digestion.
      g. Salivary glands: Sets of glands that secrete saliva, which is used to keep the inside of the oral cavity moist. This aids in speech, chewing, and the digestion process and constantly bathes the dentition to wash away debris. These glands are connected by ducts that lead into the oral cavity.

(1) Parotid: Located near the ear, this gland is the largest of the salivary glands. It secretes a serous (clear liquid) substance.
  (a) Stensen's duct is the duct that attaches to the parotid gland.

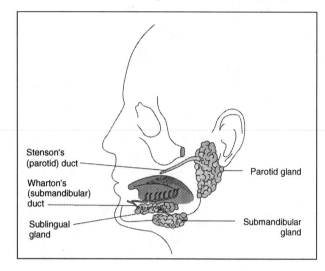

Salivary glands and ducts.

(2) Submandibular: Located on each side of the face and is irregular in shape. This gland lies beneath the mandible and secretes both a serous and mucous (slimy gluelike) secretion.
  (a) Wharton's duct is the duct that attaches to the sub-mandibular gland.
(3) Sublingual: Located beneath the mucous membrane of the floor of the mouth and is primarily mucus-secreting. It is situated on either side of the base of the tongue and is shaped like an almond.
  (a) Ducts of Rivinus are the smaller ducts that attach to the sublingual glands.
  (b) Bartholin's ducts attach to the sublingual glands.

III. CRANIAL BONES

A. There are eight cranial bones that house the brain.
  1. Frontal: Forms the forehead, frontal sinuses, and upper orbits of the eye.
  2. Parietal: Two bones joining at the top to form the roof.
  3. Temporal: Two bones forming the lower sides and floor of the cranium.
  4. Occipital: A single bone forming the inferior posterior wall of the cranium.
  5. Sphenoid: A bat-shaped bone connecting the temporal bones to the floor of the cranium.
  6. Ethmoid: A single bone that forms the superior nasal cavity and posterior orbits of the eye.

IV. FACIAL BONES

A. There are 14 facial bones that make up the maxillofacial area.
  1. Inferior nasal conchae: Two bones that lie in the nasal cavity and are processes of the ethmoid bone.
  2. Vomer: A single bone that forms the inferior portion of the nasal septum.
  3. Lacrimal: Two bones forming the medial orbits.
  4. Zygomatic: Two bones that form the arch of the cheekbone.
  5. Palatine: Two bones that form the hard palate and nasal floor.
  6. Mandible: Lower jawbone.
  7. Maxilla: Two fused bones that form the upper jaw.
  8. Nasal: Two oblong bones that form the bridge of the nose.

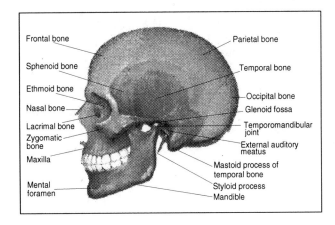

Frontal bone
Sphenoid bone
Ethmoid bone
Nasal bone
Lacrimal bone
Zygomatic bone
Maxilla
Mental foramen
Parietal bone
Temporal bone
Occipital bone
Glenoid fossa
Temporomandibular joint
External auditory meatus
Mastoid process of temporal bone
Styloid process
Mandible

Lateral aspect of the cranium.

V. MUSCLES OF THE HEAD AND NECK

A. Head and neck muscles make it possible to produce movement of the head, neck, and face through contraction and relaxation. These muscles are innervated by cranial nerves and are supplied with blood from the internal and external carotid artery. These muscles are generally suspended between an origin, a fixed structure or end, and an insertion, the movable end. Muscles may give information regarding their origin and insertion. The muscles of the head and neck are divided into eight groups.

    1. Group 1: Muscles of mastication.
    2. Group 2: Suprahyoid muscles.
    3. Group 3: Infrahyoid muscles.
    4. Group 4: Muscles of the tongue.
    5. Group 5: Muscles of facial expression.
    6. Group 6: Muscles of the neck.
    7. Group 7: Muscles of the soft palate.
    8. Group 8: Muscles of the pharynx.

B. Muscles of mastication
    1. They elevate, protrude, retrude, or cause lateral movement of the mandible.
    2. They function during chewing or mastication.
    3. They are innervated by the mandibular branch of the trigeminal nerve (V3).
    4. Blood supply is provided by the maxillary artery.

C. Temporalis muscle
    1. This powerful muscle raises and closes the jaw.
      a. Origin: Temporal fossa of the temporal bone.

      b. Insertion: Coronoid process and the anterior border of the ramus of the mandible.
      c. Innervation: Mandibular division of trigeminal nerve.

D. Masseter muscle
    1. This powerful muscle raises and lowers the jaw during eating. It can be observed when jaws are clenched and has a superficial and deep origin and insertion.
      a. Origin: The superficial part originates from the lower border of the zygomatic arch. The deep part originates from the posterior and medial side of the zygomatic arch.
      b. Insertion: The superficial part inserts on the angle and lower lateral side of the ramus of the mandible. The deep part inserts into the upper lateral ramus and coronoid process of the mandible.
      c. Innervation: Mandibular division of trigeminal nerve.

E. Internal pterygoid
    1. This muscle closes the jaw, creates lateral movement (side to side), and protrudes the jaw (brings forward).
      a. Origin: The medial surface of the lateral pterygoid plate of the sphenoid bone, the palatine bone, and the tuberosity of the maxillary bone.
      b. Insertion: Into the inner surface of the ramus and angle of the mandible.
      c. Innervation: Mandibular division of trigeminal nerve.

F. External pterygoid
    1. This muscle depresses the mandible to open the jaws. It also protrudes and moves them from side to side.
      a. Origin: Originates from two heads. The upper head originates from the greater wing of the sphenoid bone. The lower head originates from the lateral surface of the pterygoid plate of the sphenoid bone.
      b. Insertion: Into the neck of the condyle of the mandible and into the articular disc and capsular ligament of the temporomandibular joint.

c. Innervation: Mandibular division of trigeminal nerve.

G. Suprahyoid muscles
   1. The digastric muscle is a slinglike muscle that has fibers at either end and is connected in the center by an intermediate tendon or sling.
      a. Origin: Anterior belly begins on the digastric fossa of the mandible.
      b. Insertion: Intermediate tendon.
      c. Innvervation: Mandibular branch of the trigeminal nerve.

REVIEW QUESTIONS

1. The frenum is
   A. a narrow band of tissue that connects two structures.
   B. a mucous membrane that lines the entire oral cavity.
   C. the corner of the mouth where the lips join.

2. The gag reflex is the
   A. arch at the back of the mouth.
   B. protective mechanism that prevents foreign objects from entering the throat.
   C. receptor sense for taste.

3. There are _____ bones in the cranium.
   A. 15
   B. 12
   C. 8

4. There are _____ bones in the face.
   A. 15
   B. 22
   C. 14

5. The largest of the salivary glands are
   A. submandibular.
   B. parotid.
   C. sublingual.

6. The glands that lie on the floor of the mouth are the
   A. submandibular.
   B. parotid.
   C. sublingual.

7. The glands that lie on either side of the tongue are called
   A. submandibular.
   B. parotid.
   C. sublingual.

8. The duct that comes off the parotid gland is called
   A. Wharton's duct.
   B. Stensen's duct.
   C. ducts of Rivinus.

9. The duct that comes off of the sublingual gland is called
   A. Wharton's duct.
   B. Stensen's duct.
   C. ducts of Rivinus.

10. Spongy bone is also known as
   A. cortical bone.
   B. cancellous bone.
   C. crustiform bone.

11. Muscle origin is the place where the
   A. muscle ends.
   B. muscle begins.
   C. muscle inserts.

12. Muscle insertion is the place where the
   A. muscle ends.
   B. muscle begins.
   C. muscle originates.

Match the term with the correct definition.

_____ 13. Closes and puckers the lips and is also known as the kissing muscle
_____ 14. Compresses the cheeks against the teeth and retracts the angle of the mouth
_____ 15. Raises and wrinkles the skin of the chin and pushes up the lower lip
_____ 16. Draws the angles of the mouth upward and backward during laughing

   A. Buccinator
   B. Orbicularis oris
   C. Zygomatic major
   D. Mentalis

17. The portion of the tooth covered with enamel is known as the
   A. anatomic crown.
   B. clinical crown.
   C. coronal crown.

18. The substance that covers the root of the tooth is called
   A. periodontal ligament.
   B. cementum.
   C. dentin.

19. The cervix or neck of the tooth
    A. is where the enamel and cementum join.
    B. is the narrow area of the tooth where the crown and the root join.
    C. makes up the anatomical crown.

20. The root of the tooth is not
    A. embedded into the alveolar process.
    B. covered with dentin.
    C. bifurcated or trifurcated.

21. The enamel
    1. makes up the anatomical crown.
    ~~2. is the hardest substance in the body.~~
    ~~es of up to~~

25. Cuspids
    1. are designed to tear and cut food.
    2. have sharp edges.
    3. are also called canines.
    4. are referred to as the cornerstone of the dental arch.

    A. 1, 2, 3
    B. 1, 2, 4
    C. 1, 3
    D. All of the above

26. Incisors
    1. are single rooted.
    2. are located in the anterior portion of the mouth.
    3. have thin sharp edges for tearing.
    4. are located on both maxillary and mandibular arches.

    A. 1, 2, 3
    B. 1, 2, 4
    C. 1 only
    D. All of the above

27. The occlusal surface is
    A. the anterior chewing surface of the dentition.
    B. located on the molars only.
    C. the broad chewing surface of the posterior teeth.
    D. the axial surface of the posterior teeth.

28. There are _____ teeth in the primary dentition.
    A. 24
    B. 20
    C. 32
    D. 16

29. There are no _____ in the primary dentition.
    A. first molars
    B. cuspids
    C. premolars
    D. second molars

30. The permanent dentition consists of _____ teeth.
    A. 32
    B. 30
    C. 36
    D. 24

ANSWERS AND RATIONALES

1. A The frenum is a thin fold of tissue that connects two structures together. Examples include the buccal frenum, which attaches the cheek to the alveolar ridge; the maxillary midline frenum, which attaches the top lip to the maxillary ridge located between the central incisors; the mandibular frenum, which attaches the bottom lip to the mandibular ridge at the central incisors; and the lingual frenum, which is located under the tongue.

2. B The gag reflex is a protective mechanism that prevents foreign objects from being aspirated or swallowed.

3. C There are eight cranial bones. The eight cranial bones include the occipital, sphenoid, ethmoid, frontal, and two parietal and temporal bones.

4. C There are 14 facial bones. The facial bones include the mandible; the vomer; and paired bones consisting of the zygomatic, maxilla, nasal, lacrimal, palatine, and inferior nasal conchae.

5. B Parotid glands are the largest of the salivary glands, and they are located inferior and anterior to the ear.

6. A Submandibular glands are located inferior to the base of the tongue under the mucous membrane in the posterior part of the floor of the mouth.

7. C Sublingual glands are located beneath the sublingual mucosa of the mouth.

8. B Stensen's duct is the duct that comes off of the parotid gland and supplies saliva to the oral cavity.

9. C There is a group of ducts known as the ducts of Rivinus, which supplies saliva to the oral cavity. This group of ducts opens under the tongue.

10. B Cancellous bone is also known as spongy bone. It has a latticework structure that has an irregular, spongy appearance.

11. B The origin or beginning of a muscle is where the muscle attaches or originates.

12. A The insertion point of a muscle is where the muscle ends or inserts.

13. B

14. A

15. D

16. C The zygomatic major is responsible for drawing the cheeks up during laughing or smiling.

17. A The anatomic crown is that portion of the tooth that is completely covered with enamel.

18. B Cementum covers the outside of the root of the tooth. Cementum is calcified and bone-like in molecular structure.

19. C The cervix or neck of the tooth is where the anatomical crown and anatomical root join. It is not the anatomical crown only but involves the junction of those two structures.

20. B The root of the tooth is covered with cementum not dentin.

21. B The anatomical crown is covered with enamel, which is the hardest substance in the body—it can tolerate crushing strength of 100,000 pounds per square inch. Dentin is the bulk of the tooth, not enamel.

22. B Dentin makes up the bulk of the tooth and is covered by enamel.

23. C The anatomy of the pulp includes the pulp chamber, which includes the entire portion of the pulp and is located only in the crown and does not include the roots. The pulp canal conforms to the root structures. Tertiary dentin, which is reparative dentin, is formed in response to disease or trauma and is not part of the pulpal tissues.

24. A Periodontal ligaments are part of the attachment apparatus. They support and suspend the tooth in its socket.

25. D Cuspids, which are also called canines, are located in each quadrant. There is one per quadrant. They have the longest roots and are known as the cornerstones of the mouth.

26. D Central and lateral incisors have thin, sharp, biting edges. They are single rooted and are located in the anterior portion of the oral cavity.

27. C The posterior teeth are the only teeth in the human dentition that have a broad chewing surface used to grind and macerate food prior to swallowing.

28. B Primary teeth are also referred to as deciduous. There are 20 total.

29. C The primary dentition does not contain bicuspids or premolars due to the smaller size of a child's dental arch.

30. A There are 32 teeth in the human permanent dentition.

Dental Charting

CHAPTER OVERVIEW

The dental chart contains a diagram of all dental treatment that has been completed and needs to be completed. Using a red and blue pencil, the dental staff is able to keep a record of all treatment for each patient. The dentist usually recites the information and then it is recorded by the assistant. Symbols, abbreviations, and color coding are all devices used in the recording of information in the dental chart.

KEY TERMS

blood pressure	medical history	systolic pressure
clinical examination	pulse	temperature
dental history	sphygmomanometer	treatment plan
diastolic pressure	stethoscope	vital signs
intraoral examination		

I. TOOTH DIAGRAMS

  A. Geometric chart
    1. Teeth are arranged in their normal position of 1–32.
    2. Primary teeth are arranged next to the permanent teeth and lettered A–T.
    3. Teeth are represented by a circle with surfaces outlined for mesial, distal, occlusal, lingual, and facial surfaces.
  B. Anatomic chart
    1. Permanent teeth are arranged in their normal position of 1–32.
    2. Diagrams of teeth resemble the actual tooth, including the root.
    3. All surfaces of teeth are shown for charting purposes.
    4. Teeth are arranged as if you are looking into the patient's mouth. The right quadrant is on the left side and vice versa.

II. COLOR CODING DURING CHARTING

  A. Red pencil is used to chart treatment that needs to be performed.

  B. Blue pencil is used to chart treatment that has already been performed.

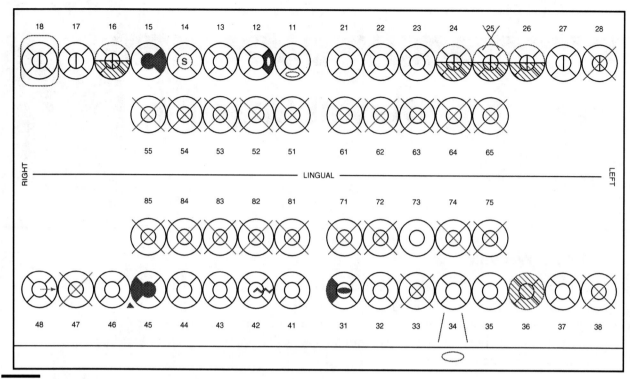

Charting using the geometric representation of the teeth and the International Standards Organization (ISO) TC 106 designation system for the teeth.

C. Black pencil is used to chart existing conditions that do not need attention at this time.

D. Green pencil is sometimes used to chart endodontic treatment.

E. Black ink is used to record treatment in the chart or notes about the patient visit.

F. Using different colors for charting enables the dental personnel to quickly and easily assess patient dental health and see where in the treatment phase the patient is.

G. Color coding during charting indicates various conditions and restorations present in the patient's oral cavity.

III. ABBREVIATIONS AND SYMBOLS USED DURING CHARTING

A. Abbreviations and symbols are used to record existing and needed treatment.

B. Abbreviations and symbols are not universal throughout the dental field.

C. Assistants should learn which symbols are preferred in their office.

Common Abbreviations Used in Charting

To be extracted	Draw a red diagonal line through the tooth.
Missing tooth	Draw a blue X through the tooth.
Impacted tooth	Draw a red or blue circle, depending on whether or not the tooth is going to be extracted, around the entire tooth.
Full gold crown	Circle the crown of the tooth and draw diagonal lines through it.
Porcelain crown	Outline the crown of the tooth.
Amalgam restoration	Outline the surfaces involved and then color in area completely.
Composite restoration	Outline the surfaces involved.
Abscess	Draw a small red circle at the apex of the tooth.
Root canal therapy	Draw a line through the root canal(s).
Fractured tooth	Draw a jagged line depicting the fracture.
Fixed bridge	Place an X on the pontic teeth and circle the abutments.
Sealant	Draw an S on the occlusal surface of the tooth.

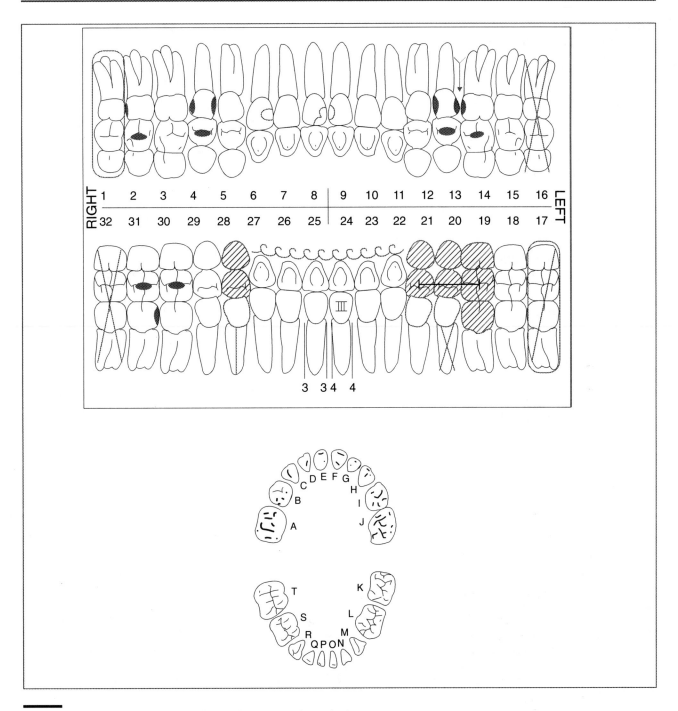

Charting using the anatomical teeth and the Universal numbering system.

Surfaces That are Charted During the Dental Exam	
Occlusal	O
Buccal	B
Facial	F
Lingual	L
Distal	D
Mesial	M
Incisal	I

Common Combinations for Different Surfaces	
Mesio-occlusal	MO
Mesio-incisal	MI
Mesio-occlusal-distal	MOD
Disto-buccal	DB
Disto-occlusal	DO
Disto-incisal	DI
Buccal-occlusal	BO
Occlusal-facial	OF

IV. ORAL EXAMINATION

A. A complete examination includes more than just charting existing treatment or treatment that is needed. An oral examination is needed to check for obvious lesions, cancerous masses, and all other soft tissues.

1. Assistant's role in the oral examination
    a. Assistant takes and records vital signs.
    b. Assistant helps the patient to complete the medical history and dental history.
    c. Assistant records all of the doctor's findings during the clinical examination.
    d. Assistant prepares the treatment room and the patient for the examination.
2. Clinical examination
    a. Dentist examines the outer soft tissue areas.
        (1) Lymph nodes for any abnormal swelling.
        (2) Facial features for any abnormalities such as cysts or lumps.
        (3) Temporomandibular joint for any abnormal clicking or popping sounds.
3. Intraoral clinical examination
    a. Dentist examines the inside of the patient's mouth and surrounding area.
        (1) Tongue
            (a) The assistant will hand the dentist a cotton 2 x 2 gauze square.
            (b) The undersurface (ventrical) side of the tongue is checked for abnormalities.
            (c) The top (dorsal) side of the tongue is checked for texture and abnormalities.
        (2) Tonsils
            (a) The assistant will hand the dentist a mouth mirror.
            (b) The dentist will check for any sign of infection or abnormality.

Procedure for Taking and Recording Vitals

Blood Pressure

1. Seat the patient and explain what you will be doing.
2. Place the blood pressure cuff on the patient's left arm and two fingers on the radial pulse of the left arm.
3. While feeling for the absence of the patient's pulse, inflate the blood pressure cuff.
4. When the pulse is no longer felt, note the reading on the dial and deflate cuff.
5. Place the stethoscope diaphragm in the anticubital area of the arm and reinflate cuff to the previously noted reading.
6. Slowly deflate the cuff, taking note when you hear the first beat and when you hear the last beat. The first reading will be the systolic and the second will be the diastolic. Note in the patient's chart the date and blood pressure reading.

Temperature

1. Using an alcohol cotton gauze square, wipe the bulb end of the thermometer and then shake the thermometer at least 5° below the normal 98.6°F.
2. Place a protective sheath over the thermometer and place under the patient's tongue for at least three minutes. If you are using a digital thermometer, wait until you hear the sound indicating that the reading is complete.
3. Read the thermometer and record in the patient's chart.

Respiration

1. Monitor the patient's breathing for at least 30 seconds and then double that reading and record in the patient's chart.

Pulse

1. Using your first two fingers, locate the patient's pulse at the radial area.
2. Count for one minute and then record in the patient's chart.

(3) Floor of the mouth
 (a) The floor of the mouth is checked for any lesions or abnormalities around the salivary ducts.

(4) Lips
 (a) The vermilion border and corners of the mouth are inspected.
 (b) The outside and inside of the lips are checked for any lesions or trauma.

(5) Gingiva
 (a) Using a periodontal probe and mouth mirror, the dentist checks pocket depths and bleeding index.
 (b) The texture, color, and appearance are evaluated.
 (c) Tissue is checked for recession or other tissue degeneration.

(6) Hard and soft palate and oral mucosa
 (a) The area is checked for any lesions or defects.
 (b) The area is checked for any trauma or abnormalities.

(7) Teeth and their occlusal relationship
 (a) The assistant will hand the dentist a mouth mirror.
 (b) Patient is instructed to bite together, and the occlusion is evaluated.
 (c) At this point, the assistant will record for the dentist any dental treatment that needs to be completed or has already been completed.

REVIEW QUESTIONS

1. All existing restorations are charted in
 A. red.
 B. blue.
 C. green.

2. Restorative work that needs to be done is
 A. charted in blue.
 B. charted in green.
 C. charted in red.
 D. not charted at all.

3. All of the following are true regarding abbreviations and symbols EXCEPT
 A. abbreviations and symbols are used to record existing and needed treatment.
 B. abbreviations and symbols can vary among offices.
 C. abbreviations and symbols are not universal throughout the dental field.
 D. abbreviations and symbols do not vary with different dentists.

Match the tooth condition with the appropriate symbol.

_____ 4. To be extracted

_____ 5. Missing tooth

_____ 6. Impacted tooth

_____ 7. Full gold crown

_____ 8. Porcelain crown

_____ 9. Amalgam restoration

_____ 10. Composite restoration

_____ 11. Abscess

_____ 12. Root canal therapy

_____ 13. Fractured root

_____ 14. Fixed bridge

_____ 15. Sealant

A. Draw a blue X through the tooth.
B. Circle the crown of the tooth and draw diagonal lines through it.
C. Circle the crown of the tooth only.
D. Draw a red diagonal line through the entire tooth.
E. Draw a jagged line depicting the fracture.
F. Draw a small red circle at the apex of the tooth.
G. Outline the surfaces involved.
H. Draw an S on the occlusal surface of the tooth.
I. Outline the surfaces of the tooth and then color in area.
J. Draw a vertical line down the center of each canal.
K. Place an X on the missing teeth and circle the abutments.
L. Draw a circle around the entire tooth.

16. The _____ surface refers to the surface that is toward the midline.
    A. distal
    B. mesial
    C. median
    D. sagittal

17. The _____ surface refers to the surface that is away from the midline.
    A. mesial
    B. distal
    C. medial
    D. incisal

18. The sharp, biting edge of the anterior teeth is referred to as
    A. facial.
    B. occlusal.
    C. incisal.
    D. buccal.

19. During an oral examination, the assistant is responsible for all of the following EXCEPT
    A. assisting the patient in completing the medical and dental history.
    B. recording all of the dentist's findings.
    C. recommending needed treatment.
    D. assisting in the preparation of the patient and room for treatment.

20. A clinical examination consists of all of the following EXCEPT
    A. the dentist examining the lymph nodes.
    B. examining facial features for any abnormalities.
    C. listening for abnormal clicking and popping of the temporomandibular joint.
    D. examining the tongue for abnormalities.

21. An intraoral examination consists of all of the following EXCEPT
    A. the dentist examining the inside of the patient's mouth.
    B. the dentist examining the patient's tongue.
    C. the assistant recording all findings by the dentist.
    D. the dentist examining the patient's tonsils.

22. Vitals include all of the following EXCEPT
    A. respiration.
    B. heart rate or pulse.
    C. weight.
    D. blood pressure.

23. Normal body temperature for an average adult is
    A. 97.6°F.
    B. 98.1°F.
    C. 98.6°F.
    D. 99.4°F.

24. PFM is the abbreviation for
    A. patient faints momentarily.
    B. porcelain-fused-to-metal crown.
    C. porcelain filling on mesial surface.
    D. porcelain finished material.

25. FGC is the abbreviation for
    A. full grown child.
    B. fine grade composite.
    C. full gold crown.
    D. first gold crown.

The following questions are based on the dental chart shown below.

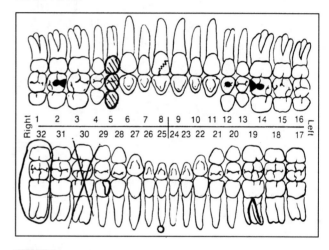

Anatomic chart with restorations

26. Tooth No. 2 has
    A. DO caries.
    B. MO caries.
    C. MO composite.
    D. MO inlay.

27. Tooth No. 5 has
    A. full gold crown.
    B. porcelain-fused-to-metal crown.
    C. full gold onlay.
    D. MOD amalgam.

28. Tooth No. 30
    A. has not yet erupted.
    B. needs to be extracted.
    C. is missing.
    D. is an abutment.

29. Tooth No. 8 has
    A. a porcelain veneer.
    B. a composite filling.
    C. a porcelain-fused-to-metal crown.
    D. an MI fracture.

30. Tooth No. 32
    A. needs to be extracted.
    B. is impacted.
    C. has been extracted.
    D. is drifting mesially.

ANSWERS AND RATIONALES

1. B Existing restorations are universally charted in blue so that the dental staff can readily recognize restorative procedures that have been performed.

2. C Restorative procedures that need to be performed are universally charted in red. Red is easy to recognize and symbolizes the need for treatment.

3. C Abbreviations and symbols are used by the dental staff to chart the dental health of the patient. Most symbols and abbreviations are universal; however, throughout different offices you may find subtle differences.

4. D
5. A
6. L
7. B
8. C
9. I
10. G
11. F
12. J
13. E
14. K
15. H

16. B The imaginary vertical line that divides the oral cavity into two halves is referred to as the midline. Any tooth surface that faces the midline is referred to as the mesial surface.

17. B Any surface that faces away from the imaginary line called the midline is referred to as the distal surface.

18. C The incisal edge is the thin, sharp, biting surface of the anterior teeth. This edge is used for tearing and piercing food.

19. C The assistant does not recommend treatment under any circumstances. This is a duty delegated only to the dentist, and the assistant is not legally permitted to perform this duty.

20. D Examination of lymph nodes, facial features, and the temporomandibular joint is part of a clinical examination. An examination of the tongue is referred to as an intraoral examination.

21. C Any examination of intraoral tissues can be collectively referred to as an intraoral examination. Recording the findings is a separate duty performed by the assistant and is referred to as collection of data.

22. C Collectively, blood pressure, respiration, pulse, and temperature are called vitals. In specialty offices and some general offices, vitals are routinely taken prior to dental treatment. The patient's weight is not considered part of the vitals.

23. C The normal body temperature for a healthy adult is 98.6°F.

24. B Universally, the abbreviation PFM is known as porcelain-fused-to-metal crown and is charted by circling the crown only on the dental chart.

25. C The universal charting symbol for FGC is full gold crown. A full gold crown is usually charted by circling the entire crown and placing diagonal lines over the outlined portion of the crown.

26. B
27. A
28. C
29. D
30. B

Infection Control

CHAPTER OVERVIEW

Pathogenic agents may be present in the mouth as a result of four conditions: oral diseases, systemic disease when oral lesions are present, respiratory diseases, and bloodborne pathogens. Contact with these pathogens can be very serious, so when working around body fluids in the dental field, precautions must be taken to minimize the risk of exposure to you and other patients. This chapter reviews universal precautions and protective barriers, minimum standards for infection control in dentistry, hazard communication, and general office safety. Sterilization and housekeeping procedures along with biological monitoring are also discussed.

KEY TERMS

biohazard
biological monitoring
critical instruments
hazard communication

incident report
noncritical instruments
personal protective
    equipment (PPE)

semicritical instruments
sharps management
single-use instruments
universal precautions

I. UNIVERSAL PRECAUTIONS

A. An approach to infection control

B. The concept states that you must treat all blood and body fluids as potentially infectious.

C. Universal precautions must be used in the care of each and every patient.

D. Use barriers for each patient.
   1. Chair covers.
   2. Light handle covers.
   3. Disposable sleeves for three-way syringe.
   4. Sterilization of handpieces after every use.
   5. Use of high volume evacuator (HVE) disposable tips and saliva ejectors.

II. PERSONAL PROTECTIVE EQUIPMENT

A. Personal protective equipment (PPE) is designed to protect the dental health-care worker from contaminated blood and saliva. PPE also protects the dental health-care worker from injury during the cleanup phase of any dental procedure.

B. Protective attire
   1. Gloves
      a. Worn when there is a potential for contacting blood, blood-contaminated saliva, or mucous membranes.
      b. Should be changed between each patient.
      c. Should not be cleaned and reused.
      d. Hands should be washed before and after donning gloves.
      e. Sterile gloves should be used for surgical procedures.
      f. Nonsterile gloves can be used during routine examinations and other nonsurgical procedures.
      g. Rubber utility gloves are used for housekeeping duties that may involve the potential contact with blood or saliva.
      h. Gloves should be changed when they have been punctured or torn.
   2. Protective gowns, laboratory coats, or uniforms
      a. Should be worn when clothing may come in contact with blood or other body fluids.
      b. Should be changed each day or when visibly soiled.
      c. Should be removed prior to leaving the work area.
      d. Must be placed in a designated area for pickup.
      e. If taken home to be laundered, must be washed in hot water with bleach.
      f. Long laboratory jackets should be worn during surgical procedures.
      g. Gloves should fit over the cuffs of the laboratory jacket.
   3. Plastic face shields or masks and protective eyewear
      a. Should be worn when there is a potential for the generation of droplets or splashing of blood or other body fluids.
      b. Surgical masks should be worn for invasive procedures.
      c. Should be changed between each patient or during treatment if the mask becomes moist or wet.
      d. Protective glasses and face shields should be disinfected after each procedure.
      e. Protective eyewear may be provided for patient to prevent debris from entering patient's eyes during procedures.

C. Barrier precautions
   1. Surface
      a. Foil, impervious backed paper, or plastic covers must be used to protect items that may become contaminated with blood or saliva.
      b. Used when cleaning and disinfecting is difficult or impossible.
      c. Must be removed with gloved hands but can be applied with clean hands.
      d. Must be discarded after each patient.
   2. Aerosols
      a. Saliva ejectors, high velocity evacuator tips, and rubber dams are used.
      b. Used to minimize the distribution of droplets or spatters during the dental procedure.
      c. Splash shields may be used to minimize exposure to the dental health-care worker during laboratory procedures.
      d. Patient positioning during certain procedures reduces the formation of droplets and spatters and aerosols.
   3. Resuscitative
      a. Ventilating devices must be available for emergency situations.
      b. After each use, they should be sterilized and bagged for next user.
      c. They can be provided as a disposable item.

D. Handwashing and care of hands
   1. Handwashing
      a. Hands should be washed before and after donning gloves.
      b. Hands should be washed before setting up the barriers for treatment.
      c. Hands should be washed after touching inanimate objects that may be contaminated with blood or saliva.
      d. Washing must be done in cool water with antimicrobial soap, and the hands should be dried completely.
      e. Antimicrobial surgical hand soap must be used prior to surgical procedures.

f. Hands should be washed before and after treating a patient.

g. After touching an object with your bare hand that is likely to be contaminated with blood or saliva, your hands should be washed.

h. If you have dermatitis or a weeping sore on your hands you should not treat a patient or touch any equipment used to treat patients until the condition is cleared up.

III. HANDLING SHARPS

A. Use and care of sharps
1. Never recap or touch a needle with hands.
2. Do not point a needle toward any part of the body.
3. Use the one-handed scoop method or other recapping devices.
4. Used disposable needles and syringes, scalpel blades, or other sharp blades should be stored in a puncture-resistant container.
5. The sharps container should be kept as close to the area of use as possible.
6. Never bend or break a needle after using.
7. When using more than one needle, do not place unsheathed needle where it may become contaminated.

IV. STERILIZATION AND DISINFECTION OF INSTRUMENTS

A. Categories
1. Critical
   a. Surgical instruments that are used to penetrate bone or soft tissue.
   b. Requires sterilization after each use.
2. Semicritical
   a. Instruments that do not penetrate bone or soft tissue.
   b. Instruments that contact soft oral tissues.
   c. Should be sterilized after each use.
   d. Can be disinfected at a high level if heat will damage the instrument.
3. Noncritical
   a. Instruments that come into contact with intact skin only.

b. Require intermediate-level or low-level disinfection.
c. Can be cleaned with detergent and water depending on what type of surface they have.
4. Single-use Disposable
   a. Must be used for one patient only.
   b. Should be discarded properly.
   c. Should never be cleaned or disinfected for a second use.

Note: Instruments that are critical or semicritical should be sterilized, packaged, and stored for use.

V. STERILIZATION METHODS

A. Sterilization is the method by which all forms of life are completely destroyed. Any living organism or pathogen is eradicated. Sterile is an absolute term. Either an item is sterile or it is not sterile. There are three accepted methods of sterilization in the dental field.
1. Autoclave
   a. Superheated steam under pressure combined with time for successful autoclaving
   (1) Pressure
       (a) 15–20 psi (pounds per square inch).
   (2) Temperature
       (a) 250°F.
   (3) Time
       (a) 20 minutes after the proper pressure and temperature are reached.
   (4) Distilled water is used in the autoclave.
   (5) Instruments are dried and wrapped in a bag or placed in a cassette for processing.
   (6) After processing, instruments are removed and allowed to dry and cool.
   (7) Examine door gaskets on a regular basis to ensure that the unit is not leaking or worn out.
2. Chemclave
   a. Similar to autoclaving except that chemical vapor is used instead of distilled water
   (1) Pressure
       (a) 20–40 psi.

(2) Temperature
(a) 270°F.
(3) Time
(a) 20 minutes.
(4) Instruments must be clean and dry before they are wrapped.
(5) Instruments can be wrapped in paper/biofilm bags or placed in cassettes or plain see-through tubing.
(6) A vapor exhaust system is recommended to eliminate harmful vapors after decompression of the chemclave.
3. Dry heat sterilization
  a. This method is used when instruments will rust in the autoclave.
  b. Instruments must be clean and dry before they are placed into the dry heat sterilizer.
  c. Procedure for sterilization
    (1) 160°F for 120 minutes.
    (2) 170°F for 60 minutes.
    (3) Instruments must be dry.
    (4) Instruments can be wrapped in foil or placed in metal and glass containers or other heat-resistant materials.
    (5) The timing of the sterilization begins when the proper temperature has been reached.

VI. BIOLOGICAL MONITORING AND PROCESS INDICATORS

A. CDC guidelines regarding proper achievement of sterilization are guaranteed only through biological monitoring.
  1. Spore testing
    a. Live spores, which are harmless but very resistant to heat, are used.
    b. Weekly monitoring is recommended.
    c. Three strips are used: two with the instruments and one kept out as the control strip. They are sent to an outside lab for evaluation.
    d. A negative report indicates sterilizer is working properly, and a positive report indicates that the sterilizer is not working properly.

B. Process indicators
  1. Process indicators are used to identify those instruments that have been processed through the sterilizer.
    a. Heat-sensitive paper located on bags, tape, or other wrapping material indicates whether the instruments were exposed to chemical vapor, steam, or other sterilization chemicals.
    b. The time that instruments were exposed to heat or chemicals is not indicated.

VII. CHEMICAL GERMICIDES

A. High level
  1. Chemicals registered as sterilant/disinfectant.
  2. Has a low surface tension
    a. Able to flow and penetrate surfaces.
  3. Example would be glutaraldehyde.
  4. Able to penetrate blood and bioburden.
    a. Bioburden is any visible organic debris.
  5. May be used as a holding solution for soiled instruments waiting to be processed.
  6. A special dipstick can be used to test its effectiveness.
  7. Can discolor skin so gloves must be worn when handling glutaraldehyde.
  8. Not suitable for disinfecting surfaces because of the slow-acting chemicals.

B. Intermediate level
  1. For surfaces soiled with body fluids.
  2. Registered as a "hospital disinfectant."
  3. Labeled as tuberculocidal.
  4. Phenolics
    a. EPA registered.
    b. Broad-spectrum disinfecting action (capable of killing a wide variety of microbes).
    c. Prepared on a daily basis.
  5. Iodophors
    a. Used for disinfecting surfaces that have been soiled with potentially infectious blood or saliva.
    b. Available as antiseptic or hard surface applications.

6. Sodium hypochlorite (household bleach)
   a. Must be mixed fresh daily at a ratio of 1:10.
   b. Fast acting.
   c. Economical and broad spectrum.
   d. Works in 3–30 minutes.

C. Low level
   1. Used for general housekeeping
      a. Cleaning floors and walls.
      b. Disinfecting and cleaning dental chairs.
      c. Cleaning countertops and units or other "splash."
   2. Labeled as "hospital disinfectant" but not "tuberculocidal."
   3. Intermediate-level and low-level disinfectants are not to be used for reprocessing critical and semicritical dental instruments.

VIII. CARE OF DENTAL EQUIPMENT

A. Handpieces
   1. Will be heat sterilized after use on each patient.
   2. Will be flushed a minimum of 20–30 seconds before and after use on each patient.

B. Valves and hoses
   1. Valves and hoses will be replaced if they are worn or contain tears or holes.
   2. Antiretraction valves shall be installed in dental unit water lines to prevent fluid aspiration.
   3. Water lines should be flushed at the beginning of the day for several minutes.
   4. Water lines should be flushed after every patient.
   5. Ultrasonic scaler and three-way syringes should be treated like all other lines.
   6. Sterile water should be used as an irrigant/coolant when surgical procedures involve the cutting of bone.

IX. LABORATORY MATERIALS

A. Contaminated materials must be cleaned and disinfected with a tuberculocidal hospital disinfectant before handling by dental laboratory personnel.
   1. Impressions
      a. Alginate.
      b. Polyvinylsiloxane.
      c. Rubber base.
      d. Hydrocolloid.
   2. Intraoral devices
      a. Partials.
      b. Dentures.
      c. Stay plates.
      d. Orthodontic appliances.
   3. Before and after being placed in the patient's mouth.
   4. Laboratory personnel who work on-site or off-site must follow protocol.

X. BIOLOGICAL MONITORING AND SPORE TESTING

A. To ensure the proper functioning of the autoclave and chemclave, weekly testing must be performed.

B. Spore testing can be sent out to independent labs for processing or can be done at the office if proper equipment and technique is used.
   1. Spore testing is accomplished by placing two strips impregnated with a bacteria that is highly resistant to heat.
   2. A control strip is kept outside of the processing cycle.
   3. All strips are processed and checked for positive or negative results.

C. Chemical indicators can be placed inside the instrument packs to verify that the packs have been through the sterilization process.
   1. Heat indicators should not be relied on alone because they do not ensure adequacy of the sterilization process.
   2. Heat or chemical indicators identify only that the instruments have been through the cycle.

D. Test strips are available to check the strength of cold sterile solutions.
   1. Dipped into the solutions, the test strips will indicate whether the solution is effective.

XI. HOUSEKEEPING AND LAUNDRY

A. Dental units and environmental surfaces
   1. Must be cleaned and disinfected after each patient.
   2. Must be cleaned and disinfected at the end of the workday.

B. Countertops and dental unit surfaces
   1. Must be cleaned with a disposable towel.
   2. Appropriate cleaning agents should be used.
   3. Surfaces must be disinfected with a germicidal solution that is "hospital disinfectant" or "tuberculocidal."

C. Walls and floors
   1. Must be cleaned routinely.
   2. Must be cleaned when visibly soiled.

D. A schedule should be posted to establish duties and frequency of those duties performed for routine housekeeping procedures.

E. Laundry
   1. Clothing is placed in an appropriate area for storage, decontamination, washing, or disposal.
   2. Clothing should never be worn outside the office.
   3. Clothing may be taken home to be laundered separately in hot, soapy water that contains bleach.

XII. BIOBURDEN SPILLS

A. Blood
   1. All blood should be removed and the area cleaned with a germicide that is approved for use as "hospital disinfectant" or "tuberculocidal."
   2. Gloves should always be worn during the cleanup procedure.

B. Waste
   1. Solid waste contaminated with blood or other bodily fluids
      a. Should be placed in a sealed bag to avoid leakage.
      b. Should be sealed and discarded under local, state, or federal regulations.
   2. Regulated medical waste
      a. Should follow local, state, or federal guidelines for disposal.

XIII. PROCESSING INSTRUMENTS

A. Cleaning and sterilizing instruments
   1. Wear heavy-duty utility or nitrile gloves.
   2. Discard all single-use items.
   3. Preclean instruments.
   4. Use an ultrasonic cleaner.
   5. Rinse and dry thoroughly before packaging.
   6. Store in packages prior to use.

XIV. EXPOSURE AND ROUTES OF TRANSMISSION

A. Autogenous infections
   1. Patient is the source of the infection.
   2. Self-produced infection.
   3. Endocarditis resulting from extensive root planing and scaling.
   4. Originating within the body.

B. Cross infections
   1. Passed from one person to the other.
   2. Common colds or flu through sneezing or coughing.
   3. Exposure from a contaminated needle or instrument.

C. Microbial transmission from secretions contacted in the dental field occurs three general ways.
   1. Direct contact
      a. Coming in contact with open sores or lesions while treating the dental patient.
      b. Bloodborne diseases such as AIDS and hepatitis.

2. Indirect contact
   a. Exposure to microorganisms from contaminated dental instruments, equipment, or dental charts.
3. Inhalation
   a. Breathing in aerosolized microorganisms from patient blood or saliva during the use of a high-speed handpiece or an ultrasonic scaler.

XV. RECORD KEEPING

A. Record keeping during an incident exposure is critical.

B. Each file should be kept for the duration of the employment of the dental health-care worker plus 30 years.

C. File must include all information regarding the employee and exposure to infectious diseases.
   1. Social Security number.
   2. Vaccination history.
   3. Informed refusal (not taking part in the hepatitis series).
   4. Incident reports.
   5. Physicians' written opinion.

D. Training records
   1. Records must be kept for three years.
   2. Training must be offered annually (done by a qualified trainer).
   3. Training must be interactive (active participation in training session).
   4. Training must be offered at the appropriate level of comprehension.

E. Material safety data sheets (MSDS) available to the employees, preferably kept in a binder for easy access in the event of an exposure.

XVI. HAZARD COMMUNICATION

A. A hazard communication or safety coordinator must be designated for the office.

B. The dental office must have a written program.

C. A list of hazardous chemicals and their quantity and location must be disclosed.

D. An MSDS book divided into categories, updated, and cross-referenced must be available.

E. Chemicals must have a registered number with the Environmental Protection Agency if they are removed from the premises.

XVII. BIOHAZARDOUS WASTE MANAGEMENT

A. Bloody gauze or tissue must be placed in a red bag labeled biohazard.
   1. Must be removed by a contract licensed hauler once a month if less than 20 pounds.

B. Sharps containers must be capped and removed when full.

C. Fixer is removed by a contract licensed hauler.

D. Amalgam scrap filling materials that contain mercury vapors must be stored under water or fixer in a sealed container and must be removed by a licensed contract hauler.

E. Mercury hygiene
   1. The management of mercury spills in the dental office can best be accomplished by using a mercury spill kit.
      a. Mercury spill kits contain chemicals and armamentarium for cleaning up a spill properly.
      b. Never use an HVE to clean up mercury because this will create an aerosol.
      c. If a mercury spill kit is not available, using PPE, gather the mercury onto a piece of paper and dispose of the mercury in a ceramic basin (i.e., lavatory commode).
   2. Mercury contamination
      a. Methods of exposure include the inhalation of vapors or airborne particles or through the skin by handling it without a glove.
      b. Prolonged exposure can cause memory loss, tremors, and kidney dysfunction.

3. Avoiding an exposure
   a. Use PPE when there is a potential for coming into contact with mercury vapors.
   b. Use premeasured capsulated amalgam.
   c. Use an HVE any time there is a procedure that generates mercury vapor.
   d. Work in a well-ventilated treatment area.
   e. Obtain a yearly urinalysis to monitor mercury exposure.

XVIII. GENERAL OFFICE SAFETY

A. A safety coordinator should be assigned.
   1. Safety coordinator should have a written plan.

B. Safety evacuation plan should be posted.

C. A building, fire, and chemical safety program should be implemented.

D. A first aid kit should be available to all employees.

E. An eyewash station should be set up for employees.

F. Pocket shields for CPR should be available for all employees.

G. Signage for radiation, safety goggle area, and equipment that may burn an employee or cause harm should be visibly posted.

H. Safety coordinator should make periodic inspections to ensure compliance.

XIX. OSHA TASK ORGANIZATION

A. OSHA categorizes tasks in order of potential exposure to contaminated blood, saliva, or bodily fluids.
   1. Category 1
      a. Tasks that have exposure to blood, body fluids, or tissues.
      b. Individuals usually classified in this category are dentists, hygienists, assistants, and laboratory technicians.
   2. Category 2
      a. Tasks that have no exposure to blood, body fluids, or tissues but may have an unplanned exposure to Category 1 tasks.
      b. Individuals classified in this category may include clerical or non-professional workers.
   3. Category 3
      a. Tasks that have no exposure to blood, body fluids, or tissues.
      b. Individuals classified in this category may include receptionists, bookkeepers, and insurance clerks.

XX. GOVERNMENT AGENCIES

A. Occupational Safety and Health Administration (OSHA)
   1. Requires that employers (dentists) maintain certain safe work practices.
   2. Policies or standards must be kept on file.
   3. Policies must be posted in full view of employees.
   4. Has the authority to conduct workplace inspections.
   5. Requires employers to provide employees with the hepatitis vaccine.

B. Environmental Protection Agency (EPA)
   1. Addresses issues that involve the environment and public safety.
   2. In the dental office, primarily concerned with the disposal of waste that is infectious or harmful to the environment.

C. Centers for Disease Control (CDC)
   1. Primary job is to track, investigate, and report the spread of diseases affecting the U.S. population.
   2. Establishes exposure guidelines for cross-contamination.
   3. Guidelines that protect the patient and the employee.

XXI. TREATMENT ROOM INFECTION CONTROL

A. Prior to the patient arriving for treatment
   1. Be sure all of the materials, equipment, instruments, and supplies are readily available so that retrieval of these items by opening drawers or cabinets is very limited. Have overgloves available.
   2. Place the patient's chart so that it will not be in danger of contamination.
   3. Place radiographs on the viewbox prior to seating the patient.
   4. Place all protective barriers on the light handles, chairs, and equipment.
   5. Leave instruments in unopened sterilization bags until just prior to the procedure.

B. After seating the patient
   1. Drape patient appropriately.
   2. Use a pretreatment antiseptic mouthwash if needed.
   3. Review the medical and dental chart carefully and interview the patient about past illnesses the patient may have had or come in contact with.
   4. Adjust the patient's chair and light prior to donning gloves.
   5. Place PPE on (mask, goggles, gown, and gloves).
   6. Open sterilized instruments.
   7. Once the procedure has started, do not break the chain of asepsis. Ask another assistant to retrieve needed items or keep a set of overgloves nearby.
   8. Control spatter by using the high volume evacuator tip.
   9. Handle sharps safely by using the one-handed scoop method for recapping or a recapping device.
   10. Do not touch your eyes or face with contaminated hands.

C. Treatment room cleanup and disinfection
   1. Prior to dismissing the patient, write procedure in chart using overgloves. Discard when finished and follow proper handwashing technique.
   2. During the cleanup phase
      a. Don utility gloves.
         (1) Utility gloves can be made of heavy rubber and autoclavable.
         (2) Hands should be washed prior to donning utility gloves and after removing them.
      b. Gather all instruments and materials that were used and take them to central sterilization.
         (1) Discard single-use items in proper receptacle.
      c. Remove all barriers and clean all contaminated surfaces and wipe with a disposable towel.
      d. Flush the handpieces with water for 10–30 seconds.
         (1) Flushing handpieces will help to eliminate the buildup of bacteria in the lines.
      e. Remove handpieces and wash, dry, lubricate, and sterilize following the manufacturer's directions.
      f. Flush the water line for at least 10 seconds.
      g. Suction the vacuum lines with water or a combination of water and bleach.
         (1) If using bleach to flush the lines, use 1 part bleach to 10 parts water.
      h. At the end of the day, flush the suction lines with an EPA-approved solution.
      i. Remove and clean the solids trap if necessary. Dispose of trap basket in a sealed bag.
      j. Nondisposable baskets are emptied into a bag and then cleaned before being put back into the trap.
      k. Discard all disposable items and any blood-soaked items such as gauze or cotton rolls. These items should go into a leak-resistant container marked biohazard.
      l. Dispose of all blades, needles, carpules, or other sharps in a clearly marked, puncture-resistant container that is leakproof.
      m. Return to treatment area and spray all surfaces with a disinfectant; wipe with a disposable towel. Spray again and let the solution air dry for at least 10 minutes (referred to as the spray-wipe-spray method).

n. Wash hands thoroughly and place barriers on appropriate areas for next patient.

XXII. HANDLING PATIENT CHARTS AND RADIOGRAPHS

A. Handling patient charts
1. During and after treatment, charts should be handled wearing overgloves.
2. Charts should be kept in an area where they can be seen easily but not in an area where they can be contaminated.
3. Charts should be looked over carefully for any changes in health or any existing health-related issues or potentially dangerous illnesses.

B. Handling radiographs
1. Gloves, mask, and goggles should always be worn when taking radiographs.
2. Overgloves may be used for processing radiographs.
3. After exposure, films should be dried off with a paper towel and stored in a plastic cup until ready to process.
4. When processing film, avoid handling the film itself.
5. Use barriers for x-ray heads, switches, door handles, and chairs.
6. After exposing radiographs and dismissing the patient, follow cleanup and disinfection procedures.

REVIEW QUESTIONS

1. When should medical gloves be worn?
A. During all dental office procedures
B. When there is a potential for contacting blood or body fluids
C. Only when working on a live patient

2. Rubber utility gloves are used for
A. cleaning up spills on countertops and floors only.
B. cleaning instruments that may be contaminated with blood only.
C. housekeeping duties that involve potential contact with blood, contaminated instruments, or decontamination procedures.

3. Protective gowns and lab coats
A. must be worn when clothing is likely to be soiled with blood.
B. should be worn if you are likely to be soiled with body fluids.
C. should be changed daily or as soon as they are visibly soiled.

4. Personal protective clothing should be
A. removed after you get home.
B. placed in a designated area to be cleaned separately when you get home.
C. removed prior to leaving the work area and placed in a separate container to be stored, decontaminated, or laundered.

5. Face shields must be worn
A. for procedures that commonly result in the generation of blood droplets.
B. during every lab procedure.
C. only when using the model trimmer or lab engines.

6. Barriers for light handles and chairs should be
A. impervious backed paper, aluminum foil, or plastic covers.
B. easy to remove.
C. adequate coverage for all items that are difficult to clean or disinfect.
D. All of the above

7. Sterilization and disinfection of critical instruments
A. is done only if the doctor requests it.
B. can be done the next day.
C. is done after each use.

8. High-level chemical germicides are registered as sterilant/disinfectant.
A. True
B. False

9. Chemical vapor sterilization
A. can be achieved with an autoclave.
B. can be achieved with a chemclave.
C. is not used in dentistry.

10. Cold sterilization can be achieved by
A. 6 hours of exposure to instruments.
B. 8 hours of exposure to instruments.
C. 10 hours or more of exposure to instruments.

11. *Single-use* instruments
    A. do not come into contact with intact skin.
    B. are not single-use disposable instruments.
    C. are designed to be used once and do not require sterilization or disinfection.

12. Steam sterilization under pressure can be achieved with a/an
    A. ultrasonic cleaner.
    B. autoclave.
    C. dry heat method.

13. Handpieces
    A. should be treated with a germicide prior to the next use.
    B. should be heat treated after each use.
    C. can be cleaned with a low-level disinfectant.

14. Lab cases such as dentures or partials should be
    A. disinfected prior to being placed in the operatory.
    B. disinfected prior to being placed in the patient's mouth.
    C. disinfected before being sent to the lab.
    D. A and B
    E. B and C

15. Biohazard trash bags are
    A. clearly visible by their red color.
    B. used in a separate trash container.
    C. labeled by the biohazard emblem.
    D. All of the above

16. Dental units and chairs should be cleaned
    A. between each and every patient.
    B. at the beginning of each day.
    C. only when visibly soiled.

17. Countertops and unit surfaces should be cleaned with disposable toweling.
    A. True
    B. False

18. Hands should be washed
    A. after donning gloves.
    B. after touching inanimate objects that may be contaminated with blood or saliva.
    C. with regular hand soap.

19. Semicritical instruments
    A. do not penetrate soft tissue or bone.
    B. contact soft oral tissue.
    C. require sterilization or high disinfection after each use.
    D. All of the above

20. Noncritical instruments
    A. come into contact with intact skin.
    B. do not require intermediate-level or low-level disinfection.
    C. do not have to be packaged prior to being used.

21. Intermediate-level germicides are for surfaces soiled with body fluids.
    A. True
    B. False

22. Low-level germicides are for general housekeeping and are usually labeled tuberculocidal.
    A. True
    B. False

23. Suction lines can be cleaned with
    A. commercial dental evacuation cleaners.
    B. bleach and water.
    C. A or B

24. Proper spore testing verification can be accomplished by
    A. reading the indicator tape on the bags.
    B. using a biological indicator.
    C. using a heat indicator.

25. Environmental surfaces such as walls and floors should be cleaned routinely.
    A. True
    B. False

26. Housekeeping or utility gloves should be worn
    A. during routine housekeeping cleanup.
    B. only when specified by the doctor.
    C. only in the lab.

27. The letters CDC stand for
    A. Center for Disease Criteria.
    B. Centers for Disease Control.
    C. Center for Dental Chemicals.

28. The letters OSHA stand for
    A. Occupational Safety and Hazard Association.
    B. Organization of Safety and Health Association.
    C. Occupational Safety and Health Administration.
    D. Office of Safety and Health Administration.

29. The chain of asepsis is best achieved by
    A. retrieval of needed instruments or materials by a circulating assistant after the procedure has started.

B. having all materials and instruments set up and ready prior to washing hands and donning gloves.

C. using an overglove when retrieving instruments from a drawer within the operatory room and then discarding it.

D. All of the above

30. When recapping an anesthetic needle, it is best to

A. use the one-handed scoop method.

B. use a recapping device.

C. leave the syringe uncapped and on the bracket tray.

D. None of the above

ANSWERS AND RATIONALES

1. B Any time a dental health-care worker has the potential to come into contact with blood or body fluids, gloves are recommended. Pathogens may invade through cuts or abrasions on the skin. Gloves should never be washed and reused and should be changed between each patient.

2. C General housekeeping duties include instrument cleaning, disinfecting countertops or bracket tables, and decontaminating the treatment area. These tasks require the dental health-care worker to wear rubber utility or nitrile gloves.

3. A Protective gowns protect your clothing from exposure to contaminated blood and must be worn for every treatment procedure.

4. C During routine dental procedures, the dental health-care worker should wear protective clothing, and it should be removed daily or when visibly soiled so that it may be decontaminated. The Centers for Disease Control recommends that protective clothing never be worn outside the treatment area.

5. A To protect the dental health-care worker, mucous membranes, which are a portal of entry for pathogenic microorganisms, should be covered with a face shield. Face shields should be decontaminated after each use with a high-level disinfectant.

6. D Light handle barriers should be placed to prevent cross-contamination and for general housekeeping purposes. An impervious backed paper, aluminum foil, or commercial barriers may be used to prevent cross-contamination and to ease cleaning of difficult or impossible surfaces following dental procedures. All barriers must be removed with gloved hands and changed after each patient.

7. C Critical instruments such as surgical instruments are instruments that penetrate bone and soft tissue. After use, they should be cleaned and sterilized.

8. A Chemical germicides such as glutaraldehydes are listed as a sterilant/disinfectant. They are an effective sterilant when instruments are soaked for up to 10 hours.

9. B A chemclave uses chemical vapor, pressure, time, and temperature to sterilize instruments.

10. C Instruments that cannot be sterilized by heat can be placed in a high-level disinfectant/sterilant for at least 10 hours. Examples include HVE tip, three-way air-water syringe tips, and plastic alginate trays.

11. C Single-use items are designed to be used once and then discarded. They are not intended to be reused.

12. B An autoclave is designed to sterilize instruments by using superheated steam, pressure, and time.

13. B Due to the potential for cross-contamination through the use of dental handpieces, OSHA recommends that all handpieces be heat treated (sterilized) after each use.

14. E Removable prosthetics should be sprayed with a disinfectant prior to being sent to the lab. Before they are placed in the patient's mouth, they may be sprayed with a disinfectant to reduce the number of pathogens that may be transmitted during the fabrication process.

15. D Biohazard trashbags are used for the disposal of articles such as gloves, blood-soaked gauze, bioburden, and other disposable items that may be soiled with blood or body fluids. They are red and have the biohazard symbol on the outside of the bag. For removal, a licensed biohazard waste disposal company must pick up these bags.

16. A   Because of the generation of aerosol droplets, all dental chairs and units should be cleaned between each patient.

17. A   Disposable toweling is used to clean countertops and units because after use, it can be disposed of immediately. If cloth towels are used, pathogens can be spread over other areas with repeated use.

18. B   Pathogens can be spread by failing to wash hands appropriately with antimicrobial soap after touching objects that may be contaminated with bodily fluids.

19. D   Semicritical instruments such as hand instruments used for restorative purposes or HVE tips must be disinfected or sterilized after each use. Because they do not penetrate soft tissue or bone, their potential for contact with blood is low. High disinfection and sterilization is adequate for these instruments.

20. B   Noncritical instruments come into contact with intact skin only. Examples may include dental dam frames, lead aprons, and protective patient goggles. These instruments require only low-level disinfection or soap and water.

21. A   Intermediate germicides are labeled "hospital disinfectant" and "tuberculocidal" and they can be used to decontaminate surfaces soiled with body fluids. Examples of intermediate-level germicides include iodophors, phonolics, and any chlorine compounds such as household bleach and water.

22. A   Low-level germicides are recommended for cleaning floors and walls. Quarternary ammonium is an example.

23. C   Because suction lines become contaminated with blood, saliva, and bioburden, suction lines are routinely flushed with commercial dental evacuation cleaners or a mix of 10 parts water to 1 part household bleach, which is proven to be a high-level disinfectant.

24. B   A biological indicator is composed of two strips impregnated with a live bacterial spore. One strip is placed in the chemclave or autoclave for sterilization cycle. After one cycle, the strip is sent with the control strip to a lab for evaluation. Indicator tapes and heat indicators state only that the instruments have been exposed to heat. Spore testing is mandatory at least once a week.

25. A   Floors, walls, and countertops should be cleaned routinely or between each patient to reduce the presence of pathogens.

26. A   During general housekeeping duties, heavy latex or nitrile gloves must be worn. Heavy latex or nitrile gloves protect hands from puncture wounds and exposure to chemicals or cleaning products.

27. B   CDC stands for the Centers for Disease Control, which tracks, investigates, and documents the spread of diseases. Its headquarters are in Atlanta, Georgia.

28. C   OSHA stands for Occupational Safety and Health Administration, which is responsible for implementing regulations regarding the safety of individuals in the workplace.

29. D   The chain of asepsis is the ability to maintain sterility of the treatment area during a dental procedure. Contact with any contaminated items breaks that chain and can contaminate the surgical area.

30. B   When recapping a needle, it is best to use a recapping device or the one-handed scoop method to avoid a needlestick exposure. Never bend or break needles or leave an uncapped needle out on the bracket tray or cabinet.

CHAPTER 5

Radiography

CHAPTER OVERVIEW

Dental radiographs are a very important component of the patient's overall dental history. They are considered a legal permanent record and should be treated as an important part of the patient's chart. Radiographs aid in the diagnostic and treatment planning phases of dentistry.

KEY TERMS

ALARA
anode
bisecting angle technique
bitewing
cathode
cephalometric
collimation
electrons

filtration
kilovoltage
maximum permissible dose
milliampere
panoramic
paralleling technique
periapical
position indicator device (PID)

rad
radiation safety
radiograph
rem
target
tubehead
x-ray

I. INDICATIONS FOR DENTAL RADIOGRAPHS

A. Detect bone loss.

B. Detect carious lesions.

C. Detect hard or soft tissue abnormalities.

D. Used in the treatment planning phase of orthodontics or restorative dentistry.

E. Prior to oral surgery.

II. CONTRAINDICATIONS FOR DENTAL RADIOGRAPHS

A. If a patient has had a full set of radiographs in the past three years.

B. If a patient has recently had radiation treatment involving other areas of the body.

C. If the patient is pregnant.

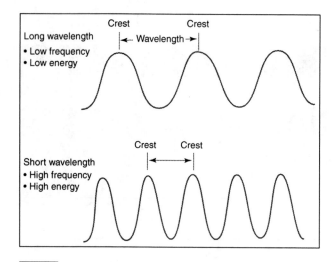

Wavelengths as they relate to energy, frequency, and x-ray. In dentistry, the shortest wavelength with high frequency and energy is used to expose dental film.

III. RADIATION PHYSICS

A. Basic atomic structure
1. An element is a simple substance that contains atoms with the same atomic number and same chemical properties.
2. An atom is the smallest particle of an element that can retain the properties of that element.
   a. A nucleus is contained in the center of an atom and stores subatomic particles called neutrons and protons.
   b. Protons are positively charged and neutrons are neutral and have no charge.
3. An electron is a negatively charged subatomic particle that travels around the nucleus.
   a. Binding energy is the force that holds the electron in place during its orbit around the nucleus.
   b. Orbiting electrons are repelled from the nucleus and the positive charge from the protons attracts them, creating a centrifugal force that causes the electron to orbit around its nucleus.
4. Molecules are considered the smallest particle of a substance that still resembles the physical and chemical makeup of that substance.

IV. TYPES OF RADIATION

A. Particulate radiation is the transmission of kinetic energy by subatomic particles emitted at a high speed by an unstable atom.

B. Electromagnetic radiation is the movement of energy through space by using electric and magnetic energy.

C. X radiation is produced when kinetic energy from high-speed electrons heats x-ray energy.
1. Primary radiation is x-rays that come from the x-ray position indicator device (PID) before they are able to interact with matter.
2. Secondary radiation is x-rays that actually interact with matter. This type of x-ray is also called scatter radiation.

V. MEASUREMENTS OF RADIATION

A. Traditional units of measurement are rad, roentgen, and rem.
1. Radiation absorbed dose (rad): The absorption of 0.01 J/kg of matter.
2. Roentgen: Amount of radiation that will produce 2.08 x 10 ion pairs in a cubic centimeter of air at a standard pressure and temperature.
3. Roentgen equivalent man (rem): One rem is equal to one rad times the qualifying factor for the type of ionizing radiation absorbed.

B. New units of measurement for radiation exposure
1. Coulomb per kilogram (C/kg) is the international unit for a coulomb of electrical charge in a kilogram of air. 1 C/kg = 3888 R.
2. The Gray (Gy) is the international unit of measurement for the absorption of J/kg of matter. 1 Gy = 100 rad.
3. Sievert is the international measurement that measures dose equivalent. 1 sievert = 1 Gy times the qualifying factor for the type of ionizing radiation absorbed.
4. Measuring dental radiation simplified: R = rad = rem and a C/kg = Gy = Sv.

VI. EFFECTS OF RADIATION

A. Direct effects of radiation
  1. Damaging effects of radiation can occur on a biological, cellular, or molecular level.
  2. Direct effects of ionizing radiation can break down the chemical bonds associated with genetic structures.
  3. Radiation exposure is cumulative and can build with each exposure.
  4. DNA damage can result in the formation of abnormal structure.

B. Indirect effects of radiation
  1. Biological damage may occur by chemicals created when water molecules are ionized.

C. Biologic damage that may occur when radiation exposure takes place
  1. Cell death may occur when embryonic tissue is exposed. Other cell damage may be a desired effect when destroying cancerous tissue.
  2. Mutation of cells may increase with the exposure to radiation.
  3. Carcinogenesis or leukemogenesis is the production of cancer-causing cells through direct exposure to radiation.

Sensitivity of Organs to Radiation Exposure

High Sensitivity
Lymph organs
Bone marrow
Gonads
Intestines

Moderate Sensitivity
Endothelial cells
Fibroblasts
Developing bone tissues
Developing cartilage tissues

Low Sensitivity
Salivary glands
Lung tissue
Muscle tissue
Brain and spinal cord

VII. EXPOSURE TECHNIQUES

A. Paralleling technique
  1. Film is placed parallel to the teeth to be exposed.
  2. The vertical position of the film should be parallel to the long axis of the tooth.
  3. The imaginary horizontal line drawn between the mesial and distal surfaces of the tooth to be exposed is the second landmark that should be parallel to the film.
  4. Vertical angulation moves the image occlusally; too much vertical angulation will result in foreshortening of the tooth, and not enough will cause elongation of the tooth.
  5. Horizontal angulation should follow the imaginary line drawn between the mesial and distal surfaces. Too much horizontal angulation will result in overlapping of mesial and distal contacts.
  6. Centering the film with the primary beam of the PID will ensure that the entire film is exposed and cone cutting will not result. Cone cutting will produce a clear image on the film in the shape of the PID being used.
  7. Film placement for the paralleling technique
    a. Central and lateral incisor.
    b. Lateral and cuspid view.
    c. First bicuspid and second bicuspid view.
    d. First, second, and third molar view.

B. Bisecting angle technique
  1. Film placement
    a. Against the incisal or occlusal edge of the teeth to be examined with no more than one-eighth to one-quarter of an inch extending beyond the edge of the incisal surface.
    b. X-ray beam should be perpendicular to an imaginary line called the bisector.
      (1) The bisector divides the angle that is formed by the tooth and film into two equal angles.

In either instance, the length of the PID determines the sharpness and resolution of the radiograph. A shorter PID gives a better image than a longer PID.

VIII. RADIOGRAPHIC EQUIPMENT

A. The x-ray machine
1. X-ray tubehead is where the primary x-ray beam is emitted.
2. The tubehead is attached to an adjusting arm, which is secured to the wall.
3. Vertical angulation is measured by a number scale located on the side of the tubehead.
4. PIDs are located at the end of the tubehead and are used to aim the primary x-ray beam at the film. They come in a variety of lengths and rectangular or circular shapes.

5. The control panel contains the controls to operate the x-ray machine.
a. On and off switches.
b. Kilovolt peak (kvp) selector controls the penetrating power of the x-ray beam.
c. The voltmeter measures kilovolts during each exposure.
d. The milliamperage (mA) controls the amount of radiation produced during each exposure.
e. The timer controls the duration of radiation production.

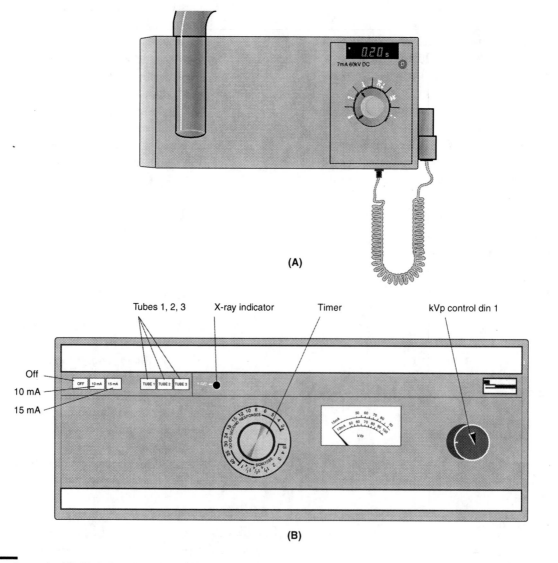

(A)

(B)

Control panels. (A) Digital settings for milliamperage, kilovoltage, and time. (B) Manual settings for milliamperage, kilovoltage, and time.

6. Deadman switch
   a. Located on the wall outside of x-ray area, on a foot pedal, or on the end of a cord and is used to activate the radiation process.
7. Aluminum filter
   a. Used to absorb low-energy x-rays that have little penetrating power.
   b. Placed in the pathway of the primary beam and used to filter out or decrease overall radiation exposure.
8. Lead diaphragm or collimator
   a. Further reduces patient exposure to radiation by limiting the area of exposure.
   b. A flat disk with a small opening that restricts the size of the x-ray beam emitted.
   c. Maximum diameter of opening by law is 2.75 cm.

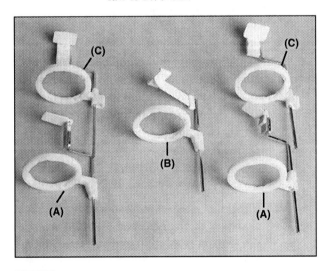

Rinn XCP components assembled correctly for (A) anterior exposures, (B) bitewing exposures, and (C) posterior exposures.

B. Intraoral equipment
   1. Rinn XCP film holder
      a. Used intraorally to align the film, teeth, and primary beam during exposure.
      b. Can be used with a rectangle or round PID.
      c. Designed to be used with the paralleling technique.
      d. Can be used with a collimating device to further reduce radiation exposure.
   2. Stabe film holder
      a. Made of Styrofoam and is disposable.
      b. Consists of a bite-block with an attached upright, which supports the film during exposure.
      c. Used intraorally and can be positioned for exposure of anterior or posterior teeth.
      d. Can be used for either the paralleling or bisecting angle techniques.
   3. Bite stick
      a. Plastic device used to hold film for periapical radiographs.
      b. Can be sterilized in the autoclave or by cold sterilization.
      c. Tolerated by patients with a sensitive gag reflex.
   4. Precision instrument
      a. One-piece stainless steel combination film holder aiming device with a built-in collimator.
      b. Used to align the teeth, film, and primary x-ray beam for exposure.
      c. Used with the paralleling technique.
      d. Can be uncomfortable for patient because of the weight of the apparatus.
   5. Bitewing tabs
      a. Are disposable and can be easily used by the operator.
      b. Foam adhesive backing type can be placed in the middle of the film.
      c. Cardboard slot type enables the operator to slip film easily into holder.

IX. PROTECTION DURING RADIOGRAPHIC EXPOSURE

A. Patient protection during radiographic exposure
   1. Patient should wear a lead-lined apron with attached thyroid collar to adequately protect the thyroid and reproductive areas of the body.
   2. Operators should follow the ALARA principle, which realizes the need for radiographs but recommends that the patient's exposure is as low as reasonably achievable.
   3. The office complies with the Consumer-Patient Health and Safety Act of 1981.

a. Requires that educational standards are set for personnel who perform radiographic procedures.

b. All dental personnel who will be performing radiographic procedures complete a recognized training program.

4. All personnel who will be performing radiographic procedures follow the U.S. Department of Health and Human Services publication regarding the selection of patients for radiographic examinations.

5. Radiography equipment is inspected and should meet federal diagnostic performance standards.

a. Head leakage.

b. Drifting of the adjusting arm.

c. Sufficient filtration for absorption of long-wave radiation.

6. Review patient's medical and dental history carefully before exposing to radiation.

7. When processing and handling film, maintain all equipment and pay close attention to technique.

B. Operator protection during exposure of radiographs

1. Follow the maximum permissible dose (MPD) level that the federal government allows radiation workers to receive.

a. Currently, guidelines are 0.05 Sv (5 rem) per year.

b. This dosage is 10 times the amount for the general population.

2. Use barriers to protect the operator and other office personnel during exposure.

a. Lead-lined walls and ceilings.

b. Closing the door to the operatory when exposing if appropriate.

3. Position of the operator during exposure.

a. Operator should stand a minimum of six feet from the patient and at a minimum 90° to 135° angle to the primary beam of radiation.

b. The operator should never hold the film for the patient.

c. The operator should never hold the tubehead.

4. Materials designed to absorb primary and secondary radiation must be used in walls, doors, and ceilings.

5. Doors must be closed while exposing radiographs and should be lined with an approved material.

6. The National Committee on Radiation Protection report number 35 lists the materials acceptable to use for radiation shielding purposes.

7. Monitoring devices

a. Dosimeter or film badges are used to monitor the amount of scatter radiation that the operatory is exposed to.

b. Dosimeter badges are routinely collected and sent out for evaluation.

c. Dosimeter badges should never be worn outside the dental office.

X. INFECTION CONTROL

A. Operatory preparation

1. All surfaces that come into contact with patient should be disinfected or covered prior to patient treatment.

a. Chairs and headrest.

b. Controls for the chair.

c. X-ray tubehead and PID.

d. Activating button.

e. Control buttons on control panel.

B. All surface disinfectants should be approved by the EPA and the ADA and recognized as an approved surface disinfectant.

C. Always wear OSHA-approved personal protective equipment when handling film packets that are contaminated with blood or saliva.

D. Protocol during the appointment

1. Take a complete medical history.

2. Treat all patients as potentially infectious.

3. Keep patient charts away from potential contamination.

4. Wear personal protective equipment when treating the patient.

5. Place required materials out prior to beginning the procedure.

6. Place contaminated films in a disposable cup after exposure.

E. Preparation of darkroom and processing techniques
1. Cover surfaces that will come into contact with contaminated films or operator gloves.
2. Use gloves when opening contaminated film packets.
3. Discard all materials in proper receptacle and disinfect work area.
4. Place film-holding devices in holding solution. After rinsing and drying completely, sterilize and leave in packet until ready to use.

XI. PATIENT MANAGEMENT DURING RADIATION EXPOSURE

A. The patient's perception of you and the procedure you are performing is vital in the management of the patient and situations in the event that difficulties arise. Your professional attitude and knowledge of the skill you are performing will make the patient and you more comfortable.
1. Remain calm and self-assured.
   a. Being calm and self-assured will convey skill and efficiency to the patient.
2. Review the patient's medical or dental history.
   a. Reviewing information will eliminate the possibility of taking unnecessary radiographs. Also, you may uncover hidden fears or anxieties that are beneficial to know beforehand.
3. Be prepared by having all of your materials and equipment out and the room set up prior to seating the patient.
   a. Having all of your equipment and materials out prior to patient seating will eliminate the need for you to leave the operatory and will cut down on time and stress to you and the patient.
4. Help the patient relax by establishing a rapport.
   a. Introducing yourself and explaining to the patient what you are about to do will minimize fear and anxiety in the patient.
5. Answer any questions with complete answers.

   a. Answering questions will minimize anxiety and will demonstrate to the patient that you are taking a genuine interest and are approachable.
6. Control the gag reflex by using breathing techniques or anesthetic spray or by having the patient concentrate on something other than what is taking place.
   a. If none of the above techniques work, reschedule the patient or on the dentist's recommendation, take a panorex (extraoral) radiograph.
7. Try other film-holding devices.
   a. Sometimes it is difficult for patients to tolerate some film-holding devices while others seem to pose no discomfort. Experiment with different devices.
8. When taking radiographs on the pediatric patient, the parent may be of help if allowed to be in the room.
   a. When handling the pediatric patient, be firm yet gentle.
   b. Keep reminding the patient about what the patient's role in the appointment is.
   c. Set clear limits for behavior during the procedure.
   d. If behavior problems persist, reschedule the appointment.

XII. PROCESSING RADIOGRAPHS

A. Darkroom design
1. Should be light leakproof.
2. Should be painted to reflect a safelight.
3. Should be resistant to chemicals and water.
4. Should contain a sink with running water.
5. Should have an overhead white light and an approved safety light
   a. Safety light should be positioned three to four feet from the work surface.
6. Should have an outside warning light that illuminates when the darkroom is occupied.
7. Should have a viewbox to view films after they have been fixed for at least three minutes.

B. Manual processing equipment
   1. Two one-gallon stainless steel tanks for manual processing
      a. Should have a circulating water bath that stays at 68°.
      b. Should have a tank for fixer and one for developer.
   2. Timer
      a. Used for accurate processing time.
   3. Film hangers for drying manual dip tank films.
   4. Drying racks to hang film hangers on.

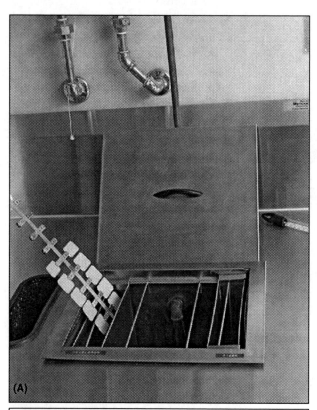

(A)

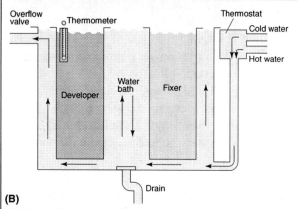

(B)

(A) Typical manual processing tank showing developer and fixer insert tanks in the water bath. (B) Line drawing of manual processing tank.

5. Solution stir sticks to circulate fixer and developer.
   6. Manual tanks should have a lid to cover the fixer and developer when dip tanks are not in use.
   7. A paper towel dispenser, a trash can, and an OSHA-approved surface disinfectant should be available for managing cleanup in the darkroom.
   8. A thermometer to measure chemical temperatures.

C. Procedure for using the manual dip tanks
   1. Uncover tanks and stir chemicals with designated stir sticks and check temperature of chemicals.
   2. Turn off overhead light and turn on safelight and close and lock door.
   3. Remove each film from package and place on film hanger clip.
   4. After all films have been loaded onto film hangers, immerse completely in developer for at least four minutes, agitating periodically.
   5. After films have been in developer for at least four minutes, remove and agitate in water bath for at least 20 seconds.
   6. Remove films from water bath and place in fixer solution for at least 10 minutes.
   7. After films have fixed for 10 minutes, remove and put in circulating water bath for at least 20 minutes.
   8. Remove films after rinsing, and allow them to dry for at least one hour before mounting.
   9. Turn overhead light on, discard film packets, and disinfect area.

Note: Handle film carefully so as not to scratch or bend it.

D. Automatic processor
   1. The processor should be placed on an even, hard surface with adequate room on all four sides.
   2. Transport system should be cleaned regularly to avoid buildup of chemicals on the rollers.
   3. Water should be changed daily.
   4. A daylight loader may be attached to most processors.
   5. Developer and fixer should be replenished on a daily basis.

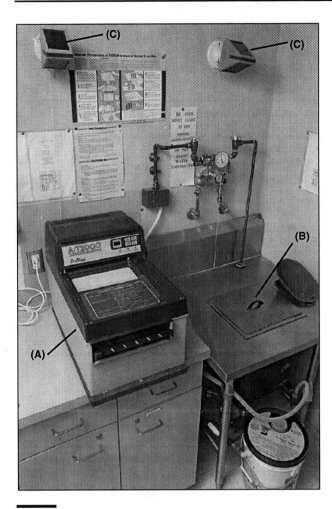

(A) Automatic film processor. (B) Manual processing tank in darkroom. (C) Safelights.

6. Processor should be turned off when not in use.

E. Procedure for using the automatic processor
   1. Turn processor on and let it warm up for approximately five minutes. The chemicals must reach at least 68° to work effectively.
   2. After closing the darkroom door, unwrap individual films and place film package contents into the trash receptacle and films back into the plastic cup used to carry films into the darkroom. This procedure will help the operator to avoid placing films in the trash receptacle along with film package contents.
   3. Place films one by one into the slots designated for each film. Only one film may be placed at a time into the slots. Any more than one film can cause the

films to stick together, and they will be rendered useless.
   4. Gently pull the lever back to drop the films into the developer and wait for the door to shut before placing any more films into the slots. If films are self-feeding, wait at least five seconds between each film.
   5. Repeat the procedure until all films are in the processor and then wait for the finished film to drop into the tray on the other end.
   6. When all films have been successfully processed, turn processor off, turn on overhead light, and mount films on film holder.
   7. Pick up all trash and disinfect the area after use.

Developing Time and Temperature Table

	Temperature	Developing Time
Lower temperatures	60°F	6 minutes
	65°F	5 minutes
Optimal temperatures	68°F	4½ minutes
	70°F	4 minutes
Higher temperatures	75°F	3 minutes
	80°F	2½ minutes

* To increase the density of the image on the duplicate, you must decrease the time of duplication.
* To decrease the density of the image on the duplicate, you must increase the time of duplication.

XIII. DUPLICATING RADIOGRAPHS

A. Many times, an assistant must duplicate radiographs for insurance purposes, other dental offices, or patients who may be leaving the practice and need a record of treatment to take with them. This process can be accomplished by using double packets when exposing films or a duplicating machine designed specifically for this purpose.
   1. Duplicating film
      a. Comes in individual periapical sizes or one long sheet.
      b. Has one side with emulsion.
      c. Becomes lighter as it is exposed to light.
   2. Duplicating machine
      a. Contains a fluorescent light source.

Common Errors and Corrections for Processing Radiographs

Mistake	Cause	Correction
Clear film	Unexposed film	Retake.
Film not completely immersed in solutions	Solution levels not adequate	Check all solutions before processing.
Light films	Underexposed Underdeveloped Exhausted chemicals Contaminated developer	Increase exposure time. Check chemicals. Change solutions.
Dark films	Overexposure Overdevelopment Light leak	Decrease exposure time. Check solution temp. Perform coin test.
Fogged film	Outdated film Exposure to heat Exposure to light	Check expiration date. Store in cool dry area. Check for light leaks.
Yellow/brown stains	Exhausted chemicals Not fixed long enough Not washed thoroughly	Change solutions. Refix. Rewash.
Streaks	Dirty rollers Dirty water bath Exhausted solutions	Clean transport rollers. Change water. Change solutions.
Black lines	Bent film	Do not bend films.
White lines	Scratched emulsion	Handle films carefully.
Two images on one film	Double exposure	Check to make sure that film was exposed only once.

   b. Has a cover that closes tightly during the duplicating process.
   c. A timer that measures the duplicating time is located on the front of the duplicator.
3. Duplicating process
   a. Turn off all lights in the darkroom.
   b. Place films on film mounts designed for duplicating.
   c. Place films on the duplicator viewing side up.
   d. Place duplicating film over the films with the emulsion side down.
   e. Close the cover securely.
   f. Set the timer and duplicate the radiographs.
   g. After timer has expired, remove films and process duplicating film in the same manner as you would any other radiographic film.

XIV. DARKROOM MAINTENANCE

   A. Safelight testing
      1. Test the darkroom safelight for effectiveness using the coin test, which can be performed by placing a piece of unexposed film out in total darkness, placing a coin on top of the film, and turning on the safelight for five to seven minutes. Process the film and check for the outline on the coin. If the outline appears, there could be a faulty safelight.
      2. Replace safelight and filters when needed.

   B. Light leaks
      1. Test the darkroom periodically for light leaks by turning off all of the lights and looking for slivers of white light coming into the darkroom.

C. Countertops and cabinets
1. Keep all countertops and cabinets clean and free from chemicals.
2. Pick up all trash after using the dark-room.

D. Darkroom equipment
1. Clean regularly and replenish chemicals as needed.
2. Check periodically for normal wear, and repair or replace as needed.
3. Clean film hangers as needed.
4. Order supplies as needed and restock on a regular basis.

XV. MOUNTING RADIOGRAPHS

A. Arrange all film with either the dots convex or concave.

B. Organize the radiographs in their natural anatomic positions.

C. Place the bitewings in the film mounts using the curve of spee as a guideline.

D. Using the bitewings as a guide, arrange the films showing the posterior teeth of the mandibular arch on the bottom of the film mount and slide into the holder.

E. Follow the same routine for the maxillary posterior teeth.

F. Place all maxillary anterior radiographs using the darkened sinus areas as a guideline in the anterior maxillary slots.

G. Place all mandibular anterior radiographs in the anterior mandibular slots.

H. Check by holding up to the light or up to a viewbox to ensure that all radiographs are in their proper position.

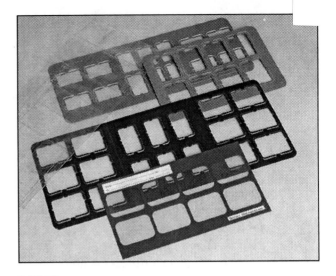

Various full-mouth, bitewing, and single-film mounts.

REVIEW QUESTIONS

1. Which of the following are indications for radiographs?
   1. To detect bone loss
   2. To detect carious lesions
   3. Done if a full set was done before two years have elapsed
   4. Done prior to oral surgery

   A. 1, 2, 3
   B. 1, 2
   C. 3 only
   D. 1, 2, 4

2. The basic atomic structure consists of
   1. atoms.
   2. neutrons.
   3. protons.
   4. electrons.

   A. 2, 3, 4
   B. 1, 3
   C. All of the above
   D. None of the above

3. Molecules are more than one atom and
   A. are considered the smallest particle of a substance.
   B. have only one atom.
   C. do not resemble the physical and chemical makeup of that substance.
   D. have only one electron.

4. The types of radiation include
   1. particulate radiation.
   2. electromagnetic radiation.
   3. x radiation.
   4. rads.

   A. 1, 2, 3
   B. 3 only
   C. 1, 3
   D. All of the above

5. A roentgen is
   A. an amount of radiation that will produce 0.01 rems of energy.
   B. a traditional unit of measurement.
   C. equal to one rad times the unit of absorbed dose.

6. Direct effects of radiation
   A. include damaging effects on a biological, cellular, or molecular level.
   B. cannot be measured.
   C. are not a factor for the patient if proper protection is worn.

7. The ALARA concept emphasizes the use of the _____ possible exposure of the patient and operator to x radiation.
   A. highest
   B. lowest

8. For safety purposes, the operator must
   A. stay out of the path of the primary beam.
   B. stand behind the protective barrier and at least six feet away from the x-ray tubehead.
   C. be positioned behind the patient and either to the left or right of the patient's head.
   D. A, B, and C

9. When the lead apron is not in use, it should be stored
   A. folded neatly on a shelf.
   B. in the darkroom.
   C. on a wooden hanger.
   D. draped over a sturdy rod.

10. Human cells and tissues most sensitive to radiation exposure are
    A. gonadal tissues.
    B. brain tissue.
    C. embryonic tissue.
    D. hepatic tissue.

11. The _____ is a lead disk that is placed over the opening of the x-ray head.
    A. anode
    B. cathode
    C. collimator
    D. primary beam

12. If a film is accidentally exposed to white light, it will be _____ when processed.
    A. black
    B. clear
    C. silver
    D. green

13. According to the international system of radiation units, a rem is expressed as a
    A. rad per kilogram.
    B. coulomb per kilogram.
    C. sievert.
    D. roentgen.

14. Milliamperage determines the _____ of potential x radiation by changing the amount of electrons in the central beam.
    A. quantity
    B. quality

15. A radiograph that captures the crown and root of a tooth is called
    A. bitewing.
    B. periapical.
    C. panoramic.
    D. occlusal.

16. The dark areas of a radiograph are referred to as
    A. contrasting.
    B. radiolucent.
    C. radiopaque.
    D. dense.

17. When placing the lead apron, which of the following areas must be covered?
    1. Reproductive organs
    2. Chest
    3. Throat
    4. Arms

    A. 1, 2, 4
    B. 1, 2
    C. 3 only
    D. 1, 2, 3

18. _____ radiation is radiation that has been deflected from its path during the contact of matter.
    A. Primary
    B. Secondary or scatter
    C. Impact

19. The shorter the wavelength, the _____ the ability of radiant energy to penetrate matter.
    A. greater
    B. weaker

20. When exposing radiographs, the operator must stand behind a
    A. lead-lined barrier.
    B. heavy plastic barrier.
    C. wooden door.
    D. folding screen.

21. Foreshortening is caused by too _____ angulation.
    A. little horizontal
    B. little vertical
    C. much horizontal
    D. much vertical

22. In one year, the maximum permissible dose (MPD) for dental personnel is _____ rem.
    A. 0.1
    B. 0.5
    C. 5.0
    D. 10.0

23. Elongation on a dental radiograph is caused by too _____ angulation.
    A. much horizontal
    B. much vertical
    C. little horizontal

24. The _____ is where the primary x-ray beam is emitted.
    A. PID
    B. tubehead
    C. collimator
    D. aluminum disc

25. The _____ is located at the end of the tubehead and is used to aim the primary x-ray beam.
    A. voltmeter
    B. PID
    C. deadman switch
    D. kvp selector

26. The control panel contains the controls that operate
    1. the on and off switches.
    2. the kvp selector.
    3. the milliamperage controls.
    4. the voltmeter.

    A. 1, 2, 3
    B. 1, 2
    C. 3 only
    D. All of the above

27. A/an _____ is used to absorb low-energy x-rays that have little penetrating power.
    A. collimator
    B. aluminum filter
    C. lead washer
    D. PID

28. A/an _____ further reduces patient exposure to radiation by limiting the area of exposure.
    A. aluminum filter
    B. collimator
    C. PID
    D. mA control

29. Dosimeter film badges
    1. are routinely used and sent out for evaluation.
    2. are used to monitor the amount of scatter radiation that the operator is exposed to.
    3. can be worn outside.
    4. are used only in radiography labs.

    A. 1, 2, 3
    B. 1, 2
    C. 1, 2, 4
    D. All of the above

30. Radiography chemicals must be at least _____ to work effectively.
    A. 76°F
    B. 82°F
    C. 68°F
    D. 61°F

ANSWERS AND RATIONALES

1. D Radiographs are instrumental in detecting bone loss, carious lesions, and impacted teeth. Bitewings are taken every year, and a full mouth series is taken every two to three years.

2. A The basic particles of an atom consist of electrons, which carry an electrical charge; the proton, which has a positive charge; and a neutron, which has no charge.

3. A Molecules are the smallest form of a substance. For example, it takes millions of H_2O molecules to create water. One H_2O molecule is considered the smallest part of that substance, and it still resembles the physical and chemical makeup of the water molecule.

4. A   The following are examples of radiation: particulate radiation is absorbed by body tissue, electromagnetic radiation is derived from gamma and ultraviolet rays, and x radiation is a form of electromagnetic radiation. A rad is a unit of measurement, not a type of radiation.

5. B   A roentgen is a traditional unit of measurement. It is used to measure the intensity of radiation to which an object has been exposed.

6. A   Direct effects of radiation are cumulative and are harmful to tissues by damaging their DNA configuration, causing normal reproduction of cells to mutate.

7. B   ALARA stands for "As Low As Reasonably Achievable" and is the standard by which radiation exposure is followed. The least exposure to get the desired results is always the objective. Lead aprons and thyroid collars are used to aid in accomplishing this.

8. C   It is in the operator's best interest to stay as far away from the primary beam as possible. Several ways to achieve this may include standing behind the patient at a 90°–135° angle, out of the path of the primary beam, or standing behind a suitable barrier or lead-lined wall.

9. D   The lead apron should never be folded or placed in an area where the operator may forget to use it. Folding the lead apron creases the lead within the lining and causes areas where radiation may penetrate the body. All aprons should be stored draped across a sturdy metal rod in the room where the x-ray machine is located.

10. C   Embryonic tissues are most sensitive to x-rays. The most sensitive period for embryonic tissue is the first three months of pregnancy. Rapidly growing tissues may mutate easier than more established or mature cells.

11. C   A collimator reduces the size of the x-ray beam and the exposure to the patient. The size of the beam increases the quality of the x-ray.

12. A   Visible light activates the silver crystals on the film and causes the film to turn black when processed.

13. B   This is a standard unit of measurement that was adopted throughout the world in 1985. One coulomb per kilogram is the international unit of measurement and one roentgen is the equivalent in traditional units.

14. B   The quantity of electricity that passes through the tungsten filament is measured as the milliamperage. The milliamperage measures the number of electrons that are available for the exposure of an x-ray film.

15. B   A periapical film is taken when the entire crown along with the root structures to include the apex are needed for diagnosis.

16. B   Radiolucent parts of the radiograph appear black or gray due to the ability of radiant energy to pass through it. Tissues that appear radiolucent on radiographs include pulpal tissues and soft tissues such as the tongue.

17. D   Tissues that are especially sensitive to radiant energy include embryonic tissues, reproductive organs, chest area, and thyroid. Close attention to these areas is important when draping the patient prior to taking radiographs.

18. B   Scatter or secondary radiation is radiant energy that is deflected from its path on impact. This radiation is deflected from its normal path and is absorbed by the patient. Dosimeter badges can register the amount of scatter radiation that the operator may be exposed to.

19. A   When the wavelength of radiant energy is shortened, the ability for it to penetrate matter increases due to the higher energy or intensity being generated.

20. A   Because radiant energy cannot pass through lead, a lead-lined wall is the safest barrier during radiation exposure. Gypsum walls have been found to be adequate in controlling exposure to the operator.

21. D   An increase in vertical angulation causes the image to become distorted and it gives the appearance that the tooth is shorter than it actually is.

22. C   Health-care workers should strive for zero exposure to radiation by observing radiation safety practices. However, 5 rems per calendar year is permissible and has been found to have no adverse effects on the body as a whole.

23. A   Elongation occurs when the PID is not positioned far enough vertically. This causes the images to appear very long and distorted.

24. A   Radiation is generated in the tubehead and is emitted from the position indicator device.

25. B   The position indicator device is used to aim the primary beam at the target. Position indicator devices come in various sizes and lengths and are lead lined to limit patient exposure.

26. A   The control panel is fixed to the wall and houses the on and off switches; the kilovoltage selector, which controls the penetrating power of the x-ray beam; and the milliamperage button, which controls the quantity of radiant energy emitted.

27. B   Low-energy wavelengths have no value in producing radiographs. An aluminum filter that is positioned between the PID and tubehead removes the low-energy wavelengths, which would otherwise be absorbed by the patient.

28. B   A collimator is a lead disc that determines the size and shape of an x-ray beam. This further reduces unnecessary exposure to the patient by restricting the beam.

29. B   Dosimeter film badges are worn to monitor dental health-care workers during exposure to radiation. These film badges should never be worn outside of the office because sunlight can affect the reading. The results may be skewed and a false reading may be returned when the badge is sent out for evaluation. The dosimeter badge may be worn in any office that exposes radiographs.

30. C   To prevent overly dark or light films, a temperature of at least 68°F should be achieved. A floating thermometer is used, and warm or cold water with the appropriate ratio of chemicals is used to adjust manual tanks. Automatic processors should be turned on for at least five minutes for the first time during the day to warm the chemicals and turned off between uses to avoid overheating chemicals.

Dental Materials and Laboratory Procedures

CHAPTER OVERVIEW

In the dental office, it is important to have a clear understanding of dental materials and their uses. This chapter reviews the many types of dental material and their role in dentistry. It is necessary to understand how each material is used and its characteristics.

KEY TERMS

alginate
amalgam
bite registration
cavity varnish

composite resin restoration
elastomeric impression
    material
glass ionomer cement

hydrocolloid impression
    material
polycarboxylate cement
zinc phosphate cement

I. ALGINATE (IRREVERSIBLE HYDROCOLLOID)

A. Used in reproducing a three-dimensional replica of the dentition and the surrounding tissues.

B. Is used when accuracy is not an issue.

C. Routinely used for opposing models, study models, temporaries, and orthodontic appliances.

D. Advantages are that it is easy to handle, relatively low cost, patient friendly, and can be used on tissue or teeth.

E. Disadvantages are that it is not as accurate as other materials, subject to dimensional changes, and subject to distortion because of its thickness.

F. Alginate is stored in airtight containers in a cool, dry place.

II. ALGINATE TRAYS

A. Trays that are used for impressions are generally metal perforated trays that allow material to flow through the holes to facilitate adherence of alginate to tray.

B. Rim lock trays can be used. They have no perforations but have a border around the rim to facilitate locking of material.

C. Both types of trays can be reused after cleaning and sterilizing.

D. Wax may be applied to the border of the tray to extend the length of the tray distally, buccally, or lingually. This method is called beading.

III. ARMAMENTARIUM NEEDED FOR THE ALGINATE IMPRESSION PROCEDURE

A. Flexible rubber bowl.

B. Mixing spatula.

C. Alginate.

D. Measuring devices.

E. Water.

F. Impression trays.

G. Beading wax if necessary.

IV. PROCEDURE FOR TAKING ALGINATE IMPRESSIONS

A. Seat and drape patient.

B. Inspect inside of patient's mouth for appropriate-size trays. Add wax to rims if needed.

C. Explain procedure to patient and ask patient to remove any retainers or partials.

D. Measure alginate onto separate paper towels for upper and lower trays.

E. Measure water according to manufacturer's recommendations and place into bowls.

F. Place powder into alginate bowl for lower tray and mix until smooth and creamy.

G. Place material in tray and seat firmly into patient's mouth, asking the patient to raise the tongue to check that tray is seated all the way down.

H. When material is set, break the suction in one motion and remove tray.

I. Repeat procedure using upper tray. If patient has a vaulted palate, apply a small amount of alginate to the palate prior to seating impression tray.

J. When both impressions are finished, disinfect, rinse, wrap in a wet paper towel, and then pour up immediately. If they cannot be poured up immediately, they may be placed in the refrigerator for up to 24 hours.

V. CUSTOM TRAYS

A. Final impression trays made from custom study models.

B. Are made only for that particular patient.

C. Used in the fabrication of partial and full dentures.

VI. ARMAMENTARIUM FOR CUSTOM TRAY FABRICATION

A. Self-cure or light-cure plastic material.

B. Study model of interest.

C. Lab knife.

D. Visible light-curing system.

VII. PROCEDURE

A. The study model is trimmed and prepared prior to the procedure.

B. Plastic material is draped over the study model and preformed over the teeth and tissues.

C. Using a lab knife, the lab person cuts the excess material from the edges.

D. The remaining material is then molded to the model, and a handle is made and attached to the end of the tray to use during the impression process.

E. The model and material are then cured according to the manufacturer's directions.

F. After the material has hardened, the rough edges are smoothed and the tray is pumiced with a pumice wheel, disinfected, and placed in a bag for use.

VIII. BITE REGISTRATION

A. Wax bite registration is used for recording the relationship of the maxilla and mandible.

B. Used when trimming study models to articulate both arches correctly.

C. Can be made of wax or other puttylike materials.

D. Used in the fabrication of cast restorations (crown and bridge and removable prosthetics).

IX. PROCEDURE FOR TAKING A BITE REGISTRATION

A. If the material of choice is wax, then a single wafer is softened under warm water and the patient is instructed to gently bring both arches together. The patient will then open, and the bite pattern in the wax will be preserved for use in the lab.

B. If the material of choice is a puttylike material with a base and catalyst, then the material is mixed and placed on the occlusal surface of the area of treatment. The patient is instructed to bite gently but until the teeth come together. The normal occlusion is held in place until the material sets.

X. HYDROCOLLOID IMPRESSION MATERIAL

A. Is reversible (can go from a gel to a solid and back to a gel).

B. Has good detail and is used for final impressions.

C. Advantages of reversible hydrocolloid material
   1. More economical than most final impression materials.
   2. Accurate.
   3. Can be used for cast crown and bridge.

D. Disadvantages
   1. Not as easy to use as other elastomeric impression materials.
   2. Requires additional equipment to prepare material in.
   3. Loses accuracy due to atmospheric conditions.

E. Procedure for using hydrocolloid material
   1. Hydrocolloid conditioner is used to prepare material in.
   2. Unit has three compartments.
      a. First compartment is used to liquefy material.
      b. Second compartment is used for storage.
      c. Third compartment is used for tray material.
   3. All compartments are filled with water.

4. Material for the tray is soft and pliable, and light-body syringe material is runny and designed to flow into the sulcular area.

XI. ELASTOMERIC IMPRESSION MATERIALS

A. Material that is used in crown and bridge for final impression.

B. Can be used with three in one disposable trays or regular perforated trays.

C. Has a base and catalyst.

D. Comes in three groups: polysulfide, silicone (vinyl polysiloxane or polysiloxane), and polyether.

E. Advantages
   1. Easy to use for operator and assistant.
   2. Very accurate.
   3. Is dimensionally stable.

F. Disadvantages
   1. Can be somewhat expensive.
   2. Prone to bubbles.

G. Procedure
   1. The mixing pads are set out (one for the base and one for the catalyst).
   2. Flexible spatulas are placed on pad.
   3. Tubes of material are put out on designated pads.
   4. Operator mixes the light body and places it in the syringe.
   5. Assistant mixes the heavy body and places it in the tray.
   6. Operator flows the light body around the area of treatment and the assistant passes the tray filled with heavy body.
   7. The operator places the tray into the patient's mouth and patient either bites down (three in one tray) or operator holds tray in place until material polymerizes (sets).
   8. The tray is removed after material polymerizes and is sent to the lab with opposing, bite registration, and lab slip.
   9. Sometimes a quick mixing gun is used by the operator to dispense the light body.

XII. PUTTY WASH METHOD

A. The putty wash method is similar to the elastomeric procedure.

B. Preliminary putty impression is taken.

C. When the putty material is set, it is removed from the mouth, and all undercuts are removed.

D. The light body is then applied, and the putty impression is passed to the operator and placed into the patient's mouth.

XIII. THE USE OF A STENT

A. A stent is used for a variety of reasons.
1. To stabilize the teeth in the arch (splinting).
2. Used following periodontal grafting to protect the graft site.
3. Used as an intermediate retainer following the removal of bands and brackets.
4. Used as trays for vital bleaching.
5. When thicker material is used, it can be an appliance for bruxating.
6. Can be used in making a temporary bridge or crown.

B. Advantages
1. Can be made right in the office.
2. Easy to fabricate.
3. Economical.
4. Comfortable for the patient because of the custom fit.

C. Disadvantages
1. Not long lasting.
2. May have to be made over again if treatment is prolonged.
3. Study models have to be stored until treatment is completed.

D. Procedure
1. An alginate impression is taken and poured up in stone.
2. The model is then separated and trimmed.
3. Wax or block out material is placed in any areas that have undercuts.
4. The desired thickness of plastic is placed in the vacuform machine and heated.
5. The softened plastic is then formed over the model and set aside to cool.
6. The plastic stent is carefully separated from the model, and all excess plastic is trimmed to fit patient's mouth.
7. The plastic stent is placed in the patient's mouth to check that soft tissue is not impinged upon.

8. The patient is instructed to wear the stent as prescribed by the dentist and to return if stent is torn or no longer fits.

E. Armamentarium
1. Patient's study model.
2. Plastic sheet of material for stent.
3. Vacuform machine.
4. Lab knife and sharp scissors.
5. Block out wax.

F. Fabricating a stent
1. A thin wafer of clear plastic material is placed into the vacuform machine.
2. The heating element of the machine is turned on, and the model is placed under the wafer and heating element.
3. When the wafer reaches the desired consistency, the vacuum portion of the machine is turned on and the sliding mechanism is slid over the model.
4. The heating element and vacuum is turned off, and the plastic is allowed to cool.
5. The stent is then trimmed with a lab knife and removed from the model. Any fine trimming is done with scissors.
6. The stent is then delivered to the patient with instructions for use and care.

XIV. GYPSUM MATERIALS

A. Products that are used to pour up impressions.

B. Can be fast setting or regular set depending on the color of the product.

C. Can be stone or plaster.

D. Vary in strength, dimension, and accuracy.

E. Types
1. Plaster
   a. Also known as "plaster of paris."
   b. Weakest of the stones.
   c. Economical.
   d. Used in areas where detail and strength are not as important.
   e. Used to pour up study models, opposing models, mounting study models and casts, and for repairing casts.
2. Class I stone
   a. Three times as strong as plaster.
   b. Used where strength is needed.

c. Used for study models and working casts for partial and full dentures.

d. Normally yellow in color.

3. Class II stone
    a. 30% stronger than class I stone.
    b. Uses less water to incorporate its small uniform parts.
    c. Used for dies or where a strong model or cast is used.

4. Orthodontic stone
    a. Mixture of plaster and class I stone.
    b. Stronger model can be used for orthodontic treatment.
    c. Used for study models for orthodontic treatment.

5. Quick set stone
    a. Usually pink in color.
    b. Used when an immediate model is needed.
    c. Can be used during treatment because of its rapid setting time.

F. Armamentarium for missing plaster and stone
    1. Flexible bowl.
    2. Spatula.
    3. Vibrator.
    4. Impression.
    5. Plaster or stone.
    6. Large piece of tile or glass slab to rest impression on.
    7. A small instrument (brush or flexible metal cement spatula).

G. Procedure
    1. According to manufacturer's recommendation, place powder and liquid ratio out.
    2. Dry impression and make sure it is free from blood or other debris.
    3. Add powder to water and begin mixing until smooth consistency has been achieved (no longer than 30 seconds). Place on vibrator to remove any bubbles.
    4. Begin adding mixture to impression while on the vibrator (set on low) and rolling beginning with the most distal area and allowing the material to flow into the anatomy of each tooth. Continue this method until the entire impression is filled with material. Pay close attention that each and every tooth is filled with no voids. A small

brush or flexible metal cement spatula can help you achieve this.

5. Set aside.
6. Take the remaining material and place on the surface that is going to be used while material is setting.
7. Invert impression and rest on top of material.
8. Bring sides up just to meet the impression material. Be careful not to attach plaster or stone to impression tray. This could cause "rim lock" and make it difficult to separate the impression without damaging it.
9. When material is set, separate.

H. Separating the impression from the plaster or stone
    1. Material should set for at least one hour (unless it is quick set).
    2. The impression should feel cool and moist to the touch.
    3. Using a lab knife, gently loosen the material from the impression.
    4. Lift impression tray straight up. Do not move from side to side because this may cause the teeth to fracture or model to break.
    5. Models may be soaked in water for three to five minutes prior to trimming. This eases the trimming process.

I. Trimming the models
    1. Wearing safety goggles, turn model trimmer and water supply on.
    2. Place models on model trimmer ledge and cut excess material from all sides, including back.
    3. Using light pressure, trim the base of the model so it is flat and approximately a half to an inch thick.
    4. Turning the model upward (teeth facing operator), trim the heels of the model at 115°.
    5. Turn model and trim the buccal aspect to the depth of the buccal sulcus, being careful not to cut the tissues or buccal frenum or shave off any portions of the tooth (angled at 55°).
    6. Using the angles for the art portion of the casts, trim the maxillary arch to a point (using a 30° angle) and the mandibular arch in a rounded fashion.

Articulate with the wax bite and trim so that casts are even.

7. After trimming is complete, turn trimmer off and remove goggles.

8. Use a lab knife to remove any bubbles or defects.

XV. DENTAL WAXES

A. Derived from bees, plants, and minerals.

B. Must be uniform and provide consistent results.

C. Used to reproduce the patient's bite, around impression trays, and constructing a prosthesis.

D. Types
   1. Pattern wax
      a. Also known as inlay wax.
      b. Has a degree of hardness and resists chipping and flaking.
      c. Will completely burn out at temperatures above 900°.
   2. Processing wax
      a. Used for impressions (box wax or utility strips for the edge of the trays).
      b. Sticky wax that is brittle at room temperature but can be melted with a flame to become pliable and sticky.
      c. Periphery wax that does not require a flame.
      d. Used in orthodontics to cover hardware that is irritating to tissues.
   3. Impression wax
      a. Used to take bite registrations.
      b. Sometimes have a sheet of aluminum in between two pieces of wax.
      c. Usually comes in the shape of a horseshoe and is red in color.

XVI. FABRICATING TEMPORARY RESTORATIONS

A. Indications for the placement of a temporary crown or bridge
   1. To protect preparation while permanent restoration is being fabricated and to decrease sensitivity.
   2. To maintain space between prep teeth and natural teeth on either side of the abutments.
   3. To maintain esthetics during the fabrication of the permanent restoration.
   4. To provide an adequate chewing surface while permanent restoration is being fabricated.

B. Types of temporaries or provisionals
   1. Aluminum posterior full coverage crowns.
   2. Polycarbonate anterior crowns.
   3. Custom acrylic coverage.

C. Temporary aluminum crowns
   1. Preformed posterior crowns.
   2. Cut and contoured to fit each tooth individually.
   3. Some have anatomy and some resemble a tin can.
   4. Can be filled with acrylic to achieve a more custom fit.

D. Armamentarium
   1. Temporary crown.
   2. Crown and bridge scissors.
   3. Crimpers or contouring pliers.
   4. Temporary cement, spatula, and paper pad for mixing.
   5. Articulating paper.
   6. Dental floss.
   7. Acrylic (optional).
   8. Finishing bur.
   9. Basic setup.
   10. Millimeter ruler.

E. Fabricating the aluminum temporary
   1. After the preparation has been cut, measure the area to be covered.
   2. Select a crown that will fit the area mesially and distally.
   3. Try the selected temporary and have patient bite down gently on a cotton roll for a preliminary seat.
   4. Take an explorer and scribe the area where the margin occurs.
   5. Remove temporary, and using the crown and bridge scissors, trim the scribed area away.
   6. Using the crimping or contouring pliers, crimp the edges inward.
   7. Try the temporary crown on the preparation to check fit and trim and contour as needed until buccal and lingual areas meet the margin and interproximal areas are not impinging on gingiva.

8. Acrylic may be placed inside the crown at this point if the operator chooses. After the acrylic is set, trim as necessary.
9. Check with floss in the interproximal and articulating paper for occlusal bite.
10. Cement the crown with desired temporary cement and remove excess.
11. Give postoperative instructions regarding wearing the temporary and taking care of the area while the temporary is on.

F. Advantages of using a preformed polycarbonate crown
1. Easy to adapt to the area of coverage.
2. Esthetically pleasing.
3. Gives appropriate shape and contour to the tooth that is being covered.
4. Can be quickly placed.

G. Disadvantages of using a preformed polycarbonate crown
1. If a patient has had periodontal disease and requires crown lengthening, these crowns are not manufactured with a long enough gingival margin.
2. Do not adapt well to teeth that are shaped other than standard-looking teeth (i.e., bell shaped, long and thin, or other irregularities).
3. Will not work for patients who have gingival recession.

H. Armamentarium
1. Temporary polycarbonate crowns.
2. Non-eugenol cement, spatula, and mixing pad.
3. Articulating paper.
4. Assorted finishing burs and sandpaper discs.
5. Temporary material.
6. Paper cup.
7. Cotton rolls and basic setup.
8. Rag wheel and pumice.

I. Fabricating the temporary polycarbonate crown
1. After the retraction cord has been removed and the final impression taken, the patient is ready to have the provisional constructed.
2. Measure the area to be covered with a millimeter ruler.

3. Choose a preformed polycarbonate crown to fit the area both mesially and distally.
4. Apply a petroleum jelly product to the preparation.
5. Mix acrylic to a homogeneous but thick consistency.
6. Fill polycarbonate crown with acrylic material.
7. While material is initially setting up, run hot water and place in a cup.
8. When acrylic has reached a rubbery consistency, remove several times on and off from the preparation to shape the inside of the crown.
9. When material begins to demonstrate an exothermic reaction, place in the water bath for 6–10 minutes.
10. Remove temporary crown and trim margins of the crown so that they do not impinge on the gingiva.
11. Contour the crown so that it fits both mesially, distally, and incisally.
12. After checking with the articulating paper, polish on the rag wheel with pumice and cement with non-eugenol cement.
13. After cement is set, clear with a scaler or explorer.
14. Give postoperative instructions to patient regarding wearing the temporary and taking care of the area while the temporary is on.
15. In some states, the assistant can fabricate and cement provisional restorations.

J. Fabricating custom acrylic restorations
1. When fabricating a custom acrylic crown, a die or matrix must be constructed.
2. Can be made of alginate or on a vacuform machine.
3. After establishing which tooth will be temporized, fabricate a die for the provisional.
4. Choose a shade that closely resembles the natural shade of the tooth to be temporized.
5. Mix enough polymer and monomer in a paper cup to adequately fill the die.
6. Place material in a plastic monoject-type syringe and extrude material into

the die, making sure that it is dry and free from moisture.

7. Place matrix (alginate impression or plastic vacuform tray) back into the patient's mouth over the area to be temporized (prep should be covered with petroleum jelly).

8. Monitor closely for the setting of material by extruding a small amount onto the patient's bib.

9. Material should come off of the preparation when it reaches the rubbery stage.

10. If material is left on too long, it could adhere to the preparation and will have to be removed with a bur and the temporary fabricating procedure started over.

11. Remove die, and using cotton pliers, remove temporary.

12. Trim excess from margins and interproximal area and place back on and off of preparation several times.

13. When the exothermic process begins, place temporary into the water bath for 6–10 minutes.

14. Remove and do final contouring and trimming with finishing acrylic burs and sandpaper discs. Polish on lathe using rag wheel.

15. Check with articulating paper and floss in between the contacts, then cement with non-eugenol cement.

16. After cement has set, remove with explorer or scaler.

17. Give postoperative instructions to patient regarding wearing the temporary and taking care of the area while the temporary is on.

18. In some states, the assistant can fabricate and cement on the provisional restoration.

19. There are two methods of fabricating a custom acrylic temporary.
    a. Direct method
       (1) The temporary is fabricated directly onto the tooth.
    b. Indirect method
       (1) The temporary is fabricated outside the mouth using a model.

20. Other materials used in the fabrication of custom temporaries
    a. Composite self-cure
       (1) Dispensed in two tubes (base and catalyst).
    b. Composite light cure
       (1) Dispensed in one cartridge.
       (2) Cured or hardened with visible light.

K. Armamentarium
   1. Die or matrix of preparation.
   2. Temporary material.
   3. Paper cup, spatula, cement, and mixing pad.
   4. Cotton rolls, basic setup, scissors, and scaler.
   5. Articulating paper, finishing burs, and sandpaper discs.
   6. Rag wheel and pumice.

L. Advantages
   1. Can be used for preparations that have irregular margins.
   2. Can be adapted to fit areas that are irregular mesially and distally.
   3. Can re-create the original shape of the crown of the tooth.
   4. Can be used to cover more than one tooth (i.e., a multiunit bridge).

M. Disadvantages
   1. Operator must have a solid understanding of tooth anatomy.
   2. Artistic ability plays a part in fabrication of custom anterior temporaries.
   3. To be efficient, operator must be experienced in the fabrication of acrylic temporaries and well versed on the use of materials.

XVII. DENTAL CEMENTS

A. Dental cements or luting agents are used for a variety of reasons. Each cement has certain characteristics that make it appropriate for different uses. The primary uses of dental cements include restoration, luting, and bases.
   1. Characteristics of cements used in restorations
      a. Used when strength is a key factor.
      b. Can be permanent
         (1) Expected to last several years.
      c. Intermediate
         (1) Expected to last about six months.

d. Temporary
  (1) Palliative (ease discomfort).
  (2) Expected to last only a few weeks.
2. Sedative purposes
  a. Used to soothe and promote healing in trauma-type situations.
  b. Can be used when the tooth has deep caries or is fractured.
3. Luting agents
  a. Hold two things together.
  b. Used to cement crowns and bridges in place.
  c. Can be used in temporary crown coverage.
  d. Can be used to cement orthodontic appliances in place.
  e. Can be used to cement posts and pins into teeth for retention.
4. Bases
  a. Protective base
    (1) Used after a tooth has been prepared for a filling.
    (2) Used to stimulate reparative dentin.
    (3) Used to protect the pulp from postoperative sensitivity.
  b. Insulating base
    (1) Used when a considerable amount of dentin is removed.
    (2) Protects the tooth from thermal sensitivity.
    (3) Used primarily under metal restorations.
    (4) Usually placed over the protective base.
  c. Sedative base
    (1) Used when a substantial amount of tooth is removed.
    (2) Zinc oxide eugenol is the material of choice.
    (3) Used to soothe the pulp.
    (4) Placed directly over the pulpal floor.
5. Zinc phosphate cement (Fleck's)
  a. Mixed on a cool glass slab
    (1) A cool glass slab dissipates the heat given off during mixing to prolong working time.
  b. Provided in a powder and liquid form
    (1) Type I (fine grain) used for the cementation of cast restorations.

c. Type II (medium grain) used as an insulating base in deep cavity preparations.
  d. Thick mixes are used for bases and thin mixes are used for cementation of cast restorations.
  e. Temperature sensitivity
    (1) Ideal glass slab temperature is 68°F.
    (2) Should not be cooled to the dew point due to condensation occurring.
6. Zinc oxide eugenol (Tempax, Tempbond)
  a. Temporary luting agent.
  b. Used as an insulating base.
  c. Sedative treatment.
  d. Cannot be used with acrylic restorations.
  e. Supplied in a powder and liquid.
  f. Soothing to the pulp.
  g. Comes in two types
    (1) Zinc oxide eugenol type I lacks strength and long-term durability.
    (2) Zinc oxide eugenol type II has reinforcing agents added and is used as a luting cement of permanent cast restorations.
  h. Eugenol precautions
    (1) Can irritate the gingiva due to the clove oil content.
    (2) Can contaminate other materials when used.
  i. Intermediate restorative material (IRM)
    (1) Is a reinforced zinc oxide eugenol cement.
    (2) Can be used for temporary cementation of permanent restorations for up to one year.
    (3) When permanent cementation is not advised, can be used as an intermediate material.
    (4) Dispensed in powder and liquid or premixed capsules.
7. Ortho-ethoxybenzoic acid cement
  a. Also known as EBA.
  b. Is the type II zinc oxide eugenol cement.
  c. Used for cementation of crowns, bridges, inlays, and onlays.

Cavity Medication Placement Sequence

1. Cavity varnish is applied in two thin coats to seal dentin tubules.
2. Cavity liner such as calcium hydroxide is placed in the deepest part of the preparation.
3. A protective base is placed to insulate the tooth from thermal sensitivity.
4. Amalgam is placed in the preparation.

8. Polycarboxylate cement (Durelon)
   a. Bonds to the tooth.
   b. Tooth surface has to be free of debris and dry before cementation.
   c. Some contain crystals that release fluoride and can be used under amalgam restorations as a base.
   d. Supplied in a powder and liquid
      (1) Must be measured exactly to manufacturer's directions.
      (2) Has a limited shelf life.
      (3) Low pH (1.7).
9. Glass ionomer (Fuji, Ketac)
   a. Powder to liquid ratio must be followed exactly.
   b. Is supplied in a capsule, light-cure, self-cure, or powder/liquid mixtures.
   c. Takes at least 24 hours for maximum strength to occur.
10. Cavity varnishes (Copalite)
   a. Used to seal dentin tubules.
   b. Can be used on a crown preparation prior to cementation of permanent crown.
   c. Flows easily and evaporates quickly.
   d. Cannot be used under resin or glass ionomers.
11. Calcium hydroxide (Dycal)
   a. Used in the deepest part of the cavity preparation.
   b. Stimulates reparative dentin.
   c. Protects the pulp by soothing it.
   d. Available in a two-paste system.
   e. Can be self-cure or light cure.

XVIII. COMPOSITE RESIN MATERIALS

A. Three major components
   1. Resin matrix.
   2. An inorganic filler
      a. Glass, quartz, or silica particles.
   3. Coupling agent
      a. Bonds the filler to the resin.

B. Provided in a paste form and after placement is either cured with visible light until material has set to a hard plastic or sets without the use of a light.
C. Used for anterior restorations.

XIX. AMALGAM

A. Used primarily for posterior restorations or as a core buildup.
B. Mixed (triturated) with mercury and a collection of alloy materials.
C. Economical and easy to use.
D. Durable and will last several years.

REVIEW QUESTIONS

1. Alginate is a/an _____ hydrocolloid.
   A. reversible
   B. irreversible

2. _____ may be applied to the edge of the alginate trays to improve the fit of the tray.
   A. Boxing wax
   B. Beading wax
   C. Orthodontic wax
   D. Pattern wax

3. A custom tray can be used only for the patient it was fabricated for.
   A. True
   B. False

4. Which of the following is true regarding a bite registration?
   1. Can be made of wax or other puttylike material
   2. Is used to articulate the relationship of the maxilla and the mandible
   3. Used when fabricating custom trays
   4. Used in the fabrication of fixed or removable prosthetics

   A. 1, 2, 3
   B. 1, 3
   C. 1, 2, 4
   D. All of the above

5. Which of the following is true regarding elastomeric impressions?
   1. Use a base and a catalyst
   2. Accurate and dimensionally stable
   3. Require a warming bath to prepare

4. Can be used with crown and bridge procedures
   A. 1, 2, 4
   B. 2, 3
   C. 3 only
   D. All of the above

6. A stent is used to stabilize the teeth in the arch or following periodontal surgery.
   A. True
   B. False

7. Gypsum materials include which of the following materials?
   1. Plaster
   2. Class I stone
   3. Quick set stone
   4. Orthodontic stone

   A. 1, 2, 3
   B. 1, 3
   C. 2 only
   D. All of the above

8. For operative dentistry, zinc phosphate cement is used
   A. to cement temporary crowns.
   B. as an alternative to a cavity liner.
   C. to cement permanent restorations.
   D. as a periodontal dressing.

9. Polycarboxylate cement is used
   A. as a base.
   B. as a liner.
   C. to cement permanent restorations.
   D. as core buildup material.

10. Cavity varnish is
    A. applied before base material but after cavity liner.
    B. applied after cavity liner but before base material.
    C. never used with base material.
    D. always used with composite resin materials.

11. Zinc oxide eugenol is used as
    A. a base under composite restorations.
    B. an insulating base material.
    C. a permanent cement.
    D. a liner.

12. Glass ionomer contains _____, which is released slowly into the tooth structures.
    A. clove oil
    B. fluoride
    C. calcium
    D. phosphorus

13. _____ is used as a cavity liner or as pulp-capping material.
    A. Zinc phosphate
    B. Zinc oxide eugenol
    C. Calcium hydroxide
    D. Polycarboxylate cement

14. Zinc oxide eugenol contains _____, which soothes tooth structures.
    A. fluoride
    B. clove oil
    C. calcium
    D. calcium hydroxide

15. When sizing an aluminum temporary crown, which of the following must occur?
    1. The crown must fit the area both mesially and distally.
    2. The crown must be trimmed and contoured to fit the preparation.
    3. The crown must not impinge on the gingiva.
    4. The crown should not be contoured on the mesial or distal surfaces.

    A. 1, 2, 4
    B. 2, 4
    C. 3 only
    D. 1, 2, 3

16. The preferred cement to use when cementing a temporary aluminum crown is
    A. zinc oxide eugenol cement.
    B. polycarboxylate cement.
    C. zinc phosphate cement.
    D. EBA cement.

17. The preferred cement to use when cementing a polycarbonate crown is
    A. zinc oxide eugenol.
    B. zinc phosphate.
    C. polycarboxylate.
    D. non-eugenol temporary cement.

18. Intermediate cements are expected to last at least _____ months.
    A. two
    B. three
    C. six
    D. nine

19. An insulating base is used for which of the following situations?
    1. After a tooth has a considerable amount of dentin removed
    2. Used primarily under amalgam
    3. When there is no danger of thermal sensitivity from a restoration

4. Usually placed over a protective base

A. 1, 2, 3
B. 2, 3
C. 4 only
D. 1, 2, 4

20. Which of the following is true of luting agents?
    1. Used to soothe and promote healing in trauma-type situations
    2. Can be used to cement crowns and bridges in place
    3. Can be used to cement orthodontic appliances in place
    4. Can be used when there is a fracture or deep caries

    A. 1, 2, 3
    B. 2, 3
    C. 3 only
    D. All of the above

21. Because of the exothermic properties of zinc phosphate, it is generally mixed
    A. on a paper mixing pad.
    B. on a cool glass slab.
    C. in a dappen dish.
    D. with a metal spatula.

22. Which of the following are characteristics of cavity varnish?
    1. Used to seal dentin tubules
    2. Used to stimulate reparative dentin
    3. Flows easily and evaporates quickly
    4. Cannot be used under resin or glass ionomers

    A. 1, 2, 4
    B. 2, 3
    C. 1, 3, 4
    D. All of the above

23. Which of the following are characteristics of calcium hydroxide?
    1. Used to stimulate reparative dentin
    2. Protects the pulp by soothing it
    3. Cannot be used under resin or glass ionomers
    4. Flows easily and dries slowly

    A. 1, 3, 4
    B. 2, 4
    C. 1, 2
    D. 2, 3, 4

24. Amalgam is
    1. used primarily for posterior restorations or as a core buildup.
    2. economical to use.
    3. durable and will last several years.

4. triturated with mercury and other alloy materials.

A. 1, 2, 3
B. 1, 3
C. 2, 4
D. All of the above

Match the following.

_____ 25. Calcium hydroxide

_____ 26. Cavity varnish

_____ 27. Zinc oxide eugenol

_____ 28. Zinc phosphate

_____ 29. Glass ionomer

_____ 30. Luting agent

A. Used to seal dentin tubules
B. Mixed on a cool glass slab
C. Contains fluoride
D. Used to stimulate reparative dentin
E. Contains clove oil
F. Used to adhere structures together

ANSWERS AND RATIONALES

1. B Due to the properties in alginate, once it has been mixed and has set, it cannot be returned to a powder/water or creamy state. Therefore, it is deemed irreversible.

2. B Utility wax ropes may be placed around the periphery of the alginate tray to extend the length of the alginate tray or provide a better fit around the vestibular areas.

3. A Because custom trays are fabricated using the patient's study models, it is a custom fit for that particular patient and can be used for that patient only.

4. C Bite registration material is used to articulate the bite between the maxillary and mandibular arches. Wax, polyvinylsiloxane impression material, or other puttylike materials may be used. A bite registration is not used in the fabrication of a custom tray because the articulation of the dental arches is not needed.

5. A Polyvinylsiloxane impression material is used to take impressions for fixed and removable prostheses. It is provided in a base and catalyst and mixed just before placement into the mouth. Polyvinylsiloxane impression material is very dimensionally

stable and does not require immediate pour up in stone or plaster.

6. A   When periodontal surgery is performed, the teeth may become temporarily mobile. During the healing phase, the dentist may fabricate a stent, which is a clear plastic retainer to stabilize the teeth in the arch.

7. D   Gypsum materials are used to create a positive reproduction created by the impression material. Gypsum products include plasters and stones.

8. C   Zinc phosphate, which is used to cement permanent crowns, is mixed on a cool glass slab. It is never used as a liner because of the irritation of phosphoric acid to the pulp. It is not suitable as a periodontal dressing.

9. A   Because of its compatibility with amalgam and composite, it may be used as a nonirritating base under either of these materials.

10. B   Cavity varnish is applied in two thin coats to seal dentin tubules and reduce thermal sensitivity. It should be placed after a cavity liner to avoid sensitivity. It can be used with zinc phosphate or zinc oxide eugenol base materials but not with resin due to the incompatibility.

11. B   Zinc oxide eugenol can be used under amalgam restorations as an insulating base material due to the eugenol (clove oil) content that is soothing to tissues and the insulating properties when the mixture is mixed to a puttylike consistency.

12. B   Fluoride is contained in glass ionomer cements. It is slowly released into the tooth structures. Glass ionomers come in powder/liquid, capsules, light cure, and paste depending on their intended use.

13. C   Because of its ability to stimulate secondary or reparative dentin, calcium hydroxide is used as a cavity liner or as a pulp cap.

14. B   The properties found in clove oil are soothing to tooth structures.

15. D   When placing a temporary crown, special care should be given to the fact that the patient will be without the permanent restoration for a short period of time. When sizing the temporary, the contacts on the mesial and distal sides should be closed to avoid drifting, and the crown should be trimmed and crimped to avoid impingement on the tissue, which could result in a periodontal problem later on.

16. A   Because of its soothing properties and limited strength, zinc oxide eugenol is used to cement temporary aluminum crowns in place.

17. D   Any non-eugenol temporary cement may be used to seat a temporary acrylic crown. The properties in eugenol retard or break down the composition of acrylic material. Zinc phosphate and polycarboxylate cements are more suited for permanent restorations.

18. C   Temporary cements are designed in strength and solubility to be effective for six months maximum.

19. D   An insulating base is used to protect a near pulpal exposure from thermal sensitivity. It can be placed after the tooth has lost a large portion of the dentin, under an amalgam, or over a protective base.

20. B   Luting agents are used to cement two things together. A luting agent can be used to cement crowns and bridges in place (polycarboxylate and glass ionomer cements) and bands for orthodontic treatment (ortho-ethoxybenzoic cement).

21. B   When mixing zinc phosphate, a cool glass slab is used to slow the setting process and give the operator extra time to manipulate it.

22. C   Cavity varnish is applied in two thin coats. It is used to seal dentin tubules, which will reduce thermal sensitivity, and because of its low viscosity, it flows easily into the cavity preparation.

23. C   Calcium hydroxide is used to stimulate reparative dentin and protects the pulp by providing a thin layer between the near pulpal exposure and other restorative materials. It is thick in nature and does not flow as easily as cavity varnish. The properties in calcium hydroxide make it suitable for use under almost any restoration.

24. D   Amalgam is a durable mix of mercury and alloy metals. It can be used as a core buildup and also as a restorative material. Amalgam is not suitable for anterior restorations because of its gray appearance.

25. D

26. A

27. E

28. B

29. C

30. F

CHAPTER 7

Restorative Dentistry

CHAPTER OVERVIEW

Dental hand instruments, handpieces, and burs are used routinely in the dental office for restorative and laboratory procedures. Knowledge of dental instruments is essential for performing dental functions with accuracy and competency. A basic understanding of how and why an instrument is used is the groundwork for performance in the field.

KEY TERMS

chisel	hoe	single-ended instrument
hand instrument	periodontal probe	stones
handpiece	rubber points	ultrasonic handpiece
high-speed handpiece	shaft	working end

I. HAND INSTRUMENTS

A. Hand instruments get their name because they are held in the operator's hand when being used without the aid of a handpiece or other device.
  1. A hand instrument is made up of three parts.
    a. Handle: The part of the instrument that the operator grasps or holds. Handles have various shapes, sizes, and textures. Manufacturers make a variety of handles to accommodate different likes.
    b. Shank: The part of the instrument that connects the handle and the working end. Shanks are designed to reach different areas of the mouth by increasing the angles for posterior areas and limiting the angles for anterior areas.
    c. Working end: The part of the instrument that is used to perform the procedure on the tooth. The working end can have a point; a blade; or a blunt tip, which is also called a nib. Hand instruments can have a single or double end.

II. BASIC SETUP

A. The basic setup is the four most commonly used instruments. The basic setup consists of a mouth mirror, an explorer, cotton pliers, and a periodontal probe.
  1. Mouth mirror: Used to see area of the mouth, retract tissue, and give light and

access to different areas of the mouth. Mouth mirrors come in a variety of sizes and types.
   a. Sizes: ¾ inch to 1⅝ inches.
   b. Types: Front surface, concave, and flat surface.

2. Explorers: Used to distinguish defects or anomalies in tooth structures. They have a thin, flexible, wirelike working end that enables the operator to use tactile sensitivity.

3. Cotton pliers: Used to place and retrieve small objects. Ends may be smooth or serrated, and handles may be locking or non-locking.

4. Periodontal probes: Used to measure pocket depths of the gingival attachment. This instrument has a long, slender working end with measurements in millimeters.

III. HAND INSTRUMENTS FOR RESTORATIVE PROCEDURES

A. Operators prefer to use certain instruments during the restorative procedure. No two operators will use hand instruments in the same manner or even at all. Some of these instruments are used for cutting enamel, smoothing or shaping preparations, or placement of materials.

1. Excavators: A hand instrument with a working end shaped like a spoon, used to remove decay from a cavity preparation. Excavators are used primarily when a dentist wants to be conservative about removing decay and when getting close to the pulp.
   a. Types of excavators include small, medium, large, and cleoid-discoid because of the scooping cutting edge that the discoid has.

2. Hatchets: Used primarily for removing weak or undermined enamel, a hatchet usually has at least one bend in the shank and a sharp cutting edge.
   a. Types of hatchets include a mesial margin trimmer and distal margin trimmer.

3. Chisels: Used to plane the enamel margins of a cavity preparation. Chisels have a cutting edge and can create sharp, crisp angles in the cavity preparations.
   a. Types of chisels include a binangle, straight, and an angle former.

4. Hoes: Used to smooth the walls of a cavity preparation prior to filling.

5. Amalgam carriers: Used to carry the triturated amalgam from the amalgam well to the patient's oral cavity.
   a. Types of amalgam carriers include the double ended with a small and large end and the single ended, which carries only one increment (*in some states, the dental assistant can place the amalgam while the dentist condenses it*).

6. Amalgam condensers: Used to condense the triturated amalgam once it is placed into the cavity preparation. The shank is angled, and the working end can be flat or have small serrations in it.

7. Amalgam carvers: Used to carve the condensed amalgam once the cavity preparation has been adequately filled. Carvers come in different types to accomplish different tasks.
   a. Types of carvers include a Tanner carver, which resembles a cleoid-discoid, and a Hollenback carver, which is used to carve the interproximal area following the removal of the matrix band and wedge.

8. Burnisher: Used to smooth the condensed amalgam or other materials after placement into the preparation. Burnishers are all-purpose tools and come in many shapes to accommodate different tasks.
   a. Types of burnishers include the ball, acorn, football, beavertail, and egg.

9. Plastic instrument: Used to move plastic or other malleable material before it sets. Plastic instruments are actually made of stainless steel. They are usually double ended and have a flat working end on one side and a condenser-like nib at the other end.
   a. One type of plastic instrument is called a Woodson.

10. Spatulas: Used to mix dental cements, alginates, gypsum products, and other impression materials. Spatulas come in different shapes and sizes depending on the task you want to accomplish.

a. Types of spatulas include the all-metal small spatula used for cements; the large metal spatula with the wooden handle for alginates and gypsum products; and plastic spatulas, which are used for other types of impression materials.

11. Crown and collar scissors: Used to trim aluminum or stainless steel crowns, trim retraction cord, remove a rubber dam, or perform other tasks that require blunt scissors. Crown and collar scissors are also called crown and bridge scissors and come with either a curved or straight cutting end.

12. Articulating paper holder: Used to hold the articulating paper in place while checking the occlusion of your patient. The handle is positioned so that it is next to the patient's cheek while the clip is on the buccal side of the patient's dentition.

Note: All instruments should be cleaned, dried, sterilized, and left in the sterilization pouch until just before they are used.

IV. DENTAL HANDPIECES

A. The dental handpiece is one of the most commonly used instruments in the dental field. Handpieces can be used in the operatory and in the dental lab. Handpieces come in two types: the high-speed handpiece and the low-speed handpiece. Dental lab engines also have a handpiece that is custom. Ultrasonic handpieces used for calculus or dental cement removal also can be considered a handpiece. After each use, any handpiece should be sterilized appropriately following the manufacturer's recommendation before it is used for another patient.

1. High-speed contra-angle handpiece
   a. Operates on compressed air.
   b. Reaches speeds of 450,000 rpm.
   c. Removes gross amounts of enamel.
   d. Equipped with water and air spray devices to cool the tooth during use.
   e. Uses a friction grip type of bur.
   f. Comes in different bur grip devices
      (1) Secured by a bur chuck.
      (2) Secured by depressing a button to insert bur into handpiece.
   g. Available in fiber optic
      (1) Mounted in the head of the handpiece.
      (2) Light source is situated so that light shines directly on the prep.
      (3) Improves visibility.

2. Slow-speed handpiece
   a. operates at speeds of up to 25,000 rpm.
   b. used for removal of soft decay.
   c. can be used to smooth tooth structures during restorative procedures.
   d. comes with a variety of attachments.
      (1) Prophy angle
         (a) Snap-on or screw type.
         (b) Disposable or autoclavable.
      (2) Contra-angle with latch.
   e. Can be used alone with straight burs.
   f. Can be used in the dental lab with long shanked straight bur.

3. Laser handpiece
   a. Used for surgical procedures.
   b. Contains a light source through a fiber-optic cable.
   c. Used to cut, cauterize, or vaporize tissue.
   d. Can be used to control bleeding during surgical procedures.
   e. Operator and assistant should be thoroughly trained prior to using laser treatment.

4. Ultrasonic handpiece
   a. Uses sound waves and water to vibrate debris from tooth structures.
   b. Used for removal of gross amounts of deposits from tooth structures.
   c. Used to clean and enlarge root canals.

5. Sonic handpiece
   a. Uses air pressure to create vibrations for the removal of deposits.
   b. Should be used on patients with pacemakers because they are safer than ultrasonic scalers due to the air-driven handpiece as opposed to the electrical source on the ultrasonic.

V. CARE OF HANDPIECES

A. Both high-speed and slow-speed handpieces must be lubricated and cleaned after each patient. Because handpieces come in contact with blood, saliva, and bioburden, they should be cleaned, sterilized, and lubricated following the manufacturer's recommendations.

VI. DENTAL BURS

A. Dental burs come in all shapes and sizes and are designed to perform different tasks. All burs, however, have the same basic anatomy.
   1. Shank: The part of the bur that fits into the dental handpiece.
      a. Can be short or long depending on where in the oral cavity it is going to be used.
      b. Straight, latch type, or friction grip.
   2. Neck: The part of the bur that connects the shank and the head.
   3. Head: The part of the bur that is used for cutting, shaping, or polishing.

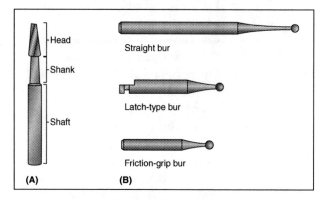

(A) Parts of a bur. (B) Different shanks: straight, latch type, and friction grip.

B. Types of carbide burs
   1. Round: Usually numbered from ¼ to 8.
   2. Inverted cone: Usually numbered from 33½ to 37.
   3. Fissure burs.
      a. Straight: Usually numbered from 56 to 58.
      b. Tapered: Usually numbered from 169 to 171.
      c. Cross-cut straight: Usually numbered from 556 to 558.
      d. Cross-cut tapered: Usually numbered from 669 to 701.
      e. Pear: Usually numbered from 330 to 333.

C. Diamond burs are used to remove gross amounts of enamel and to polish and shape restorations. Diamond burs are so named because they are impregnated with an industrial-grade diamond for cutting and smoothing performance. Diamonds are named for their shapes and classified by coarseness.
   1. Grits
      a. P (pre-stressed): Used for removing gross amounts of enamel.
      b. M (micrograin): Used for cutting and contouring.
      c. F (finishing grain): Used for removing lines and angles and smoothing.
      d. XF (super-finisher): Used for polishing and contouring composites.
   2. Types of diamond burs
      a. Round: Used to shape occlusal surfaces and make retention grooves for partials.
      b. Flat end taper: Used to remove enamel for crown preparations.
      c. Cylinder: Used to smooth and finish walls when flat sides are required.
         (1) Composite trimming and shaping burs: Used to smooth and shape composite restorations.
         (2) Flame shaped: Used when a beveled edge is needed.
         (3) Wheel shaped: Used to remove gross amounts of enamel and to shape occlusal edges.

D. Other types of rotary instruments
   1. Polishing discs: Used to polish composite materials, they have a gritty working side and are similar to sandpaper discs.
      a. Coarse.
      b. Medium.
      c. Fine.
      d. Extra fine.

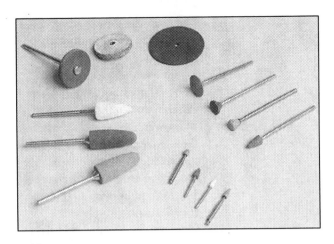

Various types and grits of stones, wheels, and points.

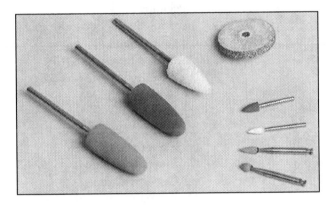

Wheel and points.

2. Stones: Used when adjusting or polishing a gold or amalgam restoration.
   a. Red: Gold and amalgam.
   b. Gray: Gold and amalgam.
   c. Black: Gold and amalgam.
   d. White: Tooth-colored restorations or enamel.
   e. Rubber points: Used to polish metallic restorations.
      (1) Brown.
      (2) Green.
   f. Mandrels: Used to attach polishing devices to the slow-speed handpiece.
   g. Lab burs: Usually shaped much the same way as ordinary burs; however, the working end is larger and they are never used in a patient's mouth. The burs are designed to take more force when pressure is applied to them.

E. Care of burs
   1. Carbide burs: Can be cleaned and sterilized but become brittle and dull after two or three uses.
   2. Diamond burs: Usually used one time and then discarded; however, some diamond burs are reused but with each sterilization become dull and lose some of the diamond texture.
   3. Discs: Used one time and then discarded.
   4. Rubber points and stones: Can be sterilized and reused.

Note: All burs should be cleaned and sterilized in between patient use. Burs should be discarded when they become dull or brittle or show any signs of rust.

VII. DENTAL DAM

A. The dental dam is used to isolate one or more teeth during dental treatment. A dental dam is thin latex rubber material that is placed over the teeth to expose only the coronal portion of the teeth. The teeth are referred to as being isolated or exposed.
   1. Dental dam application
      a. Usually applied after local anesthetic is delivered.
      b. Tooth being treated is usually free of debris or plaque.
      c. Medical and dental history are reviewed to rule out any latex sensitivity.
      d. Dental chart is reviewed to reaffirm which tooth is being treated so that the dam can be placed.
   2. Indications for placement of the dental dam
      a. Infection control protective barrier.
      b. Protects the patient from any chemicals or instrumentation used during the procedure.
      c. Prevents aspiration of foreign materials.
      d. Used to control moisture during the procedure.
      e. Retraction of gingival tissue for easier access to the tooth.
      f. Increases efficiency for the dental health team.
      g. Increases access by retracting lips, cheeks, and tongue.

3. Dental dam armamentarium
   a. Dental dam material
      (1) Comes in 6 x 6 or 5 x 5 inch sizes.
   b. Offered in different gauges (thicknesses)
      (1) Thin: Used for endodontics.
      (2) Medium: Used for its ease.
      (3) Heavy or extra heavy: Used when tissue retraction or resistance is apparent.
   c. Offered in different colors
      (1) Pastels and green.
      (2) Dark green preferred most because of good color contrast and reduces glare.
   d. Dental dam frames
      (1) Young's frame: Stainless steel U-shaped frame with sharp projections on the outer portion of the frame.
      (2) Plastic U-shaped frame: Placed under the dental dam rather than on top like the Young's frame. Plastic material is suitable for leaving in place during radiographs.
      (3) Ostby frame: Round plastic frame with sharp projections around the outer portion of the frame. Dental dam material is placed on the outside of the frame.
   e. Dental dam napkins
      (1) An option used to control moisture under the dental dam material.
   f. Dental lubricants
      (1) Used over the holes of the dam before sliding over the teeth to be isolated.
      (2) Make dam application easier.
      (3) Can be any water-soluble lubricant.
      (4) Lubricate patient's lips with petroleum jelly prior to dam placement.
   g. Dental dam punch
      (1) Used to create holes in the dental dam needed to isolate the teeth to be treated.
      (2) Holes on the punch are graduated in size to accommodate tooth size.
   h. Dental dam stamp and templates
      (1) Dental dam stamp is a rubber stamp with a standard upper and lower arch template on it.
      (2) Flexible templates are available so that they can be moved around to accommodate arches that have malpositioned teeth.
   i. Dental dam clamp forceps
      (1) Used to place dental clamps onto the cementoenamel junction of the anchor tooth.
   j. Dental clamps
      (1) Used for the anchor tooth in dam placement.
      (2) Come in different varieties
         (a) Anterior double bowed.
         (b) Bicuspid.
         (c) Molars.
         (d) Winged or wingless.
         (e) Flat pronged.
         (f) Inverted pronged.
         (g) Cervical clamps.
      (3) Made of chrome or nickel plated steel.
      (4) Anchor tooth is the tooth distal to the tooth being treated.
      (5) Come in pediatric sizes.
4. Dental dam application
   a. Armamentarium
      (1) Precut dental dam material.
      (2) Dental dam stamp and ink pad or template and pen.
      (3) Dental dam punch.
      (4) Dental dam clamp with floss ligature (for retrieval in the event of aspiration).
      (5) Dental dam clamp forceps.
      (6) Dental dam frame.
      (7) Dental floss or tape.
      (8) Lubricant for patient's lips.
      (9) Lubricant for dam.
      (10) Burnisher (beavertail) for inverting dental dam.
      (11) Scissors.
      (12) Coronal polish setup if needed.
   b. Dental dam application
      (1) Multiple tooth isolation method

(a) Choose the teeth to be isolated (3 or 4 teeth in addition to treatment tooth; 8 to 10 teeth are used for optimum stability).

(2) Stamp dental dam and punch appropriate holes.

(3) Choose appropriate clamp and tie ligature floss around bow of clamp.

(4) Place lubricant on patient.

(5) Place clamp on anchor tooth (one tooth distal to tooth being treated).

(6) Place dental dam material over anchor tooth and walk dental dam material along arch, exposing crowns of teeth to be isolated.

(7) Using a beavertail burnisher, invert dental dam into sulcus of gingiva.

(8) Place dental napkin over dental dam material.

(9) Place frame on dental dam material.

(10) Pull floss ligature through.

(11) Ligate through all isolated teeth with floss.

(12) Readjust dental dam material to remove any wrinkles or folds.

c. Single tooth isolation method

(1) Used for endodontic treatment.

(2) Class V restorations.

(3) One tooth or two teeth are isolated only.

d. One-step method

(1) Clamp and dental dam material are placed at the same time.

e. Two-step method

(1) Clamp is placed and then dental dam material over clamp.

f. Dental dam removal

(1) Remove any ligatures that may have been used to stabilize the dental dam.

(2) Using dental dam forceps, remove dental dam clamp.

(3) Using scissors, cut between the septum of each isolated tooth and remove dental dam material, frame, and dental dam napkin.

(4) Check dental dam and patient's oral cavity for any retained pieces of dental dam material.

(5) Rinse patient's mouth and any residual debris from the patient's face.

g. Alternative dental dam techniques

(1) Quickdam

(a) Used instead of traditional dam.

(b) Dental dam and frame combination.

(c) Quicker and easier to use than traditional dam.

(2) Placing a dental dam around a fixed bridge

(a) Stamp hole for pontic.

(b) Place ligating floss in the mesial and distal interproximal of the pontic for stability.

(c) A surgical needle may be used to aid in the ligation and securing of the dental dam around the pontic of the bridge.

REVIEW QUESTIONS

1. The _____ is the part of the instrument where the operator grasps or holds the instrument
   A. shank
   B. handle
   C. nib
   D. working end

2. The basic setup consists of
   A. mouth mirror, periodontal probe, and explorer.
   B. mouth mirror, explorer, and pocket marker.
   C. cotton pliers, mouth mirror, and explorer.
   D. mouth mirror and explorer.

3. Explorers have which of the following characteristics?
   1. A thin flexible, wirelike working end
   2. Are useful in detecting subtle anomalies in tooth structures
   3. Can be single or double ended

4. Are designed to give the operator tactile sensitivity when using

   A. 1, 2, 3
   B. 2, 3
   C. 3 only
   D. All of the above

4. A spoon excavator
   1. is a hand instrument with a working end that is shaped like a spoon.
   2. is used to remove soft decay.
   3. comes in one size.
   4. is used when the operator does not want to create a pulpal exposure.

   A. 1, 2, 4
   B. 2, 3
   C. 3 only
   D. None of the above

5. Amalgam condensers are used to
   A. carry amalgam to the preparation.
   B. pack amalgam into the preparation.
   C. mix mercury and alloy together to create amalgam.
   D. are used to remove old amalgam material.

Match the following.

_____ 6. Hatchet

_____ 7. Hoe

_____ 8. Chisel

_____ 9. Carver

_____ 10. Burnisher

_____ 11. Plastic instrument

   A. Used to smooth the walls of a cavity preparation prior to filling with amalgam
   B. Used to plane the enamel margins of a cavity preparation
   C. Used for removing weak or undermined enamel
   D. Used to smooth condensed amalgam
   E. Used to carve condensed amalgam after the preparation has been filled
   F. Used to move resin material prior to curing

12. Ultrasonic handpieces are used to remove calculus and dental cements from the oral cavity.
    A. True
    B. False

13. The high-speed contra-angle handpiece reaches speed of 450,000 rpm.
    A. True
    B. False

14. Which of the following is true about the slow-speed handpiece?
    1. Operates at speeds of up to 25,000 rpm
    2. Can be used to smooth tooth structures during restorative procedures
    3. Used for removal of decay on hard enamel structures
    4. Comes with a variety of attachments

    A. 1, 2, 4
    B. 3, 4
    C. 2 only
    D. All of the above

15. Laser handpieces have which of the following characteristics?
    1. Used for surgical procedures
    2. Contains a light source through a fiber optic cable
    3. Used to cut, cauterize, or vaporize tissue
    4. Can be used to control bleeding during surgical procedures

    A. 1, 2, 3
    B. 1, 3
    C. None of the above
    D. All of the above

16. The high-speed contra angle handpiece should be cleaned, lubricated, and sterilized after each patient use.
    A. True
    B. False

17. Which of the following are types of carbide burs?
    1. Round fissure
    2. Tapered cross cut fissure
    3. Straight cross cut fissure
    4. Inverted cone fissure

    A. 1, 2, 3
    B. 2, 3
    C. 4 only
    D. All of the above

18. A mandrel is used to
    A. extend the bur length by 2 mm.
    B. attach polishing devices to the slow-speed handpiece.
    C. sharpen polishing stones.
    D. remove gross amounts of enamel.

19. Stones are used when adjusting or polishing a gold or amalgam restoration.
    A. True
    B. False

20. A white stone is used when polishing an amalgam restoration.
    A. True
    B. False

21. Which of the following is true regarding a dental lab bur?
    1. Usually shaped much the same way as ordinary burs
    2. Can be used in the patient oral cavity
    3. Should be cleaned and sterilized the same way ordinary burs are
    4. Are designed to take more force when being used

    A. 1, 2, 4
    B. 2, 3
    C. 4 only
    D. 1, 3, 4

22. Rubber points and stones can be
    A. used one time and then discarded.
    B. used only outside the patient's mouth.
    C. sterilized and reused.
    D. sharpened when they become dull.

23. Finishing discs come in x-fine, fine, medium, and coarse grits.
    A. True
    B. False

24. High-speed handpieces generally use a _____ bur.
    A. latch type
    B. friction grip
    C. static
    D. concentrated

25. Finishing strips are used to smooth the _____ surfaces of the finished restoration.
    A. buccal and lingual
    B. mesial and distal
    C. facial and distal
    D. incisal and lingual

Place in order of use starting with A and ending with E.

26. _____ Burnisher

27. _____ Condenser

28. _____ Carver

29. _____ Articulating paper

30. _____ Amalgam carrier

ANSWERS AND RATIONALES

1. B The handle of an instrument is designed for operator comfort. It can be round or have several sides. It connects the shank to the working end.

2. C The three most common instruments that will appear on the bracket tray are the mouth mirror, cotton pliers, and explorer, which comprise the basic setup. The back office team will use these three instruments the most.

3. D An explorer is used to detect defects in tooth structures. Because of its thin flexible end, it can be used when subtle anomalies such as decay or fractures need to be detected. They are always included on any restorative or exam setup tray.

4. A Spoon excavators are used to scoop out soft decay from cavity preparations. They come in a variety of sizes and have a semisharp cutting edge.

5. B Amalgam condensers, which come in different sizes, are used to condense or pack soft amalgam into the cavity preparation.

6. C
7. A
8. B
9. E
10. D
11. F
12. A Ultrasonic handpieces operate by converting high frequency current into vibration. These vibrations are felt at the tip of the ultrasonic handpiece. Ultrasonic handpieces are ideal for removing tenacious calculus or orthodontic cement.

13. A The high-speed contra-angle handpiece travels at revolutions of 450,000 per minute. It is ideal for removing decay from enamel surfaces. The speed of the handpiece generates frictional heat and so a fine mist of water and air are generated at the end of the handpiece to keep the operative site cool.

14. C Slow-speed handpieces operate slower than the high-speed contra-angle. They are ideal for removing soft decay and smoothing composite material during restorative procedures. The speed is too slow to be effective for removing enamel.

15. 4   Laser handpieces are generally used for surgical procedures. They may be used to cut or cauterize tissues during surgery. Care when using the laser handpiece should always be a concern because any dirt or contaminate may damage the fiber-optic cables.

16. A   The Centers for Disease Control recommends that all handpieces that come into contact with blood or saliva be cleaned and sterilized following each patient use. When lubricating the handpiece, you should always follow the manufacturer's recommendations. Handpieces should also be flushed for at least 20–30 seconds before and after each patient use.

17. 4   Carbide steel burs are used for cutting tooth structures. They come in several different shapes to achieve different types of cuts. The most common shapes are round, inverted cone, tapered and straight cross-cut, and tapered and straight plain. Carbide steel burs are numbered for the size and shape of the head of the bur.

18. B   A mandrel is an attachment that connects onto the latch-type contra-angle. It is used to attach different types of discs, rubber cups, and other polishing devices onto the slow-speed handpiece.

19. A   Stones are routinely used for polishing amalgam restorations to a shiny finish. Red, gray, and black stones are used to finish metallic surfaces.

20. A   White stones are primarily used to finish amalgam or tooth-colored restorations.

21. D   Dental lab burs are used in the dental lab only. They look much like regular dental burs except that they are larger in size and are designed to withstand heavier forces. They are never used in the patient's mouth and are sterilized between each use.

22. C   Because of the abrasive nature of the rubber points, they can be sterilized and used several times before they have to be replaced. They cannot be sharpened because the abrasive material is impregnated into the rubber point itself.

23. A   Finishing discs are small circular discs used to smooth or finish tooth surfaces. They are usually used on resin or plastic restorations.

24. B   Burs that do not require a latch are defined as friction grip. Friction grip burs generally require a bur chuck to release and tighten the bur in the handpiece. Some high-speed handpieces have a quick release button for the friction grip burs and do not require a bur check.

25. B   Finishing strips and lightening strips are used to smooth overhangs in the interproximal areas between the teeth.

26. C

27. B

28. D

29. E

30. A

Endodontics

CHAPTER OVERVIEW

Endodontics is the branch of dentistry concerned with the diseases, injuries, and treatment of pulpal tissues. Endodontics is sometimes referred to as root canal therapy. Root canal therapy provides the opportunity to save a tooth that may otherwise be lost to extensive decay or trauma to the pulp. This chapter covers the instrumentation and materials used in endodontic therapy, procedures routinely performed by the endodontist, and infection control during endodontic therapy.

KEY TERMS

apicoectomy	mobility test	root amputation
broach	necrotic	root canal therapy
endodontic explorer	non-vital	rubber stops
endodontic file	obturate	spreaders
Gates-Glidden burs	paper points	transillumination test
gutta-percha	Peeso reamer	vitality
hemisection	percussion test	vitalometer
irrigating solution	pulpitis	working length
Lentulo spiral		

I. ANATOMY OF THE PULP

A. The pulp chamber is the part of the pulp that follows the anatomy of the entire tooth. The pulp as a whole is called the pulp chamber.

B. The coronal pulp is located within the crown of the tooth.

C. Pulp horns are located in the coronal portion and extend upward toward the occlusal or incisal edges.

II. COMPOSITION OF THE PULP

A. Nerve tissue
 1. Receives and transmits stimuli.
 2. Travels through the apical foramen.
 3. Can necrotize through disease or trauma.

B. Blood supply
 1. The pulp connects to the dental arteries and travels through the apical foramen.
 2. Contains nutrients that feed the tooth.
 3. Provides protection from bacterial invasion.

C. Other components of the pulp
   1. Lymph
      a. Provides an infection control mechanism for the tooth.
   2. Fibroblasts
      a. Provide cellular substances needed for valuable fluid exchange.
   3. Tissue fluid
      a. Provides moisture and nutrients to the pulpal tissues.

III. ENDODONTIC PULP TESTING

   1. Exploratory procedures and testing
      a. Subjective: Recording all symptoms explained by the patient.
      b. Objective: Pulp vitality readings, radiographs, visual, and clinical examination.
   2. Testing individual teeth
      a. Tooth must not already have had endodontic treatment.
      b. Have a full crown.
      c. Restorations that prevent the testing instrument from coming into contact with enamel.
   3. Pulp vitality testing: Testing the pulp using a battery-operated instrument that delivers a mild electrical pulse. This pulse will establish the vitality of the dentition.
   4. Mobility testing: A technique used to test the degree of movement of a tooth within the socket.
   5. Percussion: Gently tapping on the coronal portion of the suspected tooth to establish unusual sensitivity.
   6. Heat: Applying a heated instrument or heated gutta-percha to the suspected tooth to establish unusual sensitivity.
   7. Ice stick: The application of an ice stick or chilled instrument to the dentition to determine the degree of sensitivity to cold.
   8. Anesthesia: The doctor may inject anesthesia into the area when the suspected tooth cannot be determined through routine testing. The process of elimination during the individual anesthesia of each tooth will isolate the tooth in question.
   9. Transillumination: Using a strong light source (fiber optic or visible light) to illuminate each tooth and examine for potential fractures relating to tooth sensitivity.
   10. Radiographs: Used to identify any suspicious activity around the apex and surrounding tissues.

IV. ENDODONTIC PROCEDURES

   A. Root canal therapy
      1. Complete removal of the coronal and root portion of the pulp.
      2. Requires more than one appointment.
      3. Procedure
         a. Tooth in question is examined and a radiograph taken.
         b. Local anesthetic is administered if necessary and dental dam is placed.
         c. An accessory canal or opening is made.
         d. The pulp is removed from the pulp chamber and root canals. Instrumentation of the canals using broaches, files, and reamers are used.
         e. A pellet containing medication along with temporary material is placed and the tooth is sealed until the next appointment.
         f. Subsequent appointments are needed to completely clean out the pulp chamber and root canals.
         g. On the final appointment, the canals are obturated or filled and a final radiograph is taken.
         h. A temporary is placed and a final restoration will be placed at a later date by the general dentist.
   B. Pulpotomy
      1. Usually performed on primary teeth.
      2. Is indicated when there is trauma or injury to the pulp.
      3. Two treatments are available when considering a pulpotomy.
      4. Partial removal of the pulp
         a. Apexification: This procedure is performed on an immature permanent tooth needing root canal therapy. Calcium hydroxide is then placed into the canal and the accessory canal is then closed with temporary or permanent cement.

b. Apexogenesis: Treatment of the pulp by extirpating the diseased portion of the pulp and leaving the rest of the pulp intact so that the roots may continue to form.

C. Pulpectomy
   1. Performed when the pulp cannot be saved.
   2. Complete removal of the pulp chamber and root canal pulpal tissues.
   3. Canals on primary teeth may or may not be filled.

D. Root amputation
   1. Removal of one or more roots on a multirooted tooth.
   2. Performed when an existing root canal has failed.
   3. Can be performed on a vital tooth but will require endodontic therapy on remaining roots.

E. Apicoectomy
   1. The surgical removal of the apex of the root of a tooth.
   2. Usually performed when there is inadequate sealing of the apex following a root canal.
   3. Can also be performed when there is a fracture of the root of a tooth.
   4. Usually performed on endodontically treated teeth.

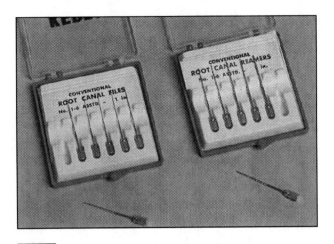

Reamers showing standardized numbers.

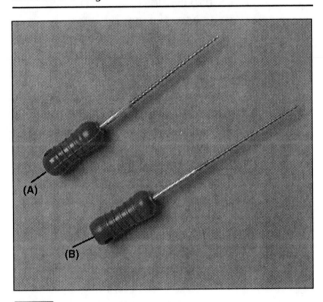

(A) K-type file. (B) Hedström file.

V. ENDODONTIC INSTRUMENTATION

A. Hand instruments
   1. Broach: Used to remove the bulk of the pulp from the canal.
      a. Sizes range from coarse to xxxx-fine.
   2. Files: Used to clean and shape canals.
      a. Sizes range from 8–140 mm.
      b. Come in two varieties
         (1) K-type, which have a spiral shape.
         (2) Hedström, which have sharp blades for quick cutting.
      c. Can be shaped to accommodate irregular canals.
   3. Finger plugger: Used to condense gutta-percha into the canals.

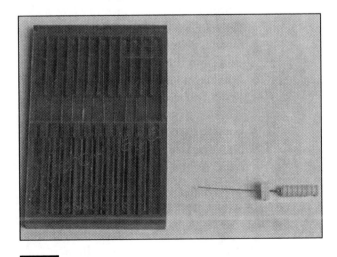

Barbed broach.

4. Endodontic explorer: Hand instrument used to probe and locate position of endodontic canals.
5. Endodontic spoon excavator: Hand instrument used to remove debris from the coronal aspect of the tooth.
6. Plastic instrument: Hand instrument used to place temporary filling material into the accessory canal.

B. Apex locater
1. Instrument used to locate the apex of the tooth during endodontic therapy.

C. Ultrasonic cleaning device
1. Used to debride the canals during endodontic therapy.
2. Uses high frequency and water to break down material within the canals.

D. Rotary instruments
1. Slow-speed contra-angle: Fits on slow-speed handpiece and is used to hold instrumentation needed for endodontic therapy.
   a. Lentulo spiral: Used to place canal sealer into clean and dried canals.
   b. Peeso reamer: Used to enlarge and shape canals.
      (1) Comes in six sizes.
      (2) Spiral in shape and made of tungsten carbide.
   c. Gates-Glidden: Used to enlarge and shape canals prior to filling.
      (1) Fits on a latch-type contra-angle attachment.
      (2) Comes in six sizes and resembles a Peeso reamer but has an elliptically shaped barbed cutting end.

VI. MATERIALS USED IN ENDODONTICS

A. Obturating materials
1. Paper points: Used to dry canals that have been irrigated.
2. Gutta-percha: An inert material used to fill clean and dried canals.
3. Accessory points: Used in conjunction with master cones in obturating canals. Made of gutta-percha material and used to fill the space after the master cones have been placed.

B. Irrigants
1. Sodium hypochlorite (household bleach and water).
2. 70% isopropyl alcohol
   a. Used in the final stages prior to obturation.
3. Anesthetic
   a. Used in the beginning stages to anesthetize and irrigate simultaneously.
4. Hydrogen peroxide
   a. Used for its effervescent qualities.

C. Medicaments
1. Formocreosol.
2. Camphorated monochlorophenol.
3. Calcium hydroxide.
4. Most medications are applied using a cotton pellet and placed in the coronal portion of the tooth and temporary cement is placed over the area until the next appointment.

D. Other armamentarium used during endodontic therapy
1. Heat source: Used to heat an instrument for gutta-percha condensing.
2. Irrigating syringe: Used to irrigate canals during endodontic procedures.
3. Dental dam setup: Used to isolate the tooth that endodontic therapy will be performed on.
4. Millimeter ruler: Used to establish a working length and measure files during root canal therapy.
5. Cotton pellets: Used to place medications into the accessory canal.
6. Spatula and mixing pad: Used to mix sealer and temporary cements.
7. Locking hemostats: Used for transporting items to and from the canals.
8. Scissors: Used to cut gutta-percha and paper points.

VII. INFECTION CONTROL DURING ENDODONTICS

A. Infection protocol during endodontic therapy
1. Personal protective equipment must be worn, and protocol must be followed.
   a. Gloves, mask, protective eyewear, and lab coat must be worn.

b. A complete medical and dental history must be taken on the patient prior to treatment.

2. Follow general sterilization guidelines regarding hand instruments and rotary instruments.

3. Dispose of all single-use items.
   a. Paper points and all other paper products.
   b. Saliva ejectors.
   c. Broaches.

4. Files that have become fatigued through excessive sterilizing should be disposed of.

5. All files, reamers, hand instruments, and any other items that are autoclavable must be put into a holding solution, rinsed and dried, and placed into an autoclave or chemclave after being bagged or placed in a sterilizing cartridge.

6. Glass bead sterilizer
   a. Used to sterilize files and reamers at chairside.
   b. Small heated container filled with tiny glass beads or salt and used during endodontic therapy.
   c. Heated to 270°F.

B. During endodontic therapy, aseptic conditions are very important due to the nature of the procedure. The goal during endodontic therapy is to remove all traces of bacteria from the canal. It is imperative that during the procedure there is no introduction of bacteria or other contaminants into the canal.

VIII. RADIOGRAPHS DURING ENDODONTIC THERAPY

A. Radiographs are an important component of the overall endodontic procedure.
   1. Establish nature and extent of the infection.
   2. Used to establish a working length by which to set the canal cleaning instruments at.
   3. Used by the insurance company for billing purposes.

B. Exposing and processing radiographs during endodontic therapy
   1. Important points to follow
      a. Never bend or crease the film. This will cause elongation or foreshortening and can distort the image on the film.
      b. Placement of film to include apex is critical to completely debride and fill the canal.
      c. Processing times must be followed closely to provide a clear and readable image.

IX. ISOLATION OF OPERATIVE SITE DURING ENDODONTICS

A. During endodontic therapy, a dental dam is used to aid in maintaining visibility and aseptic conditions.

B. A plastic frame is used to avoid artifacts on the radiographs.

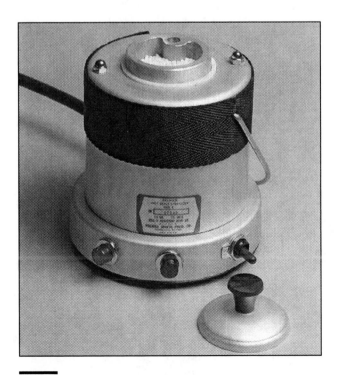

Glass bead sterilizer.

REVIEW QUESTIONS

1. A pulpectomy is
   A. the partial removal of the pulp while the tooth remains non-vital.
   B. the complete removal of the pulp and the tooth is no longer vital.
   C. the partial removal of the pulp while the tooth remains vital.
   D. the complete removal of the pulp while the tooth remains vital.

2. A pulpotomy is
   A. the partial removal of the pulp while the tooth remains vital.
   B. the complete removal of the pulp while the tooth remains non-vital.
   C. the partial removal of the pulp while the tooth remains non-vital.
   D. the complete removal of the pulp while the tooth remains vital.

3. The film taken during endodontic therapy to establish the length of the canal during instrumentation is called a _____ radiograph.
   A. panorex
   B. periapical
   C. working length
   D. cephalometric

4. Which of the following are accepted methods of sterilization for endodontic files?
   1. Glass bead sterilizer
   2. Autoclave
   3. Ultrasonic
   4. Chemclave

   A. 1, 2, 3
   B. 1, 2, 4
   C. 1, 2
   D. All of the above

5. An apicoectomy would be indicated if
   1. inadequate sealing of the canal is present.
   2. fractured roots are present.
   3. accessory canals are present.
   4. canals are calcified.

   A. 1, 2, 3
   B. 1, 2
   C. 1, 2, 4
   D. None of the above

6. Methods for testing the sensitivity of the pulp include which of the following?
   1. Transillumination test
   2. Vitalometer
   3. Cold test
   4. Percussion test

   A. 1, 2, 3
   B. 1, 2, 4
   C. 2, 3, 4
   D. All of the above

7. Radiographs taken during endodontic therapy include which of the following?
   1. Working length
   2. Final periapical
   3. Diagnostic periapical
   4. Bitewing

   A. 1, 2, 3
   B. 1, 2, 4
   C. 2, 4
   D. All of the above

8. _____ is the part of the pulp that follows the anatomy of the entire tooth.
   A. The pulp horn
   B. The pulp canal
   C. The pulp chamber
   D. The coronal pulp

9. Nerve tissue in the pulp does which of the following?
   1. Receives and transmits stimuli
   2. Travels through the apical foramen
   3. Promotes bone regeneration
   4. Can necrotize through disease or trauma

   A. 1, 2, 3
   B. 1, 2, 4
   C. 1, 2
   D. All of the above

10. Subjective responses regarding tooth sensitivity include which of the following?
    1. Observation during transillumination testing
    2. Patient's perception of where the pain originates
    3. Sensitivity to chewing
    4. Evaluation of the radiograph

    A. 1, 2, 3
    B. 2, 3
    C. 1, 2, 4
    D. 4 only

11. Mobility testing is
    A. a technique to evaluate unusual sensitivity of a tooth.
    B. a technique used to evaluate the movement of a tooth within the socket.
    C. a technique used to evaluate the ability of a tooth to move into a new position.
    D. used only in endodontics.

12. Root canal therapy
    1. is the partial removal of the root portion of the pulp.
    2. is the complete removal of the coronal portion of the pulp.
    3. is the complete removal of the coronal and root portion of the pulp.
    4. is indicated when there is trauma or injury to the pulpal tissues.

    A. 1, 2, 3
    B. 1, 2, 4
    C. 3, 4
    D. All of the above

13. A root amputation
    1. is removal of one or more roots on a multi-rooted tooth.
    2. is performed when an existing root canal has failed.
    3. can be performed on a vital tooth.
    4. is also referred to as a hemisection.

    A. 1, 2, 3
    B. 1, 2, 4
    C. 1, 3
    D. 1 only

14. An apicoectomy
    1. is the surgical removal of the apex of the root of a tooth.
    2. is usually performed when there is inadequate sealing of the apex following a root canal.
    3. can be performed when there is a fracture of the root of a tooth.
    4. is usually performed on endodontically treated teeth.

    A. 1, 2, 3
    B. 1, 2, 4
    C. 1, 4
    D. All of the above

15. An ultrasonic cleaning device
    A. debrides the canals of foreign material.
    B. can be used in a slow-speed handpiece.
    C. does not require the use of water.

Match the following.

_____ 16. Broach

_____ 17. Gates-Glidden

_____ 18. K-type file

_____ 19. Hedström

_____ 20. Gutta-percha point

_____ 21. Paper points

_____ 22. Lentulo spiral

    A. Used to enlarge and shape canal walls
    B. Inert material used to obturate the canals
    C. Used to remove soft tissue from the canals
    D. Used to dry canals during root canal therapy
    E. Used to plane the walls of the canal
    F. A drill used to enlarge and straighten the canal
    G. Used to place canal sealer prior to filling

23. The dental dam in endodontics is used to prevent patients from breathing through their mouth.
    A. True
    B. False

24. Radiographs, vitality readings, a clinical examination, and input from the patient regarding symptoms are needed for evaluating a tooth for endodontic therapy.
    A. True
    B. False

25. Accessory points are used during the obturation of a tooth.
    A. True
    B. False

26. Paper points can be sterilized and reused.
    A. True
    B. False

27. A broach is considered a single-use item.
    A. True
    B. False

28. A glass bead sterilizer is used to
    A. store files and broaches during endodontic therapy.
    B. sterilize small instruments at chairside during endodontic therapy.

...ercha.
... medications prior to placement
...nal.

...gs are pulp vitality readings and the
... of a radiograph.
   ...ve
   B. Subjective

30. A Hedström file has a _____ cutting edge.
    A. twisted
    B. barbed
    C. rigid
    D. blunt

ANSWERS AND RATIONALES

1. B A pulpectomy is the complete removal of the pulp and is generally performed on primary teeth when a traditional root canal cannot be performed.

2. A When the partial removal of the pulp is indicated, a pulpotomy may be performed. A pulpotomy is generally performed when there is extensive decay to the coronal portion of the tooth.

3. C A working length film is taken to establish the length of the canal during endodontic therapy.

4. B A glass bead sterilizer can be used at chairside. An autoclave and chemclave can be used to effectively sterilize endodontic files.

5. B When a canal has not been adequately sealed or a fractured root is present, an apicoectomy may be performed to alleviate chronic infection or discomfort.

6. C Several methods are used to evaluate the health of a pulp. A vitalometer, which uses electrical current to establish the vitality of the tooth; an ice stick to test sensitivity to cold; and lightly tapping, which is called a percussion test, are routinely used.

7. A Several radiographs are taken during the course of endodontic therapy. A diagnostic periapical is taken to diagnose the tooth, a working length is taken to establish length, and a final periapical is taken to confirm treatment.

8. B The pulp canal follows the anatomy of the root structures within the tooth.

9. B Pulpal tissue fills the pulp canals and coronal pulp and is responsible for transmitting stimulus. Pulpal tissue also nourishes the tooth by providing blood and lymph via the apical foramen and can necrotize through disease or trauma.

10. B Subjective responses are those observations or reactions that are felt by the patient and communicated to the dentist and staff. Sensitivity to chewing and where the pain originates are all responses that can be answered only by the patient.

11. B Mobility is the degree of movement detected within the alveolar socket. These readings are recorded during the examination and used in the overall diagnosis.

12. C A traditional root canal consists of the complete removal of the coronal and root canal portion of the pulp and is usually indicated when there is trauma or disease to the pulpal tissues.

13. B A hemisection or root amputation can be performed to remove one or more roots or when an existing root canal has failed in one canal but is successful in any of the other treated canals.

14. D Following root canal therapy, inadequate sealing of the apex of a canal may occur or a root canal may fracture. When this occurs, an apicoectomy is sometimes performed. It is never performed on a vital tooth.

15. A An ultrasonic device uses high frequency to create vibration along with an irrigant such as sterile saline or water. This vibration debrides the canals of necrotic tissues and helps to prepare the canal for obturation (filling).

16. C
17. F
18. A
19. E
20. B
21. D
22. G
23. B A dental dam is used to improve infection control, prevent the patient from aspirating small instruments or materials, and improve visibility by retracting tissues and decreasing saliva content in the area.

24. A Information gathered by the dental team is vital in evaluating and treating a tooth for endodontic therapy.

25. A Accessory points resemble gutta-percha points but are thinner and are used to aid in the filling of a tooth.

26. B Paper points cannot be reused because they are made of paper. They are a single-use item and are discarded after each use.

27. A Broaches are very small and have barblike cutting edges. Tissues are easily retained in the barbs, and therefore broaches cannot be adequately sterilized.

28. B A glass bead sterilizer is a small containe filled with heated salt or tiny glass beads and is used to sterilize small instruments during endodontic therapy.

29. A Objective findings are those findings that are found through the examination by the dentist or assistant.

30. B Unlike a K-type file, which is twisted in nature, a Hedström file has a barbed appearance.

Periodontics

CHAPTER OVERVIEW

Periodontal diseases, which involve the bone, gingiva, and gingival fibers that support the teeth, are the leading cause of tooth loss in adults. Periodontics concentrates on the prevention, detection, and treatment of periodontal diseases. Oral hygiene and preventive care are also stressed in the periodontal practice.

KEY TERMS

curettage
debridement
flap surgery
gingivectomy

graft
osseous surgery
periodontal dressing
periodontal probe

recession
root planing
scaling

I. PROGRESSION OF PERIODONTAL DISEASE

A. Gingivitis
   1. Inflammation, bleeding, and tenderness of gingival tissues.
   2. Can be reversed.
   3. Is usually corrected with a thorough prophylaxis.
   4. Periodontal probings at 4 mm.

B. Mild periodontitis
   1. Gingival inflammation and bleeding.
   2. Involves mild degeneration of the alveolar bone.
   3. Some calculus formation on the roots of the teeth.
   4. Periodontal probings at 5–6 mm.

C. Moderate periodontitis
   1. Gingival bleeding and some recession.
   2. Involves moderate degeneration of the alveolar bone.
   3. Periodontal probings at 6–8 mm.

D. Advanced periodontitis
   1. Moderate recession.
   2. Very mobile teeth.
   3. Probings at 8 mm and above.

II. INSTRUMENTATION USED IN PERIODONTICS

A. Hygiene instruments
   1. Scaler
      a. Instrument used to remove large deposits of a supragingival calculus

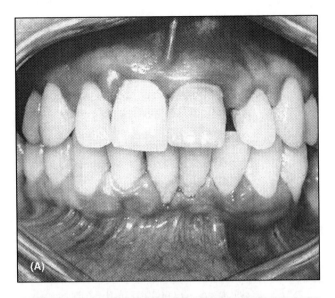

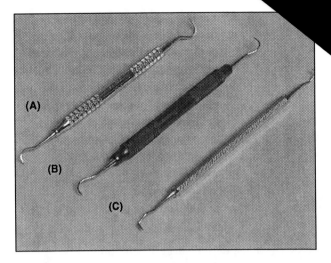

Types of periodontal scalers. (A) Combination instrument with a sickle on one end and a Jacque on the other. (B) The Shephard's hook. (C) A Jacque.

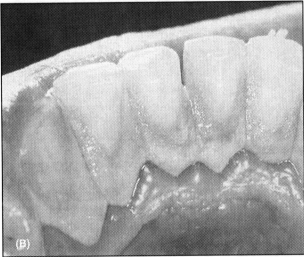

(A) View of patient with unhealthy gingival tissues—advanced gingival inflammation. (B) Unhealthy gingival tissues and lingual calculus.

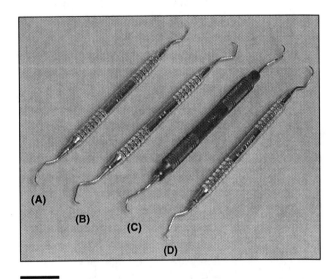

Types of periodontal curettes: Gracey curettes. (A) No. 5-6. (B) No. 7-8. (C) No. 9-10. (D) No. 13-14.

(1) Sickle scaler: Removal of calculus from anterior areas of mouth.
(2) Chisel scaler: Removal of calculus from the contact areas of the anterior teeth.
(3) Hoe scaler: Removal of heavy calculus on buccal and lingual surfaces of the posterior teeth.
(4) Universal curette: Has two cutting surfaces and adapts to all tooth surfaces.

2. Curette
   a. Instrument used after scaler to complete calculus removal, clean periodontal pockets, and plane the roots of the teeth.

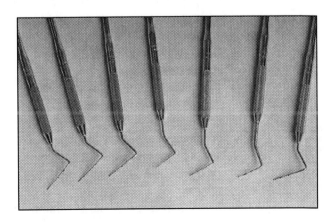

4 Variety of periodontal probes.

onic scaler or Cavitron
trument used for root planing,
rettage, and scaling. It electroni-
lly generates 29,000 vibrations per
econd. It uses water to cool the
area while ultrasonic waves vibrate
debris from the tooth structures.

b. Tips come in various shapes and
sizes to accommodate areas of
cleaning.

4. Periodontal probe
   a. Long, thin instrument used to measure pocket depth.

B. Periodontal surgical instruments
1. Retractor
   a. University of Minnesota: Used to
   reflect tissue during periodontal
   surgical treatment.
   b. Bishop: Used to reflect tissue during
   periodontal surgical treatment.
2. Periosteal elevator
   a. Instrument used to release the
   periosteum from the alveolar bone.
3. Surgical curette
   a. Instrument with a sharp, spoonlike
   end used for debridement.
4. Bard-Parker blade and blade handle
   a. Instrument used to create releasing
   incisions or for tissue removal during periodontal surgery.
5. Periodontal knives
   a. Orban: Used to remove tissue from
   the interdental areas. These instruments are shaped like spears and
   have a cutting edge on both ends.
   b. Kirkland: A very common type of
   knife used in periodontal surgery. It
   has a spadelike end and is used for
   cutting.
6. Suture scissors and tissue scissors
   a. Scissors designed to cut tissue or
   suture material.
   b. Very thin cutting blades and usually
   very sharp working ends.
7. Needle holder
   a. Hemostat-type of instrument used
   to hold the needle during suture
   placement following surgery.
8. Hemostat
   a. Used as an all-purpose instrument.

III. PERIODONTAL THERAPY

A. Complete prophylaxis
1. Also referred to as a prophy.
2. The complete removal of plaque, calculus, and debris from the supragingival and subgingival surfaces.
3. Oral hygiene instruction is given to
   patient with an appointment for a
   recall.

B. Root planing and scaling
1. The complete removal of the calculus
   from all subgingival areas to include
   the root surfaces.
2. Root surfaces are planed to resist adhe-
   sion of any calculus in the future.
3. Recommended for moderate to
   advanced periodontitis.

C. Gingival curettage
1. The mechanical scraping of dead or
   dying tissue of the gingival walls.
2. Usually done in addition to root planing and scaling.

IV. PERIODONTAL SURGICAL TREATMENT

A. Gingivectomy
1. Surgical removal of diseased gingival
   tissue from the soft tissue wall of the
   periodontal pocket.
2. Indicated when periodontal disease has
   damaged the gingival pocket beyond
   repair.
3. Indicated for gingival enlargements.
4. Indicated for abscesses that occur
   above the suprabony periodontal areas.

B. Gingivoplasty
1. Periodontal surgery involving the gingiva to correct any gingival abnormalities.
2. Performed in the absence of diseased
   periodontal pockets.
3. Indicated for abnormal growths such as
   pregnancy tumors or hyperplastic
   tissue.

C. Flap osseous surgery
1. Periodontal surgery involving the
   reduction of periodontal pockets and
   reshaping of the alveolar ridge. The

flap of gingiva or oral mucosa of the oral cavity is separated from the underlying tissues.
2. Indicated for pocket reduction of 5 mm or above.
3. During the reflection of tissue, the roots of the teeth are planed and the subgingival areas are scaled free of calculus.
4. Following a flap osseous surgical procedure, a periodontal pack is placed.

D. Frenectomy
1. Surgical procedure involving the removal of the frenum.
2. Can involve lingual, maxillary midline, or mandibular midline frenum.
3. Most common is maxillary midline to correct a diastema.
4. Second most common is a lingual frenectomy to free tongue for improved speech function and eating ability.

E. Osteoplasty
1. The surgical reshaping of the alveolar ridge.
2. Recontouring or remove defects of the alveolar bone.
3. Can be done prior to denture fabrication.
4. Can be subtractive osseous surgery
   a. Removal of bone.
   b. Removal of exostosis or torus.
5. Can be additive osseous surgery
   a. Bone grafting procedures.
   b. Ideal for patients who are missing bone.

F. Periodontal abscess treatment
1. The accumulation of infection within a periodontal pocket
   a. Chronic: Ongoing and usually without symptoms.
   b. Acute: Sudden onset of pain, which can be accompanied by tooth mobility.
   c. Treatment includes cleaning the area and prescribing antibiotics.

G. Free gingival graft
1. The removal of tissue, which is placed in an area where the gingiva is weak.

2. Can be performed for recessed areas of the mouth.

H. Crown lengthening
1. The removal of gingiva and sometimes bone tissue to accommodate the fabrication of a new crown. The margin of the new crown will extend below its original margin.

V. PERIODONTAL DRESSINGS

A. Periodontal dressings are used to give coverage to periodontal surgical sites during the healing phase, minimize postoperative pain, and protect the surgical site from trauma.
1. Types of periodontal dressings
   a. Non-eugenol based: Made by mixing a powder base with a catalyst. Contains clove oil but can cause an allergic reaction with patients.
   b. Eugenol based: Supplied in tube form; one base and an accelerator mixed together and applied to the surgical site.
   c. Light-cured material: Supplied in a single-dose system. Can be applied directly to the surgical site, molded, and then cured with a visible light.

VI. SPLINTING

A. Splinting is used to stabilize mobile teeth in their position during periodontal surgical therapy.
1. Splints may serve a temporary function or a permanent one.
2. Splints enable the patient to chew more easily.
3. A temporary splint is manufactured out of flexible plastic material and can be taken on and off easily.
4. A permanent splint may be manufactured in the form of many crowns or onlays soldered together to provide arch support for many periodontically compromised teeth.

VII. PERIODONTAL CHART

A. Periodontal probings may be taken to aid in the evaluation of a patient's dentition and surrounding tissues by inserting a periodontal probe into the sulcus around a tooth until it touches the alveolar ridge. A millimeter reading is then recorded.
   1. These readings are used to evaluate the health of the surrounding tissues of the teeth.
   2. One to 3 millimeters is considered healthy gingiva.
   3. Four millimeters is considered gingivitis.
   4. Five millimeters and above is active periodontitis.
   5. Six probing depths are recorded.
      a. Mesiofacial.
      b. Facial.
      c. Distofacial.
      d. Mesiolingual.
      e. Lingual.
      f. Distolingual.

B. Mobility readings may be recorded to evaluate the mobility of individual teeth.
   1. Mobility scale is used to evaluate.
      a. 0: Normal.
      b. 1: Slight mobility.
      c. 2: Moderate mobility.
      d. 3: Extreme mobility.

C. Medical and dental history
   1. Review any systemic diseases.
   2. Evaluate patient health for periodontal treatment.
   3. Evaluate dental health to uncover any reasons for periodontal problems.

VIII. CORONAL POLISHING

A. Coronal polishing is a procedure in which plaque and extrinsic stains are removed. Some states allow their registered dental assistants or expanded-functions dental assistants to perform this procedure. Otherwise, the dentist or hygienist would take this responsibility. Coronal polishing is limited to polishing only those portions of the clinical crown. The clinical crown is the portion of the crown that is visible in the mouth. When performing coronal polish on small children with no evidence of calculus, this procedure is called a prophylaxis. If removal of calculus is involved, this may be performed only by a licensed dentist or hygienist. Coronal polish may be performed prior to other procedures, which will be outlined in this chapter.

B. Indications for coronal polishing
   1. To remove plaque or stain.
   2. Before placing a dental dam.
   3. Before the placement of temporary or permanent crowns.
   4. Before cementing orthodontic bands and brackets.
   5. Before using any acid etch solution.

C. Contraindications for coronal polishing
   1. Lack of stain or debris.
   2. Patients at high risk for dental caries.
   3. Patients at risk for transient bacteremia who require a prophylactic antibiotic.
   4. Sensitive teeth.
   5. Newly erupted teeth.
   6. Patients with an active disease such as hepatitis or tuberculosis.

D. Stains
   1. Stains are deposits that occur in or on teeth. Because of their appearance, stains can be bothersome, and certain types of stains can be removed through coronal polish. Other stains that occur within the tooth cannot be removed.

E. Types of stains
   1. Intrinsic: Stains that occur within the tooth. These stains cannot be removed by coronal polishing.

a. May be endogenous and occurring during tooth development
   (1) Tetracycline antibiotics.
   (2) Dental fluorosis.
   (3) Other systemic conditions.
b. Silver amalgam.
c. Non-vital teeth.
d. Endodontic treatment.

2. Extrinsic: Stains that occur on the outside of the tooth.
   a. Black stain.
   b. Brown stain.
   c. Chlorhexidine.
   d. Green stain.
   e. Orange stain.
   f. Tobacco stain.
   g. Stains from food.
      (1) May be exogenous—occurring after tooth has erupted.

F. Armamentarium
   1. Low-speed handpiece and prophy angle, either autoclavable or disposable.
   2. Prophy bristle brush and cup, either screw type or snap-on.
   3. Prophy paste.
   4. HVE and saliva ejector.
   5. Dental tape and/or floss.
   6. Fluoride trays (if needed).
   7. Disclosing agent.

G. Patient preparation
   1. Check patient's medical and dental history for any contraindications to the coronal polish procedure.
   2. Set up armamentarium, drape patient, and don personal protective equipment.
   3. Explain the procedure to the patient.
   4. Identify plaque area with disclosing agent and begin polish procedure.

H. Coronal polish procedure
   1. Begin with the upper right maxillary quadrant and work around to the left maxillary quadrant staying on the buccal/facial aspect.
   2. Continue in the same manner on the lingual surfaces.
   3. Begin on the mandibular lower right quadrant and work around to the left mandibular buccal/facial surface.
   4. Begin on the mandibular right lingual area and work around to the mandibular right in the same manner as for the maxillary arch.
   5. Rinse and suction the patient as needed.
   6. Use fulcrum and positioning as warranted.
   7. Floss and final rinse.
   8. Document procedure in chart and apply fluoride if applicable.

I. Abrasive agents
   1. Dental abrasive agents are used to remove stains and polish teeth, restorations, and prosthetic appliances such as dentures.
   2. They are available in many grits. The coarser the abrasive, the more grit or abrasiveness it has. Abrasives come in extra coarse, coarse, medium, fine, and extra fine. Abrasive agents will remove very small amounts of enamel over time, so the finest grit available to do the job required is recommended. The rotation speed of the handpiece and the pressure applied to the tooth surface are also considered when polishing. Abrasive powders should be mixed with water to create a slurry. Slurry should be thick enough to stay on the brush or in the cup.
   3. Common abrasives used for polishing natural teeth
      a. Silex: Used for heavily stained teeth.
      b. Super-fine silex: Used for removal of light stains.
      c. Fine pumice: Mildly abrasive and may be used for tobacco stains.
      d. Zirconium silicate: Less likely to abrade tooth enamel.
      e. Chalk (calcium carbonate): Used to whiten teeth.
      f. Commercial preparations: Most commonly used in coronal polish. Sold by the box and packaged in individual cups with added flavoring and fluoride.
   4. Common abrasives and polishes used for non-natural teeth
      a. Tripoli: Used to smooth and add whiteness to temporary polycarbonate or acrylic crowns.
      b. Rouge: Used to polish gold.

J. Fulcrum or finger rest
1. Used to stabilize operator's hand during the procedure.
2. Repositioned throughout the procedure to accommodate polishing areas of the mouth.
3. Usually the ring finger on the hand that holds the handpiece.
4. Should always be used to limit fatigue and stress on operator's wrist and ligaments of the hand and to prevent slipping and possible injury to patient's oral tissues.

REVIEW QUESTIONS

1. A/an _____ measures pocket depth during a periodontal evaluation.
    A. explorer
    B. pocket marker
    C. periodontal probe
    D. curette

2. An extrinsic stain occurs
    A. on composite filling only.
    B. on the outside of the tooth.
    C. inside of the tooth.
    D. on non-vital teeth only.

3. Scaling is the
    A. removal of plaque only.
    B. removal of rough and diseased cementum.
    C. flushing of debris from a pocket using a syringe.
    D. the debridement of plaque and calculus deposits from tooth surfaces.

4. Osseous surgery is
    A. the reduction of addition of bone.
    B. the reduction of gingival tissue.
    C. the initial step in periodontal therapy.
    D. not part of periodontal therapy.

5. A gingivectomy is
    A. the removal of gingiva.
    B. done to improve visibility for root planing and scaling.
    C. done when there is hyperplastic tissue growth.
    D. All of the above

6. Common abrasives used for non-natural teeth include which of the following?
    1. Prophy paste
    2. Tripoli
    3. Rouge
    4. Fine pumice

    A. 1, 2, 3
    B. 1 only
    C. 2, 3
    D. None of the above

7. Intrinsic stains include which of the following?
    1. Tetracycline stain
    2. Fluorosis
    3. Tobacco stain
    4. Death of the pulp

    A. 1, 2, 4
    B. 2, 3
    C. 1 only
    D. All of the above

8. An example of an extrinsic stain would include which of the following?
    1. Tobacco stain
    2. Green stain
    3. Chlorhexidine stain
    4. Exogenous stain

    A. 1, 2, 4
    B. 2, 3
    C. 4 only
    D. All of the above

9. Gingivitis is characterized by
    A. inflammation.
    B. bleeding.
    C. tenderness.
    D. All of the above

10. Curettes
    A. are used to remove large deposits of supragingival calculus.
    B. are used to clean debris from periodontal pockets.
    C. are not sharpened.
    D. have a blunt tip.

11. The sequence of events for traditional periodontal therapy is which of the following?
    1. Complete prophylaxis
    2. Root planing and scaling
    3. Gingival curettage
    4. Surgery if indicated

    A. 1, 2, 4, 3
    B. 1, 3, 2, 4
    C. 3, 2, 4, 1
    D. 1, 2, 3, 4

12. A frenectomy
    A. is periodontal surgery involving the removal of periodontal pockets.
    B. is the removal of the frenum attachment.
    C. is the detachment and reattachment of the frenum.
    D. can be performed only on patients with a diastema.

13. Gingivoplasty is
    A. periodontal surgery performed for abnormal or hyperplastic tissue growths.
    B. periodontal surgery involving the reshaping of the alveolar bone.
    C. indicated for pocket reduction of 6 mm or more.
    D. usually followed by osseous surgery.

14. Periodontal disease that is ongoing and usually without symptoms is referred to as
    A. acute.
    B. chronic.
    C. temporary.
    D. None of the above

15. A periodontal abscess
    A. causes bone loss.
    B. can be acute.
    C. is the accumulation of infection within a periodontal pocket.
    D. All of the above

16. A free gingival graft is
    A. not indicated for recession.
    B. the removal of tissue, which is placed in a weaker area for reinforcement.
    C. performed when there is a pocket depth of 8 mm or more.
    D. done when there is extensive bone loss in the area.

17. A splint is
    1. used when there is extensive bone loss.
    2. used when mobile teeth need to be stabilized during periodontal therapy.
    3. used when the patient cannot tolerate traditional periodontal dressings.
    4. usually permanent.

    A. 1, 2, 3
    B. 1, 2
    C. 3, 4
    D. All of the above

18. Healthy gingival tissue has probing depths of
    A. 1–3 mm.
    B. 4–5 mm.
    C. 6–7 mm.
    D. 9–10 mm.

19. A tooth that has little mobility would be charted using the Roman numeral
    A. I.
    B. II.
    C. III.
    D. IV.

20. When performing periodontal probing, _____ surfaces for each tooth are probed.
    A. 3
    B. 5
    C. 6
    D. 12

21. Indications for coronal polishing include which of the following?
    1. To remove plaque or stain
    2. Before the placement of a dental dam
    3. After using acid etch solution
    4. Before cementing orthodontic bands and brackets

    A. 1, 2, 3
    B. 1, 2
    C. 2 only
    D. None of the above

Match the following.

_____ 22. Tetracycline stain

_____ 23. Green stain

_____ 24. Tobacco stain

_____ 25. Chlorhexidine stain

_____ 26. Fluorosis

_____ 27. Black stain

_____ 28. Orange stain

_____ 29. Necrotic pulp

_____ 30. Brown stain

    A. Extrinsic stain
    B. Intrinsic stain

ANSWERS AND RATIONALES

1. C Periodontal probes have a thin straight edge that has marked gradations of millimeter measurements. The probe is inserted into the free gingiva and used to measure pocket depth.

2. B Extrinsic or exogenous stains occur on the outside of the tooth enamel. Examples of extrinsic stains include tobacco, coffee, and chlorhexidine stains.

3. D Scaling is performed by using a sharp scaler or curette to scrape or debride the supragingival surfaces. Plaque and calculus are removed supragingivally using a scaler.

4. A Osteoplasty is periodontal surgery that involves removal of bone from the alveolar ridge. Subtractive osteoplasty is the removal of bone, and additive osseous surgery is the addition of bone to an area by performing bone grafting procedures.

5. D A gingivectomy is performed to give the operator better visibility during scaling procedures. The removal of hyperplastic tissue improves esthetics, and the removal of diseased tissue improves overall oral health.

6. C Tripoli and rouge are not used on natural teeth. They are primarily used in the lab.

7. A An intrinsic stain occurs within the tooth. It is usually laid down during developmental stages but can also occur when the pulp is traumatized and becomes necrotic.

8. D Extrinsic stains occur on the outside of the tooth. Tobacco and chlorhexidine stains leave a brown stain, while green stains are most commonly found in children.

9. D Gingivitis is the first stage of periodontitis. Red, inflamed, and bleeding gums with no bone loss are characteristic of gingivitis.

10. B Curettes are similar to scalers in appearance. A curette has a blunt end and sharp edges, which are used to scrape or debride periodontal pockets to remove necrotic material.

11. D Traditional periodontal therapy begins with a thorough cleaning involving root planing and scaling. It is then followed by a second evaluation, and new probing depths are recorded, at which time the dentist will determine whether periodontal surgery is indicated.

12. B A frenectomy is the removal of the frenum attachment. Maxillary midline, buccal, or lingual frenum are examples of areas where a frenectomy may be performed.

13. A Abnormal tissue growth from medications or patients with diabetes can be accomplished by performing a gingivoplasty to remove hyperplastic tissue.

14. B Periodontal disease takes time to manifest. During that time patients may not know that slowly their gingival and bone tissues are degenerating. This type of ongoing destruction is known as chronic.

15. D A periodontal abscess is a localized infection in the periodontal pocket. Curettage of the area followed with an antimicrobial rinse is usually the first course of action.

16. B When there is a lack of attached gingiva, a free gingival graft is indicated. A thin strip of tissue is completely removed and then reattached to the weak or unattached area. This provides a hard band of gingival tissue to prevent further recession.

17. B A fixed splint, which is attached to the lingual surface of the teeth, can be done when there is extensive bone loss due to periodontal disease resulting in mobility. A splint attaches mobile teeth to stronger teeth to extend the useful life of the dentition.

18. A Healthy gingiva when measured with a periodontal probe reads 1–3 mm. In the first stages of periodontal disease, the probing depths increase.

19. A Roman numeral I is the symbol used for teeth that have little mobility. As mobility increases, the Roman numeral increases. Readings can range from I–III.

20. C When measuring periodontal pockets, there are six readings for each tooth. Mesiobuccal, mesiolingual, buccal, lingual, distobuccal, and distolingual are the six measurements.

21. A Coronal polishing is the cleaning or polishing of tooth surfaces using pumice or prophylaxis paste. Coronal polishing removes extrinsic stains and should be performed before placement of a permanent restoration or orthodontic bands to remove plaque and debris prior to cementation.

22. B

23. A

24. A

25. A

26. B

27. A

28. A

29. B

30. A

Oral and Maxillofacial Surgery

CHAPTER OVERVIEW

Oral and maxillofacial surgery is the field of dentistry that is concerned with the diagnosis and surgical treatment of diseases, injuries, and deformities of the face and oral cavity. Oral and maxillofacial surgery procedures may be practiced in a private office (outpatient) or in a hospital for more serious cases.

KEY TERMS

anesthesiologist
biopsy
conscious sedation
elevator
exfoliative cytology
exodontics
extraction

hemostats
needle holders
nitrous oxide
orthognathic surgery
periosteal elevator
rongeur

scalpel
surgical aspirating tip
surgical curette
surgical dressing
suture
tissue forceps

I. ORAL SURGEON

A. Has a DDS or DMD degree.

B. Has spent two to four additional years studying oral surgery.

C. Has served a hospital residency during those two to four years of study.

D. Must pass a state, regional, or national exam in oral surgery.

II. DENTAL ASSISTANT IN ORAL SURGERY

A. Preoperative duties
1. Take and record vitals.
2. Interview the patient regarding medical and dental health.
   a. Any premedication that may be indicated.
   b. Any health problems that should be noted by DDS prior to surgery (takes nitroglycerine, blood thinning medications, and so on).

3. Give preoperative instructions regarding medications that will be prescribed, oral hygiene following surgery, and what to expect after surgery.
4. Obtain appropriate radiographs.
5. Confirm transportation for patient following surgery.

B. Assisting duties during surgery
   1. Monitor patient activity during the surgical procedure.
   2. Stabilize the jaw and neck during treatment.
   3. Maintain chain of asepsis.
   4. Pass and receive instruments.
   5. Perform all chairside duties such as aspirating and maintaining a clear field.
   6. Recognize and respond appropriately to any medical emergency.
      a. Anaphylaxis due to allergy.
      b. Respiratory failure.
      c. Cardiac arrest.
      d. Syncope.
      e. Diabetic episode.

C. Postoperative duties
   1. Give postoperative instructions to patient.
      a. Medications.
      b. Oral hygiene.
      c. How to control bleeding once patient is at home.
      d. Inflammation.
      e. Diet and smoking.
      f. Other complications that may arise following surgery
         (1) Dry socket.
         (2) Discomfort.
         (3) Excessive bleeding.
         (4) Signs of infection.
         (5) Reactions to medications.
   2. Manage all biohazard and maintenance of equipment and instruments following the procedure.
   3. Handle records management.
      a. Record all treatment and other pertinent information regarding the treatment in patient's chart.
         (1) Amount of anesthetic used.
         (2) Any unusual findings.
         (3) How many sutures placed and what type.
         (4) Medications distributed.

III. SURGICAL INSTRUMENTS

A. Surgical instruments are used for all dental surgical procedures. These instruments are unique to surgery and are not used for restorative or other aspects of dentistry. Surgical instruments are deemed critical instruments and must be cleaned, dried, and sterilized before each use. Most surgical setups are wrapped in surgical towels and sterilized. They remain in the sterilized towel until just before use.

B. Surgical instrumentation
   1. Made of polished stainless steel.
   2. Textured handles for ease in establishing a secure grasp.
   3. Can be sterilized or discarded after a single use.
   4. Disposable instrumentation is designed for a single use.
      a. Suction tips.
      b. Suture needles and suture material.
      c. Anesthetic needles.

C. Types
   1. Aspirating syringe
      a. Used with local anesthetic carpules to administer local anesthetic.
      b. Prevents the injection of local anesthetic into blood vessels.
   2. Elevators
      a. Periosteal elevator
         (1) Used to reflect tissue from bone.
         (2) Detaches gingival tissue from around the cervix of the tooth.
      b. Extraction elevator
         (1) Also called straight elevators.
         (2) Used to apply leverage against a tooth to loosen it from the periodontal ligament.
         (3) Passed to the operator using the palm grasp technique.
         (4) Sterile cotton 2 x 2 used by assistant to keep ends clean during the surgical procedure.
      c. Root tip pick
         (1) Also called root tip teaser.
         (2) Used to ease broken or retained roots from alveolar socket.
         (3) Long, angled, slender tips to reach into small spaces.

3. Surgical curette
   a. Double ended with a scoop shape at the tip.
   b. Resembles a spoon excavator.
   c. Used to clean or curette the interior of the socket following extraction of abscessed or diseased teeth.
4. Rongeur
   a. Resembles extraction forceps with a sharp cutting edge.
   b. Has a spring handle and is used in the same manner as nail nippers.
   c. Has sharp cutting edges that can trim alveolar bone and eliminate sharp, bony projections.
5. Bone file
   a. Resembles a rasp or file.
   b. Available in a variety of shapes and sizes.
   c. Used in a sawing motion to smooth the alveolar bone following an extraction.
6. Scalpel
   a. Also called a surgical knife.
   b. Used to cut soft tissue with little or no trauma.
   c. The scalpel blade comes with a handle and disposable blades that are attached to the end.
7. Hemostat and needle holder
   a. Used to grasp or hold items.
   b. Can be sterilized.
   c. Usually have locking handles.
   d. Handles resemble scissors.
   e. Have straight or curved tips.
8. Scissors
   a. Delicate scissors used to cut tissue or suture material.
   b. Suture scissors have a notch at the end to aid in the removal of sutures by grasping the knot of the suture material and gently tugging through the site.
   c. Can have smooth or serrated cutting edges.
9. Tissue retractor
   a. Used to reflect or retract soft tissue during surgery.
   b. Resembles cotton pliers with a straight end.

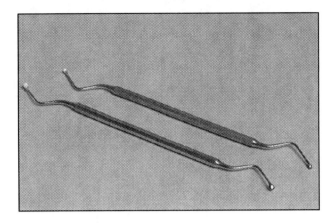

Surgical curettes.

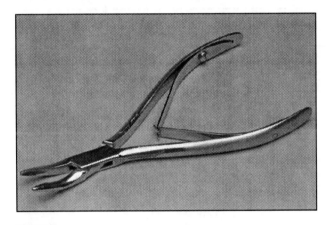

Rongeurs.

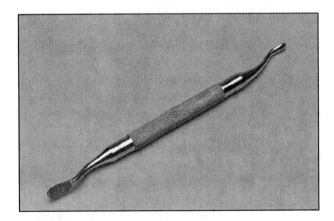

Surgical bone file.

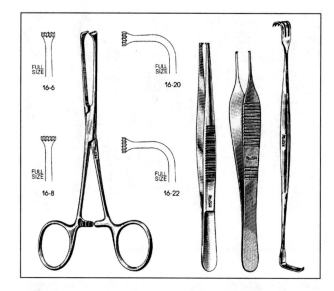

Tissue retractors. *(Courtesy of Miltex Instrument Co., Inc., Lake Success, NY)*

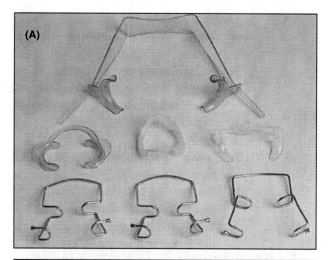

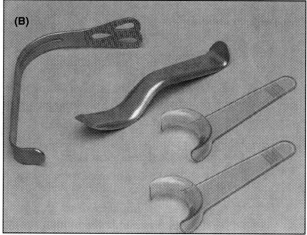

(A) Tongue and cheek retractors. (B) Lip, tongue, and cheek retractors.

10. Tongue, lip, or cheek retractor
    a. Designed to hold the tongue, lip, or cheek out of the area during surgical procedures.
    b. Can be stainless steel or plastic.
    c. Comes in large or small, curved or angled.
    d. Types
       (1) University of Minnesota
       (2) Bishop
       (3) Columbia
11. Mouth prop or gag
    a. Allows the patient to rest or relax the jaw during long surgical procedures.
    b. Used during local and general anesthesia.
    c. Comes in different sizes and shapes.
    d. Made of rubber material and is autoclavable.
    e. Mouth gags are attached to a scissor-type handle and have a clicking mechanism to achieve the correct mouth sizes.
    f. Mouth props come in adult small, medium, and large and also pediatric sizes.
12. Surgical chisel and mallet
    a. Used to remove bone.
    b. Used to reshape the alveolar ridge.
    c. Can be used to section multirooted teeth.
    d. Used with a small mallet with a rubber end.

13. Aspirating tip
    a. Used to remove debris, saliva, and blood from the surgical site.
    b. Smaller tip than the regular HVE tip.
    c. Used in a wiping motion.
    d. Fits easily into the socket or around surgical area.
    e. Can be disposable or autoclavable.
14. Forceps
    a. Extraction forceps are available in many different shapes and sizes.
    b. Each size and shape is designed to remove specific teeth in specific areas.
    c. Beaks are shaped to grasp the crown of the tooth.
    d. Extraction forceps are passed in the palm grasp position.
    e. Pediatric forceps are designed the same except they have a smaller head to accommodate the smaller dentition.

15. Miscellaneous surgical items
    a. Blades used to cut soft tissue
       (1) Come in several shapes, with numbers 12 and 14 the most common.
       (2) Disposable and must be discarded after each use in the sharps container
    b. Sutures
       (1) Come in various sizes and made of different types of material
           (a) Silk.
           (b) Polyester.
           (c) Gut.
    c. Gauze 2 x 2 or 4 x 4 squares
       (1) Come in presterilized packaging or can be sterilized in package before use.
       (2) Used to absorb blood and debris removal from instruments.
       (3) Used in the control of bleeding following surgery.
    d. Anesthetic carpules
       (1) Disposable carpules filled with anesthetic designed for single use.
       (2) Used with an aspirating syringe.
    e. Surgical drapes
       (1) Bibs.
       (2) Sterile towels.
       (3) Plastic isolating drapes.
    f. Kidney basin and irrigating bulb
       (1) Used with sterile saline solution to irrigate surgical area.

IV. ASSISTANT'S ROLE DURING OPERATIVE PROCEDURES

A. The assistant must always follow the chain of asepsis.
   1. The instruments, surgical drapes, and surgery materials must be kept in a sterile environment.
   2. Contact with anything that is not sterile will break the chain of asepsis and allows contamination of the surgical area.
   3. Set up instruments in order of use, set up the operatory barriers, and perform all preparatory duties prior to the surgical scrub and gowning.

4. Place patient chart out with radiographs prior to surgery.
5. Set up operatory with all instrumentation and materials needed for surgical procedure.
6. Patient preparation
   a. Perform medical/dental health history review.
   b. Give all necessary preoperative and postoperative instructions.
7. Manage all biohazard waste as prescribed by your state and OSHA guidelines.
8. Review all medications that will be given out.
   a. Antianxiety medications prior to surgery.
   b. Antibiotics for patients with mitral valve prolapse or joint replacement.
9. Ask the patient to empty bladder.
10. Seat and drape the patient.
11. During the surgical procedure
    a. Maintain chain of asepsis.
    b. Keep field clear by using the aspirating tip and gauze as needed.
    c. Steady the patient's head and mandible if needed.
    d. Monitor equipment that registers blood pressure, pulse, and respiration.
12. Following the surgical procedure
    a. Monitor patient for bleeding.
    b. Record all data regarding treatment in chart.
    c. Redeliver postoperative instructions to patient if possible.
    d. Monitor patient in recovery bay and dismiss to designated transportation person.
       (1) Patients should be dismissed only when they are ambulatory.
       (2) All bleeding should be under control before the patient is released.
    e. An ice pack may be placed on the site to keep inflammation down.
    f. All pain medications or antibiotic therapy should be explained to patient or transportation person if patient has had general anesthesia.

13. Postoperative visit
    a. A postoperative visit is scheduled five to seven days following routine surgical treatment.
    b. Sutures are removed, and the site is irrigated with saline solutions.
    c. The site is then evaluated for any abnormalities or infection.
    d. Look for signs of infection such as redness, swelling, pain, and heat.

V. POSTOPERATIVE COMPLICATIONS

A. Infection
    1. A course of antibiotics is given along with pain medication, if needed.
    2. Alveolitis (dry socket or loss of blood clot)
        a. Symptoms include extreme pain, foul odor, and exudate (pus).
            (1) Treatment
                (a) The doctor anesthetizes the area, irrigates with an antibiotic rinse, and uses a curette to stir up bleeding within the socket to create a new blood clot.
                (b) The doctor irrigates with an antimicrobial rinse and places Nugauze or dry socket paste.
    3. Periodontal dressing dislodged
        a. Area may or may not be sensitive to hot and cold.
        b. If sensitivity is an issue, then site must have dressing replaced, and pain medication should be given if needed.

VI. ORAL AND MAXILLOFACIAL SURGICAL PROCEDURES

A. Simple extraction
    1. Removal of an erupted tooth.
    2. Patient is anesthetized. The assistant assists during the anesthetic procedure.
    3. Dentist begins by reflecting the tissue away from the tooth and elevating it out of the socket. The assistant assists by passing the designated elevator to the dentist.
    4. After the tooth has been elevated to the desired height, then the extraction for-

ceps are used. The assistant passes the desired forceps and aspirates as needed.
    5. After the tooth has been luxated and removed, the assistant aspirates and receives the beak of the forceps along with the extracted tooth and places it on the surgical tray for disposal into the sharps container.
    6. The dentist irrigates and places sutures if necessary.

B. Multiple extractions
    1. The same procedure is followed as for single extraction.
    2. If an immediate denture is going to be placed, the prosthesis must be out and ready to place directly following the last extraction.

C. Complicated or bony impaction
    1. Doctor anesthetizes the patient. The assistant attends during the anesthetizing procedure.
    2. In many cases, a flap will be laid using the scalpel, and a surgical bur in the high-speed handpiece may be used to remove bone so that the tooth may be exposed. The assistant attends by aspirating and using sterile saline to irrigate.

Basic Post-operative Instructions Given to the Surgical Patient

1. Consume a soft diet for the next 24–48 hours.
2. Apply pressure with gauze until bleeding has subsided. Saliva will be blood tinged for the next 48 hours.
3. Rinse with warm salt water rolling your head in a figure eight motion after each meal.
4. An irrigating syringe may be used to gently flush the area after initial healing has been established.
5. Do not exert pressure on the surgical site by smoking or using a straw. This may dislodge the clot that is forming and lead to "dry socket."
6. Ice packs may be used for 15 minutes on and 15 minutes off to control swelling.
7. An over the counter analgesic or prescription may be used to control discomfort.

Note: Each office may have their own set of post-operative instructions and the above are just a sample of some of the more commonly dispensed.

3. The doctor uses the desired instruments to remove the tooth (elevators, forceps, chisel and mallet, and so on).

D. Alveoplasty
 1. Surgical reduction of bone to contour the ridge.
 2. The doctor makes an incision in the tissue along the crest of the alveolar ridge. The assistant passes the scalpel and aspirates blood from the site as the doctor makes the incision.
 3. The doctor may use rongeurs or a bone file to contour the ridge.
 4. Site is irrigated with saline solution and sutures are placed. The assistant attends during suture placement.
 5. A gauze pack of periodontal dressing is placed if an immediate denture is not used.

E. Biopsy
 1. Excisional biopsy
   a. Removal of entire lesion.
   b. Ideal for small growths or lesions.
   c. Does not usually create an esthetic or functional deformity.
 2. Incisional biopsy
   a. Indicated when a lesion is larger than 1 cm.
   b. A wedge or sample of tumor or lesion is sectioned and evaluated under a microscope.
   c. A complete removal is not made until a diagnosis is reached.
 3. Exfoliative cytology
   a. Nonsurgical technique.
   b. Cells are gathered by scraping a sample off of lesion.
   c. Evaluated microscopically.
 4. Biopsy results
   a. Nonmalignant
     (1) Nonthreatening to the patient and removal can be postponed.
   b. Malignant
     (1) Can be life threatening to the patient and should be removed immediately by a qualified specialist.
 5. Specialty surgery
   a. Dental implants
     (1) Endosteal implants
       (a) Surgically embedded in bone.
       (b) Made of titanium.
       (c) Bone attaches to implant and then a permanent restoration is attached to the top of implant.
     (2) Subperiosteal implant
       (a) Metal frame that lies under the periosteum but on top of the alveolar ridge.
       (b) Dentures may be attached to the implant.
       (c) Ideal for patients who have limited alveolar bone.
     (3) Advantages
       (a) Restores chewing function.
       (b) Esthetically pleasing.
       (c) More stable than a conventional denture.
     (4) Disadvantages
       (a) Large financial investment.
       (b) Treatment can be lengthy.
       (c) Risk of infection.
       (d) Patient must be in good physical health.
   b. Dental assistant's role in patient education following implant surgery
     (1) Oral hygiene
       (a) Home care should be stressed.
       (b) Special implant cleaning tools are needed for adequate home care.
       (c) Tools should be demonstrated so that patient can use them with ease and confidence at home.

REVIEW QUESTIONS

1. Postoperative instructions given to the patient include which of the following?
 1. Medications prescribed for pain
 2. Oral hygiene
 3. Premedication for joint replacement
 4. Diet following surgery

 A. 1, 2, 3
 B. 1, 2, 4
 C. 2, 3
 D. All of the above

2. Medical emergencies that may arise during oral surgery include which of the following?
 1. Anaphylaxis

2. Cardiac arrest
3. Syncope
4. Diabetic episode

A. 1, 2, 3
B. 1, 3
C. 2, 3, 4
D. All of the above

3. Treatment that should be recorded in the patient's chart should include which of the following?
   1. Amount of anesthetic carpules used
   2. Amount of sutures placed
   3. Medications given to patient prior to and following surgery
   4. Any unusual findings

   A. 1, 2, 3
   B. 1, 3
   C. 4 only
   D. All of the above

4. Extraction elevators
   1. are used to apply leverage against a tooth.
   2. are passed to the operator using the palm grasp technique.
   3. come in many different sizes.
   4. are also called extraction forceps.

   A. 1, 4
   B. 1 only
   C. 1, 2, 3
   D. All of the above

5. Bone files are
   1. used to cut soft tissue during surgery.
   2. used in a sawing motion to smooth alveolar bone.
   3. used much the same way rongeurs are used.
   4. are also called root tip picks.

   A. 1, 2, 3
   B. 1 only
   C. 2 only
   D. 3, 4

6. Tissue retractors
   A. are used to grasp or hold tissue.
   B. are used to smooth rough edges of bone.
   C. are used to reflect or retract soft tissue.
   D. usually have locking handles.

7. Dry socket is also known as
   A. condylitis.
   B. alveolitis.
   C. erosion.
   D. avulsion.

8. Oral surgery would be performed for which of the following reasons?
   1. To remove teeth that are beyond restoring
   2. To remove impacted third molars
   3. To remove teeth prior to orthodontic treatment
   4. To remove retained roots

   A. 1, 2, 3
   B. 1, 4
   C. 3, 4
   D. All of the above

9. The term _____ means to move the tooth back and forth within the socket.
   A. displace
   B. festoon
   C. luxation
   D. capitation

10. The surgical instrument that has a sharp cutting edge and is capable of trimming alveolar bone and eliminating sharp, bony projections is referred to as
    A. a bone file.
    B. a rongeur.
    C. forceps.
    D. a chisel and mallet.

11. During the postoperative visit,
    1. sutures are removed.
    2. the tissue is checked for any signs of infection.
    3. a periodontal pack is placed over the surgical site if sensitivity is present.
    4. all information is recorded in the patient's chart.

    A. 1, 2, 3
    B. 1, 4
    C. 1, 2, 4
    D. All of the above

Match the following.

_____ 12. Root tip pick

_____ 13. Scalpel

_____ 14. Surgical curette

_____ 15. Tissue retractor

_____ 16. Scissors

_____ 17. Hemostat or needle holder

_____ 18. Mouth prop

   A. Double ended with a scoop shape at the tip
   B. Used to reflect or retract soft tissue during surgery
   C. Delicate instrument used to cut tissue or sutures
   D. Used to remove broken or retained roots
   E. Used to grasp suture needles or other items
   F. Used to aid the patient in relaxing the jaw during long procedures
   G. Used to cut soft tissue

19. An excisional biopsy is
   A. the removal of an entire lesion.
   B. the partial removal of a lesion.
   C. not recommended for small growths.
   D. indicated when a lesion is larger than 1 cm.

20. Exfoliative cytology is
   A. a surgical technique.
   B. evaluated visually for abnormalities.
   C. the process by which cells are scraped from a lesion.
   D. done only in a hospital setting.

21. Malignant means that a growth is
   A. nonthreatening and removal can be postponed.
   B. life threatening and should be removed immediately.

22. Disadvantages when considering implants may include which of the following?
   1. Treatment can be lengthy
   2. Risk of infections
   3. Large financial investment
   4. Oral hygiene is very difficult

   A. 1, 2, 3
   B. 1, 4
   C. 4 only
   D. All of the above

23. Alveoplasty
   A. is the surgical reduction of bone to contour the ridge.
   B. is the removal of gingiva prior to denture placement.
   C. is the contouring of the gingiva.
   D. can be done after an implant is placed.

24. A simple extraction consists of
   A. the removal of a tooth with a bony impaction.
   B. the removal of an erupted tooth.
   C. always placing sutures following removal of the tooth.
   D. more than one appointment.

25. When surgical instruments cannot be cleaned immediately, they are
   A. placed on the towel until the procedure is over.
   B. wiped with alcohol.
   C. placed in a holding solution.
   D. sprayed with disinfectant.

26. Before sterilizing surgical instruments, it is important to
   A. tightly seal them in a sterilizing pouch.
   B. dry them thoroughly with a clean towel before wrapping or bagging.
   C. wrap them in a sterile towel and let them dry.
   D. air dry them on a tray.

27. It is necessary to _____ hinged instruments prior to sterilizing.
   A. open
   B. close

28. Ice packs are used to relieve
    A. pain.
    B. swelling.
    C. bleeding.
    D. All of the above

29. When a blood clot is dislodged due to the exertion of forces such as sucking on a straw and as a result, the patient experiences extreme discomfort it is referred to as
    A. ankylosis.
    B. acidosis.
    C. alveolitis.
    D. osteosis.

30. _____ forceps are designed to grasp the bifurcation of the root of a mandibular molar.
    A. Universal
    B. Curved
    C. Cowhorn
    D. Bayonet

ANSWERS AND RATIONALES

1. D Prior to surgery, common postoperative instructions include going over medications that are being prescribed, special diet following surgery, and keeping the area clean following surgery. Premedication for joint replacement is discussed prior to surgery.

2. D Any time a surgical procedure is performed, there is always a possibility that a medical emergency may occur. Heart attack, fainting, allergic reaction to anesthetics, and diabetic episodes are some of the most common. The assistant needs to be prepared at all times to respond to any and all emergencies.

3. D Any time patient contact is made, whether or not treatment is rendered, any information should be recorded. Amount of anesthetic used, sutures placed, all medications, and any unusual findings should be recorded in the patient's chart.

4. C Extraction elevators are instruments with a straight handle and various types of tips. Tips vary depending on the tooth or tooth fragments to be removed. They apply pressure to the tooth to elevate it out of the alveolar socket so that extraction forceps may grip and remove it.

5. C A bone file is used to smooth alveolar irregularities following the removal of one or more teeth.

6. C Tissue retractors are used to retract the tongue and soft tissues during surgical procedures. Minnesota and Bishop retractors are examples.

7. B Dry socket is also referred to as alveolitis. Alveolitis is characterized by extreme pain, foul odor, and inflammation.

8. D Oral surgery procedures would be performed for the following reasons: to remove teeth that are badly broken down or decayed and cannot be repaired, to remove impacted wisdom or third molars, to remove teeth prior to orthodontic treatment, and to remove roots that have been broken off and are retained in the alveolar socket.

9. C To luxate a tooth means to move it back and forth in an attempt to dislodge it from the alveolar socket.

10. B Rongeurs are similar in appearance to cuticle clippers and have a sharp edge that is used to cut or nip pieces of bone.

11. D A postoperative visit is indicated following a surgical procedure. Activities that may take place during a postoperative visit include checking for signs of infection; removal of sutures and irrigation of the area with sterile saline solution; and if sensitivity is present, placing a periodontal pack over the area. Everything should be recorded in the patient's chart.

12. D

13. G

14. A

15. B

16. C

17. E

18. F

19. A. When suspicious growths appear in the patient's mouth, the dentist may elect to do an excisional biopsy, which is the complete removal and inspection under a microscope of the lesion.

20. C When cells are scraped from an area and inspected under a microscope, it is referred to as exfoliative cytology.

21. B   A life-threatening growth or tumor may be malignant, which means that it should be evaluated immediately for removal.

22. D   Implants involve lengthy treatment and a high risk of infection and require a substantial financial commitment and motivation toward maintaining better than average oral hygiene.

23. A   Surgically reducing the bone to contour the ridge prior to denture placement is called alveoplasty.

24. B   When the tooth is not completely embedded in soft tissue and bone, it is referred to as a simple extraction and can be removed without using a surgical bur.

25. C   Surgical instruments should be placed in a disinfecting holding solution if they cannot be cleaned immediately. The holding solution should completely cover the instruments and should not take the place of sterilization.

26. B   Instruments should be completely dry before sterilizing. This will diminish the possibility of rust forming on the instruments.

27. A   When sterilizing scissors or any instruments that have a hinge, they must be open during the sterilization process. This procedure enables the instruments to be sterilized in all areas that may be hidden if they were allowed to remain closed.

28. B   Ice packs are used immediately following surgery for 15 minutes on and 15 minutes off for an hour to reduce swelling. Pain and bleeding are controlled with other methods.

29. C   Alveolitis occurs when the blood clot has been lost due to forces such as sucking on a straw or smoking. It usually occurs in the first 24 hours following surgery.

30. C   Cowhorn forceps have curved beaks that are designed to grasp the tooth at the furcation for easier manipulation and removal.

Pediatric Dentistry

CHAPTER OVERVIEW

Pediatric dentistry is the identification, prevention, and treatment of dental diseases in children. The pedodontist usually sees children from infancy through adolescence. Procedures performed by the pedodontist are very similar to the services performed for older patients. The pedodontist takes the patient's age and future dental implications into consideration before performing any treatment. The pediatric dental office is designed for the younger patient by design and staffing.

KEY TERMS

behavior management	child abuse	pediatric dentist (pedodontist)
behavior modification	papoose board	premedication
techniques	pediatric dental office design	preventive dentistry

I. SERVICES PROVIDED BY THE PEDIATRIC DENTIST

A. Restorative procedures
  1. Amalgam fillings
  2. Stainless steel crown placement
  3. Pulpotomy
    a. Partial removal of the pulpal tissues.
  4. Palliative treatment
    a. Relieving patient of immediate discomfort.
  5. Composite fillings
  6. Direct and indirect pulp capping
  7. Classifications of fractures
    a. Class I: Enamel is fractured only.
    b. Class II: Enamel and dentin are exposed but not pulpal tissue.
    c. Class III: Extensive fracture involving the pulp.
    d. Class IV: Entire crown is fractured off.

B. Endodontic procedures
  1. Pulpectomy
    a. The complete removal of all pulpal tissues from a primary tooth canal.
  2. Root canal therapy on permanent teeth
    a. If root canal therapy is performed on a permanent tooth, the tooth is then filled with an inert material and a permanent restoration is placed.

C. Oral surgery
  1. Treatment of avulsed teeth (teeth that are completely removed from the alveolar socket).

2. Removal of retained roots from fractured teeth.
3. Removal of retained deciduous teeth.
4. Frenectomy.
5. Luxation injuries (teeth are dislodged from their original place).
6. Removal of teeth prior to orthodontics.

D. Orthodontics (preventive or interceptive)
  1. Space maintainers.
  2. Palatal expanders.
  3. Mouth guards
  4. Correcting oral habits (i.e., tongue thrusting, thumb sucking)
  5. Placing bands, brackets, and arch wires for minor orthodontic cases

E. Preventive dentistry
  1. Complete prophylaxis
    a. May include scaling for some older patients.
  2. Application of topical fluoride
    a. Usually to the age of 13 years old.
  3. Oral hygiene education
    a. Interact with the patient to examine the technique and frequency of brushing and flossing.
  4. Radiographs
  5. Sealant placement
  6. Patient education
    a. Diet and nutrition.
    b. Fluoride intake.
    c. Emphasize regular visits.
    d. Reinforce importance of completing all needed restorative procedures.

F. Pediatric dental office design
  1. Waiting room
    a. Designed with smaller chairs and a table for coloring or drawing.
    b. Puzzles, games, and books designed for younger patients.
  2. Operatory
    a. Usually an open concept.
    b. Assistant is always with the child or close nearby.
    c. Activities such as reading or listening to music while child is waiting.
  3. Back office staff
    a. Always cheerful and friendly.
    b. Willing to explain procedures and demonstrate the use of instruments so as not to frighten the patient but inform.

    c. Uniforms are usually fun and bright along with bibs to ease intimidation.
  4. Managing behavior
    a. Be patient and listen to the fears or concerns your young patients may have.
    b. Reinforce good behavior and manage inappropriate behavior.
    c. Explain exactly what you expect from the child.
    d. Build a rapport with your young patients by getting to know them and their interests.
  5. Behavior modification techniques
    a. Premedication.
    b. Tone of voice by dentist or assistant to gain control.
    c. Papoose board.
    d. Hand-over-mouth technique.
    e. Reward good behavior with a new toothbrush or other small gift.

G. Child abuse
  1. Signs of child abuse
    a. Shaking.
    b. Bite marks.
    c. Missing hair.
    d. Burned areas or trauma in the mouth from forced feedings.
    e. Signs of sexual abuse.
  2. The dental team and its role in child abuse
    a. It is your responsibility to report all suspected child abuse.
    b. You are legally required to report suspected abuse, and if you are aware that abuse is evident and do not report it, you may have a legal suit brought against you.
    c. Many states have laws protecting you and shielding your identity when you report suspected child abuse.
    d. If abuse is suspected, report it to your dentist, and let the dentist report it to the proper authorities.

REVIEW QUESTIONS

1. Which of the following procedures are performed by the pediatric dentist?
   1. Orthodontics
   2. Oral surgery
   3. Endodontic therapy
   4. Restorative procedures

   A. 1, 2, 4
   B. 2, 3
   C. 3 only
   D. All of the above

2. If a deciduous primary molar has gross caries, which type of restoration will probably be used?
   A. Composite filling
   B. Acrylic filling
   C. Stainless steel crown
   D. Cast porcelain crown

3. A pulpectomy is
   A. the partial removal of the pulpal tissues.
   B. the complete removal of the pulpal tissues.
   C. the partial removal of pulpal tissues in the coronal portion of the tooth.
   D. the complete removal of pulpal tissues in the coronal portion of the tooth.

4. Signs of child abuse may include which of the following?
   1. Trauma to oral tissues
   2. Bite marks
   3. Various bruises in stages of healing
   4. Mild shyness

   A. 1, 2, 3
   B. 1, 3
   C. 4 only
   D. All of the above

5. The natural loss of teeth is called
   A. eruption.
   B. resorption.
   C. exfoliation.
   D. extraction.

6. Which of the following techniques are used in behavior management?
   1. Hand over mouth
   2. Premedication
   3. Voice control
   4. Rewarding good behavior

   A. 1, 2, 3
   B. 2, 3
   C. 3 only
   D. All of the above

7. The pediatric office is designed for the child by
   1. providing reading and entertainment catered to specific age groups.
   2. providing treatment specific to children.
   3. maintaining open communication with the caregiver regarding the patient's treatment.
   4. paying special attention to attitudes and behavior of staff toward the patients.

   A. 1, 2, 3
   B. 4 only
   C. 2, 3
   D. All of the above

8. Subjective fears are
   A. fears learned from others.
   B. fears learned from actual experience.
   C. fears that have no basis.
   D. fears that occur only in certain age groups.

9. A child's behavior toward dental treatment largely depends on
   A. the child's impression of the dentist.
   B. the degree of friendliness the staff shows toward the child.
   C. the caregiver's attitude toward dentistry.
   D. the extent of the child's knowledge of dentistry.

10. Validation of a child's feelings toward dentistry requires
    A. the dentist explaining all procedures.
    B. the front office staff allowing a caregiver to accompany the child to the treatment room.
    C. denying or playing down fears to control behavior.
    D. the dentist to acknowledge and confirm the child's concerns before moving forward with the treatment.

11. Stainless steel crowns are usually cemented with
    A. glass ionomer cement.
    B. polycarboxylate cement.
    C. zinc phosphate cement.
    D. attention being paid to the length of time that the crown will remain on the tooth.

12. _____ crowns are used on primary teeth in the anterior areas of the mouth.
    1. Stainless steel
    2. Porcelain
    3. Composite resin
    4. Polycarbonate

    A. 1, 2, 3
    B. 1, 3
    C. 3, 4
    D. All of the above

13. In a Class I fracture, _____ is/are lost, and the treatment involves _____ the area for comfort.
    A. enamel/repairing
    B. dentin and enamel/repairing
    C. enamel/smoothing
    D. enamel, dentin, and pulpal tissue/pulp capping

14. The material most commonly used in direct pulp capping is
    A. zinc phosphate cement.
    B. polycarboxylate cement.
    C. calcium hydroxide.
    D. glass ionomer cement.

15. Apexification and apexogenesis are treatments that involve
    A. the development of pits and fissures.
    B. the permanent teeth that have not erupted.
    C. the status of root development.
    D. trauma to the surface of deciduous teeth.

16. An avulsed permanent tooth requires
    A. reimplantation and root canal therapy.
    B. immediate reimplantation and possible splinting.
    C. removal and space maintainer placed.
    D. reattachment through periodontal surgery.

17. A _____ is used to provide space when deciduous teeth are lost prematurely.
    A. palatal expander
    B. space maintainer
    C. removable retainer
    D. Both B and C

18. _____ are routinely used on pediatric patients to increase visibility and patient comfort and to aid in patient management.
    A. Dry angles
    B. Dental dams
    C. Slow-speed handpieces
    D. Saliva ejectors

19. A _____ is an appliance that is cemented into place and with the use of gentle force, gradually widens the palate.
    A. face bow
    B. temporary crown
    C. rapid palatal expander
    D. space maintainer

20. Before the clinical examination, the caregiver provides a _____ for the staff regarding the child's health and background.
    A. medical history
    B. immunization record
    C. previous dental treatment record
    D. MD release for treatment

21. Methods of fluoride application include which of the following?
    1. Tray application
    2. Brush on
    3. Oral rinse
    4. Fluoridated water

    A. 1, 2, 4
    B. 2, 3
    C. 1, 2, 3
    D. All of the above

22. _____ material bonds to tooth surfaces and acts as a barrier to protect pits and fissures of the posterior teeth.
    A. Resin
    B. Sealant
    C. Composite
    D. Polycarbonate

23. A fabricated _____ is used during contact sports.
    A. Hawley retainer
    B. mouth guard
    C. vacuform retainer
    D. stent

Place the following procedures in order of operation, with the first being A and the last being E.

_____ 24. Sealant material is placed.

_____ 25. Acid etch is placed, rinsed, and tooth is dried.

_____ 26. Cotton rolls are placed for isolation.

_____ 27. Coronal polish is performed with fine pumice.

_____ 28. Material is cured with a light or isolated to allow setting if material is self-cure.

29. _____ requires re-etching of the tooth prior to sealant placement.
    A. Overdrying
    B. Salivary contamination
    C. Light exposure
    D. Application of a dental dam

30. A/an _____ restoration is placed following a pulpectomy.
    A. permanent
    B. calcium hydroxide
    C. amalgam
    D. zinc oxide eugenol

ANSWERS AND RATIONALES

1. D Routine procedures performed in the pediatric dental office include orthodontics, routine oral surgery, endodontic therapy such as a pulpectomy or pulpotomy, and other restorative procedures such as amalgams and stainless steel crowns.

2. C A stainless steel crown is used after large amounts of decay are removed from the posterior teeth of primary molars. Stainless steel crowns provide an adequate chewing surface for the pediatric patient.

3. B A pulpectomy is the complete removal of the pulp from a primary tooth. The root is not filled but left open due to the future loss and resorption that will be taking place.

4. A The dental assistant should be sensitive to the signs of child abuse. Some of those signs may include trauma to oral tissues from forced feeding, bite marks that resemble human dentition, and bruises in various stages of healing. Severe shyness could be a symptom, but mild shyness is normal for most children when they are in an unfamiliar environment.

5. C The process of losing primary teeth in preparation for the eruption of permanent teeth is referred to as exfoliation.

6. D To effectively manage a pediatric patient, several methods may be employed, including the hand-over-mouth technique (which is rarely used), premedication with antianxiety medications, using your voice to control the situation, and rewarding the patient for good behavior.

7. D The pediatric dental office is designed with the child in mind. Entertainment geared toward children and good communication with the caregiver are key. Procedures that are specific to pediatric dentistry are also provided so that the child can rely on the primary pediatric dentist for all procedures.

8. B Fears learned through actual experience are referred to as subjective fears. These are experiences that the child has encountered through previous visits to the dental office.

9. C The caregiver is the person who instills ideas into the child when dental treatment is needed. The way the child's caregiver sees dental treatment and the need for good oral health depends largely upon the caregiver's past experiences. Those ideas are passed on to the child.

10. D By acknowledging the child's fears and validating the child's concerns, the dentist is able to move past the initial fear and to stress the importance of completing the procedure; the child in turn trusts the dentist, and a sense of understanding can be established between them.

11. D The type of cement used to cement a stainless steel crown depends on the length of time that the crown will be on the tooth. Temporary cement may be used on a primary tooth while permanent cement may be used on a permanent tooth.

12. C Composite resin and polycarbonate crowns are used on primary anterior teeth for esthetic purposes. Porcelain-fused-to-metal crowns are not placed on primary teeth.

13. C In a Class I fracture, in which the enamel is lost or chipped, smoothing with a white stone or fine diamond will usually alleviate any roughness.

14. C Calcium hydroxide, which is soothing to the pulp, is used for a direct pulp cap.

15. C During apexogenesis and apexification, treatment is dependent on the stage of root development.

16. B An avulsed tooth is a tooth that has been dislodged from the alveolar socket. Immediate reimplantation is critical. Endodontic therapy is evaluated if the tooth does not respond on its own.

17. B A space maintainer is used to maintain the space between two teeth where another tooth was prematurely lost. This prevents drifting while the patient is waiting for the permanent tooth to erupt.

18. B Dental dams are used to maintain a dry field, aid in retraction of tissues, and aid in the management of the pediatric patient during routine restorative procedures.

19. C A rapid palatal expander is placed to enlarge the palate prior to orthodontics. The pediatric dentist may take the impression, seat the appliance, and oversee treatment.

20. A The caregiver must provide the office with a medical history before any treatment can be rendered. Known allergies, medications, and other medical information must be noted and discussed prior to treatment.

21. C To apply fluoride to the dentition, the assistant may employ several different methods. The traditional trays may be used, or the patient may brush the fluoride on. An oral rinse may be provided. With any fluoride treatment, the patient should wait at least 30 minutes before eating or drinking anything.

22. B Sealant material is routinely used to fill the deep pits and fissures of the posterior teeth. Sealants prevent plaque from becoming trapped in the grooves of the teeth, which can cause decay through plaque acid attacks and the inability to completely remove it.

23. B A custom mouth guard is used during contact sports to prevent the patient from experiencing trauma to the teeth and tissues of the oral cavity.

24. D

25. C

26. B

27. A

28. E

29. B During the sealant procedure, if saliva contaminates the tooth surface after etching, the tooth must be re-etched.

30. A Following a pulpectomy, a permanent restoration is placed to maintain the integrity of the tooth.

CHAPTER 12

Prosthodontics

CHAPTER OVERVIEW

Prosthodontics is the branch of dentistry that deals with the replacement of missing teeth with removable or fixed appliances. These prosthetic restorations are fabricated by a dental lab technician and then cemented or delivered by the dentist to the patient. This chapter reviews fixed and removable prosthodontics, including inlays, onlays, veneers, cast crowns and bridges, and partial and complete dentures.

KEY TERMS

abutment	full denture	opposing model
cast crown	gingival retraction	partial denture
core buildup	inlay	pin retention
extraoral factors	intraoral factors	post buildup
fixed bridge	onlay	unit
framework		

I. FIXED PROSTHODONTICS

A. Fixed prosthodontics are placed for a variety of reasons.
   1. Restore esthetics to the dentition.
   2. Aid in the ability to masticate.
   3. Prevent adjacent teeth from drifting.

B. Indications for the placement of fixed prosthesis
   1. One or two adjacent teeth are missing in the same arch.
   2. Surrounding bone and gingival tissues are healthy enough to support a fixed crown or bridge.
   3. Abutment teeth are suitable enough to support the fixed bridge.
   4. Patient can maintain good oral hygiene and has the motivation to take care of the area postoperatively.

C. Contraindications for placing a fixed prosthesis
   1. Supporting tissues are diseased or inadequate.
   2. No abutment teeth are present.
   3. The patient is not motivated to restore missing teeth.
   4. Cost is prohibitive.

5. Patient has poor oral hygiene habits and could not take care of a fixed prosthesis.

D. Assistant's role in fixed prosthodontics
1. Set up the operatory.
2. Prepare the patient.
3. Assist during the preparation of the teeth for the abutments.
4. In some states the assistant is licensed to place retraction cord and take impression.
5. Assist during the retraction of cord and choosing the shade of the prosthesis.
6. Assist in the mixing and taking of elastomeric impressions and bite registration.
7. Take opposing impressions if needed.
8. In some states the assistant can fabricate, seat, and clear the cement from the temporary prosthesis.
9. Fill out the laboratory slip and bag the impressions.
10. Document information in the patient's chart.
11. Schedule the patient for the seating of the permanent prosthesis.

E. Assistant's role in the seating of the permanent prosthesis
1. Check to see that prosthesis is back from the lab.
2. Seat and drape the patient.
3. Place all instrumentation out for seating appointment.
4. Remove temporary. In some states the assistant may pumice around prep area if sensitivity is not present.
5. Assist dentist in the try-in phase of the seating appointment.
6. Mix cements as needed by dentist.
7. Pass instrumentation for seating prosthesis.
8. In some states the assistant is trained to remove cement supragingivally.
9. Floss and check the area for unremoved cement.
10. Dismiss patient and document procedure in patient's chart.

F. Armamentarium
1. Large spoon excavator
   a. Used to remove any carious debris from prep area.

2. Additional hand instruments (each dentist will have a preference)
   a. Used to refine margins or preparation.
3. Burs, diamond stones, and discs (each dentist will have a preference)
   a. Used to cut the bulk of the prep and refine prep margins.
4. Gingival retraction setup (retraction cord and retracting instrument)
   a. Used to condense into sulcus surrounding preparation for gingival retraction.
5. Cotton rolls and gauze sponges
   a. Used to absorb moisture and isolate the oral cavity during the preparation phase.
6. High volume evacuator (HVE) tip
   a. Used to keep area free of saliva and debris during the procedure.
7. Elastomeric impression material and appropriate tray
   a. Used to take the impression for the permanent restoration.
8. Bite registration material
   a. Used to record the relationship of the patient's occlusion.
9. Alginate material and tray for opposing impression (if three in one tray is not used)
10. Basic setup

G. Instrumentation for seating appointment
1. Cast restoration
   a. The assistant should make sure that the prosthesis is in the office before patient shows for appointment.
2. Towel clamps or hemostats
   a. Used to remove the temporary restoration.
3. Large spoon excavator or sickle scaler
   a. Used to remove excess cement from prep area.
4. Cavity varnish and applicator (operator's choice)
   a. Sometimes cavity varnish is used to seal the entire prep before cementation occurs to reduce sensitivity after seating.
5. Cements or other luting agents to seat crown (operator's choice)
   a. Used in the final setting of the prosthesis.

6. Articulating paper and holder
   a. Used to register the bite after initial placement has been made.
7. Bite stick or cotton rolls
   a. Used to aid the operator in seating the prosthesis completely.
8. Saliva ejector or HVE tip.
   a. Used to keep area free of saliva and debris during the procedure.
9. Dental floss or sickle scaler
   a. Used to remove excess cement from preparation site.

H. Preparation of a cast crown or fixed bridge
   1. Preparation appointment
      a. The dentist reduces the height and contour of the tooth.
      b. Height reduction is done to provide adequate clearance for the cast crown.
      c. Contour of the tooth is achieved by removing bulk from the proximal, lingual, and buccal aspects of the tooth.
   2. Shade selection
      a. Sometimes done before the preparation is cut.
      b. Must be as close as possible to achieve maximum esthetics.
      c. Shade guide available for matching anterior teeth.
      d. The dentist will inquire whether gold or other material is to be used. The rule of thumb is that gold should not oppose porcelain because of the abrasiveness of the porcelain.
   3. Impressions
      a. Retraction cord is placed and hemostasis is achieved.
      b. Elastomeric and opposing impressions are taken.
      c. Bite registration is taken.
   4. Fabrication of the temporary
      a. In some states the assistant is licensed to fabricate, seat, and clear cement.
   5. Reappoint patient and send case to the laboratory for processing.
      a. It is important to make sure that the patient returns in a timely fashion to have permanent restoration seated to avoid changes in tissue or tooth position.
      b. Lab should have all pertinent information and materials to fabricate prosthesis.

I. Delivery appointment
   1. Temporary crown is removed and prep area is cleared of debris; a polishing of the prep with pumice is sometimes performed to ensure the prep is clean (sometimes sensitivity is a problem, so an anesthetic setup should be available).
   2. Permanent restoration is fitted and adjusted as needed.
   3. The dentist uses his or her choice of luting agent to permanently cement crown to prep.
   4. The assistant mixes the cement and passes the cement-filled crown to the dentist.
   5. Bite sticks or cotton rolls are passed to aid the dentist in seating the crown while the area is kept dry and free of moisture.
   6. In some states the assistant is licensed to remove excess supragingival cement.

J. Other procedures involved with single unit preparations
   1. Core buildup
      a. Used when a tooth is vital.
      b. Used in conjunction with a post when a tooth has been endodontically treated.
      c. Supports the cast and crown when substantial amounts of tooth are missing.
      d. Provides a larger area of retention.
      e. Can be of amalgam or plastic self-curing or light-curing material.
   2. Pin retention
      a. May be necessary to add strength to core buildup.
      b. Placed before the core buildup.
      c. Provides added retention to the restoration overall.
   3. Post and core
      a. Can be done only on endodontically treated teeth.
      b. Provides strength and stability to the post and crown.

    c. Placed at least the height of the clinical crown down into the canal.

    d. A canal is drilled to receive the post.

    e. Cement is placed into the canal with a Lentulo spiral.

    f. Core buildup may follow after post is cemented into place.

K. Gingival retraction methods

  1. Cord retraction

    a. Retraction cord comes in a variety of thicknesses.

    b. Condensed with a plastic instrument or other retraction device.

    c. Removed just prior to taking the impression.

  2. Electrosurgery

    a. Tissue is removed using an electrosurgery unit.

    b. Thin looped wire that removes tissue at a high rate of heat.

    c. Advantages are that the tissue is cauterized while being removed.

  3. Surgical knife

    a. Done when there is a high rate of hypertrophic tissue.

    b. Hemostasis must be achieved before impressions are taken.

  4. Mechanical retraction

    a. Forces tissue from the tooth.

    b. Temporary crown is placed that extends beyond the margin and into the sulcus.

    c. Patient wears crown for several days and then it is removed just prior to the impression.

L. Temporary or provisional coverage methods

  1. Aluminum preformed crowns

    a. Used for posterior teeth.

    b. Easily trimmed and adapted to fit preparation.

    c. Can be cemented on with a variety of cements.

  2. Preformed polycarbonate crowns

    a. Used for anterior teeth.

    b. Sometimes filled with acrylic for better retention.

    c. Cannot use eugenol-based products with this temporary if acrylic is used in the fabrication.

  3. Custom acrylic crowns

    a. Can be used for anterior or posterior teeth.

    b. Usually made from acrylic monomer and polymer.

    c. Custom vacuform trays or alginate impressions are used in the fabrication.

    d. Shade should be chosen carefully and final trimming and polishing to match esthetically is important.

    e. Cannot use any eugenol-based cements for cementation.

M. Inlays, onlays, and veneers

  1. When a full crown is not needed, an inlay or onlay may be used. These are fixed restorations that are cast from gold or other metallic alloys.

    a. Inlays

      (1) Used to restore one, two, or three surfaces of the prepared tooth.

      (2) Used when the occlusal, mesial, or distal walls have to be replaced.

    b. Onlays

      (1) Designed to restore the occlusal and some proximal surfaces of a posterior tooth.

      (2) Similar to an inlay but restores the proximal walls and marginal ridge.

    c. Veneers

      (1) Placed to improve the appearance of the anterior teeth.

      (2) Shade of luting agent used for cementation is similar to that of the natural tooth.

      (3) Facial and incisal areas are reduced only.

      (4) Can be used to mask structural defects of anterior teeth.

N. Components of a fixed bridge

  1. Pontic

    a. A pontic is the "dummy" tooth or artificial tooth that replaces one or more missing natural teeth. The pontic is attached to the abutments, which are cemented on to the preparations.

2. Abutment
   a. Also known as a retainer.
   b. A natural tooth that serves as the support for the replacement teeth.
   c. Usually a cast crown or inlay.
   d. Can be more than two teeth.
3. Units
   a. Total parts of the fixed bridge.
   b. Include the abutments and pontics.
   c. The single units that make up a total bridge.

II. REMOVABLE UPPER OR LOWER PARTIAL DENTURE

A. Replaces one or more missing teeth in an arch.

B. Underlying tissues and existing teeth are used for support.

C. Made of acrylic and alloy metal.

D. Improves esthetics, restores mastication process, and supports remaining teeth.

E. Indications for partial denture
   1. Multiple teeth are missing in one arch.
   2. Patient has the ability to maintain good oral hygiene.
   3. Patient is mentally and physically able to follow through during fabrication.

F. Contraindications for partial dentures
   1. Patient is unable to maintain adequate oral hygiene.
   2. Patient does not have adequate bone and tissue support.
   3. Patient does not have proper muscle tone or is not in good health.

G. Fabrication of the removable partial denture
   1. First appointment is for a consultation.
      a. Study models are obtained.
      b. Radiographs are placed on the viewbox.
      c. Patient photographs are available.
      d. Examples of removable prosthetics are shown to the patient.
      e. The treatment plan is presented to the patient along with the financial obligation and time involved.
   2. Dental assistant's role during the first appointment
      a. Have all above items prepared and set out for the dentist to go over.
      b. The cost estimate is prepared by the front office assistant and available for review with the patient prior to the start of treatment.
      c. If the plan is accepted and financial arrangements are secured, the assistant may go ahead and take alginate impressions for the custom trays.
   3. Steps in the fabrication of the removable partial denture
      a. First appointment
         (1) Alginate impressions are taken and sent to the lab for custom trays.
      b. Second appointment
         (1) Final impressions are taken by the dentist.
            (a) The assistant places an alginate setup out for the dentist to take final impressions.
      c. Third appointment
         (1) Try-in of framework is made and occlusal bite registration is taken.
            (a) The assistant places materials out for the above procedure to be completed.
      d. Fourth appointment
         (1) Framework with wax bite is delivered, and try-in is done.
         (2) Shade of replacement teeth is chosen.
         (3) The assistant places materials for above procedure.
      e. Fifth appointment
         (1) Try-in of wax teeth with framework is done, and any adjustments are made.
         (2) The case is then sent to the lab to be processed.
         (3) The assistant places materials for above procedure.
      f. Sixth appointment
         (1) Final delivery of partial denture to patient and any last adjustments are made.
         (2) The assistant places materials for the above procedure.

H. Full upper or lower denture
   1. Constructed of acrylic and either plastic or porcelain teeth.
   2. Used to replace a missing arch of teeth.
   3. Indications for a full denture
      a. Patient must have proper musculature and alveolar ridge to support a full denture.
   4. Patient must be motivated to keep a full denture clean and repaired.

I. Contraindications for a full denture
   1. Musculature and bone level are not adequate.
   2. Mentally or physically the patient cannot tolerate a removable prosthesis.
   3. Patient does not have a realistic idea of what a prosthesis entails.

J. Steps in the fabrication of a full upper or lower denture
   1. First appointment
      a. Alginate impressions are taken and sent to the lab for custom tray fabrication.
      b. The assistant takes alginate impressions and sends them with the completed lab slip to the dental lab.
   2. Second appointment
      a. Final impressions are taken with custom trays for the construction of baseplates and occlusal rim construction.
      b. The assistant puts custom trays and alginate setup out for the dentist to take custom impressions. Assist patient in dismissal.
   3. Third appointment
      a. Try-in of baseplates and occlusal rims. Bite registration is taken and shade of replacement teeth is chosen.
      b. The assistant puts the needed materials out for the dentist to perform the above procedure.
      c. Baseplates, occlusal rims, and shade are sent to lab so teeth may be set.
      d. Lab slip is set out for the dentist to complete. Assistant contacts lab for pickup.

   4. Fourth appointment
      a. Try-in of the completed wax-up is done, and any adjustments are made by the dentist. The try-in is sent to lab for processing.
      b. The assistant places the appropriate setup out for the dentist to perform the above function. Assistant contacts lab for pickup.
   5. Fifth appointment
      a. The completed dentures are delivered to patient, and minor adjustments are made.
      b. Appropriate items are placed out for the dentist to perform above procedure.
   6. Sixth appointment
      a. Adjustments to the new partial denture are made as needed.
      b. Appropriate items are placed out for the dentist to perform above procedure.

K. Parts of a partial denture
   1. Framework
      a. The cast metal skeleton that provides support for the saddle and the connectors.
   2. Major connector
      a. Also known as a bar.
      b. Piece of rigid metal that joins the right and left quadrant framework of the partial denture.
      c. Helps to form support for the remaining teeth
         (1) Palatal connector.
         (2) Lingual connector.
         (3) Stress breaker.
      d. Saddle
         (1) Mesh extension of the connector that is covered with the acrylic.
         (2) Rests on the alveolar ridge.
      e. Retainer
         (1) Also known as a clasp.
         (2) Supports and provides stability to the partial denture.
         (3) Circles the abutment tooth
            (a) "I" bar retainer.
            (b) Circumferential retainer.

f. Rests
  (1) A metal projection on or near the clasp.
  (2) Designed to control the extent of the seating of prosthesis.
  (3) Aid in distributing the retention load of the partial denture to several teeth and not just one.
  (4) Occlusal rests
    (a) Located on the occlusal surface of the tooth.
    (b) Minimize trauma by transmitting stress along the long axis of the tooth.
  (5) Lingual rests
    (a) Placed on the cingulum of the lingual surface of the tooth.
  (6) Artificial teeth
    (a) Constructed from acrylic or porcelain.
    (b) Tube teeth are posterior teeth prepared with a recessed hole in the base of the crown.
g. Intraoral factors
  (1) Facial muscles must be able to retain functional control with removable prosthesis in place.
  (2) Salivary flow must be adequate for prosthesis to be comfortable. Too much saliva, however, could present other problems.
  (3) There must be an adequate alveolar ridge.
  (4) Oral mucosa must have adequate attachment to avoid irritation.
  (5) Oral habits must be minimal or under control to avoid extreme stress on the ridges and remaining teeth.

h. Extraoral factors
  (1) Physical health must be optimal so that patient is able to tolerate the many appointments needed to fabricate the prosthesis.
  (2) Mental health is an important factor when deciding on a removable prosthesis for your patient.
  (3) Social and economic factors must be taken into consideration. How important is replacing missing teeth to the patient?
  (4) Occupation is taken into consideration. Will the new prosthesis fit into the patient's occupational activities?

III. INFECTION CONTROL

A. Prior to sending lab cases out, all impressions, bite registrations, and other items that have been in the patient's mouth must be disinfected.

B. Receiving area
  1. Should be separate from the production area.
  2. Should be cleaned and disinfected daily.
    a. Countertops and equipment.
    b. Floors, walls, and chairs.
  3. All cases should be disinfected before sending them to the production area.

C. Production area
  1. Personnel working in the production area should wear a lab jacket and personal protective equipment when working with patient lab cases.
  2. All instruments should be kept separate and sterilized every day.
  3. Rag wheels can be washed and sterilized daily.

D. Outgoing cases
  1. Each case should be disinfected prior to delivery to patient.
  2. A mixture of 1:10 parts bleach and water can be used.
  3. All cases are sealed in a plastic bag with sterilized water for delivery.

REVIEW QUESTIONS

1. Fixed prosthetics are placed for which of the following reasons?
   1. To prevent adjacent teeth from drifting
   2. To replace dentition for an entire arch
   3. To aid in the ability to masticate
   4. To restore esthetics to the dentition

   A. 2 only
   B. 1, 2, 4
   C. 1, 2
   D. 1, 3, 4

2. Contraindications for placement of fixed prosthetics include which of the following?
   1. Supporting tissues are diseased or inadequate.
   2. No abutment teeth are present.
   3. The patient is not motivated toward restoring missing dentition.
   4. One or two teeth are missing in the same arch.

   A. 1, 2, 3
   B. 3, 4
   C. 2 only
   D. All of the above

Match the following.

_____ 3. Core buildup
_____ 4. Pin retention
_____ 5. Pontic
_____ 6. Abutment
_____ 7. Porcelain-fused-to-metal crown
_____ 8. Veneer
_____ 9. Onlay
_____ 10. Inlay
_____ 11. Immediate denture
_____ 12. Full upper denture
_____ 13. Framework

A. Designed to restore the occlusal and some proximal surfaces of a posterior tooth
B. Used when a substantial amount of tooth structure is missing
C. Restoration used to cover the facial and incisal surfaces of a tooth
D. Used to replace an entire arch of missing teeth
E. Artificial tooth that replaces one or more teeth in a bridge
F. Placed at the time the final extractions are completed; the prosthesis is fabricated prior to extractions
G. Adds strength and retention to overall buildup
H. Cast restoration that covers complete anatomical crown of a tooth
I. The cast metal skeleton that provides support for the saddle and the connectors
J. Used when occlusal, mesial, or distal walls of a tooth have to be replaced
K. Attached to the pontics of a cast bridge restoration

14. A diamond bur is used to remove gross amounts of enamel and refine margins during the preparation of a cast crown.
    A. True
    B. False

15. A luting agent is used to cement onlays, inlays, and veneers.
    A. True
    B. False

16. A finishing diamond is used to remove excess cement from a cast crown after final seating.
    A. True
    B. False

17. Pumice is used to remove excess temporary cement prior to final cementation.
    A. True
    B. False

18. Amalgam or self-curing plastic can be used as a core buildup.
    A. True
    B. False

19. A core buildup is performed only on a non-vital tooth.
    A. True
    B. False

20. Retraction cord is placed
    A. prior to cementing the temporary crown.
    B. only after hemostasis is achieved and just prior to the final impression.
    C. before the bite registration.
    D. after the opposing impression.

21. During the preparation appointment for a cast crown,
    A. the bulk of the tooth is reduced and contoured.
    B. the shade of the prosthesis is chosen.
    C. impressions are taken of the preparation and opposing teeth.
    D. All of the above.

22. Gingival retraction methods include
    A. cord retraction.
    B. surgical reduction using a Bard-Parker.
    C. electrosurgery.
    D. None of the above

23. Parts of a partial denture include which of the following?
    1. Baseplate
    2. Saddle
    3. Framework
    4. Retainer

    A. 1, 2, 3
    B. 1, 4
    C. 2, 3, 4
    D. All of the above

24. Contraindications to placing a full denture include which of the following?
    1. Patient does not have adequate bone level.
    2. Patient does not have a realistic view of wearing a denture.
    3. Patient is not of sound mind and physical well-being.
    4. Patient does not have adequate musculature to support prosthesis.

    A. 1, 4
    B. 2, 3, 4
    C. 2, 3
    D. All of the above

Place the following steps in order for a cast restoration, beginning with No. 25 as the first step and No. 30 as the last step.

_____ 25.

_____ 26.

_____ 27.

_____ 28.

_____ 29.

_____ 30.

    A. Retract gingiva.
    B. Prepare tooth.
    C. Fabricate temporary and cement in place.
    D. Take final impression.
    E. Administer anesthetic.
    F. Dismiss patient and schedule for seating appointment.

ANSWERS AND RATIONALES

1. **D** Fixed prosthetics such as crowns and bridges are placed to prevent drifting of adjacent teeth either mesially, distally, or vertically. They are also placed to restore chewing function and esthetics.

2. **A** Contraindications for placement of a fixed prosthesis would include the patient not having adequate bone support to make the prosthesis successful, when there are no abutment teeth, and when the patient is not motivated either emotionally or financially toward replacement of lost teeth.

3. **B**
4. **G**
5. **E**
6. **K**
7. **H**
8. **C**
9. **J**
10. **A**
11. **F**
12. **D**
13. **I**

14. **A** A diamond bur, due to its texture, is able to remove large amounts of enamel during the preparation phase of a full coverage crown. Diamonds come in various textures, and the finer textures are used to refine margins following the removal of the bulk of the tooth.

15. **A** A luting agent is any agent or cement that is used to adhere two substances together. Luting agents are suitable for cementing most fixed prosthetics.

16. **B** An explorer or scaler is used to remove excess cement following the cementation of a fixed prosthesis. A diamond may interrupt the finish on the cast restoration and weaken the porcelain or damage the gold.

17. **A** Pumice may be used to remove temporary cement that has adhered to the preparation of the crown. It also cleans the surface of any other debris prior to cementation of the permanent restoration.

18. **A** A core buildup adds bulk to a preparation that is missing a large portion of tooth structure. Amalgam and self-cure plastic are suitable for use as buildup material.

19. **B** A core buildup can be performed on a vital as well as non-vital tooth. Sometimes old amalgams are left in the tooth and the preparation is incorporated into the existing restoration.

20. **B** Retraction cord is the tiny string that is wedged in between the gingival tissue that separates the gingiva from the tooth. By doing this, an adequate impression that captures the entire margin as well as the preparation can be achieved.

21. **D** The preparation appointment consists of removal of the bulk of the tooth, choosing a shade, and taking the final and opposing impressions.

22. **A** Using retraction cord is a suitable method for retracting tissue prior to taking impressions. Using a Bard-Parker and electrosurgery are examples of tissue reduction not retraction.

23. **C** The partial denture includes the framework, saddle, and retainer. A baseplate is part of the construction of a full denture.

24. **D** Reasons why a full denture would not be fabricated would include inadequate bone level to support a denture, patient feels that a denture is an answer to their dental health and does not take into consideration the drawbacks of wearing a denture, or the patient is not of sound mind and mentally cannot wear or maintain a denture.

25. **E**
26. **B**
27. **A**
28. **D**
29. **C**
30. **F**

CHAPTER 13

Orthodontics

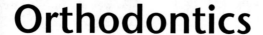

CHAPTER OVERVIEW

Orthodontics is the specialty in dentistry that is concerned with the diagnosis and treatment of malocclusion within the dentofacial structures. The orthodontic office is primarily concerned with the jaws and surrounding facial structures. Recognizing and treating malocclusion or the prevention of malocclusion is also a responsibility of the orthodontic office. This chapter covers the classes of malocclusion, orthodontic treatment procedures, appliances, and armamentarium used in orthodontics.

KEY TERMS

alginate
Angle's classification of
    malocclusion
bracket
distocclusion

malocclusion
mesioclusion
neutroclusion
open bite
orthodontic radiography

overbite
overcrowding
overjet
protrusion
retrusion

I. ORTHODONTIC TREATMENT

A. Conditions that may indicate the need for orthodontic treatment
   1. Difficulty with speech.
   2. Esthetics.
   3. Temporomandibular joint disorders.
   4. High susceptibility to dental caries or periodontal disease due to crowding.
   5. Difficulty with mastication.

B. Conditions that may contraindicate orthodontic treatment
   1. Patient apathy or disinterest.
   2. Lack of alveolar support.
   3. Rampant caries or periodontal disease.
   4. Poor oral hygiene.
   5. Poor mental or physical health.
   6. No financial means.

C. Malocclusion, or the abnormal relationship between the maxilla and mandible, is divided into three different categories.
   1. Angle's classification of malocclusion
      a. Class I: Neutroclusion
         (1) When the jaw is at rest, the dentition is considered normal.

Class name	Molar relationship	Description	Illustration	Facial profile
Neutrocclusion	Mesiobuccal cusp of maxillary first permanent molar occludes with the buccal groove of mandibular first permanent molar.	Similar to normal occlusion with individual teeth or groups of teeth out of position.	Class I	Mesognathic
Distoclusion	Buccal groove of the mandibular first permanent molar is distal to mesiobuccal cusp of maxillary first permanent molar.	Division 1—maxillary teeth in labioversion.	Class II, Division 1	Retrognathic
		Division 2—linguoversion of mandibular teeth	Class II, Division 2	Retrognathic
Mesiocclusion	Buccal groove of the mandibular first permanent molar is mesial to mesiobuccal cusp of maxillary first permanent molar.	Mandibular teeth mesial to normal position.	Class III	Prognathic

Angle's Classifications of Malocclusion and Facial Profiles

(2) The mesiobuccal cusp of the first right maxillary molar occludes in the buccal groove of the mandibular first molar, and the mesiolingual cusp of the maxillary permanent first molar occludes with the occlusal fossa of the mandibular permanent first molar.

b. Class II: Distocclusion

(1) The mesiobuccal cusp of the maxillary first molar occludes between the mandibular second premolar and first molar.

(a) Division 1: Labioversion is characterized by a protruding upper lip over the facial aspect of anterior teeth with the lower lip tucked under the lingual surface.

(b) Division 2: Linguoversion is characterized by the maxillary lateral incisors being tipped labially and mesially.

The anterior maxillary central incisors may be tipped inward but positioned correctly.

c. Class III: Mesiocclusion

(1) The mesiobuccal cusp of the maxillary first molar occludes between the mandibular first and second mandibular permanent molars.

(2) This abnormality usually positions the mandible in front of the maxilla.

(3) The maxillary teeth retrude or are set back behind the anterior teeth.

d. Other malocclusions

(1) Overbite: Excessive overlap of the maxillary anterior teeth over the mandibular anterior teeth.

(2) Overjet: Excessive protrusion of the maxillary anterior teeth over the mandibular anterior teeth.

(3) Overcrowding: Teeth are crowded due to overlapping in an arch.

(4) Congenitally missing teeth: Teeth are due to erupt but never appear, causing diastemas and tipped or drifting teeth.

(5) Open bite: There is no vertical overlapping of the anterior teeth.

II. ORTHODONTIC TREATMENT PHASES

A. Four categories of orthodontic treatment enable the office to deliver care in a more specific mode.

1. Preventive orthodontics
   a. Using space maintainers to maintain the space when primary teeth are lost prematurely and permanent teeth have not yet erupted.
   b. Correcting bad oral habits such as finger or thumb sucking.
   c. Supervision of the primary and permanent dentition during eruption and exfoliation.
   d. Early detection of possible abnormalities that may arise due to hereditary or developmental factors.

2. Limited orthodontics
   a. Can be used when there is not a need for complete orthodontic treatment.
   b. Retainers to correct minor crowding.
   c. Treatment that is focused on one area of the dentition and completed for the benefit of the entire dentition.

3. Interceptive orthodontics
   a. Usually performed during the mixed dentition stage when a tooth erupts out of position.
   b. Correction of crowding through extractions of primary or permanent teeth.

4. Corrective orthodontics
   a. Bands, brackets, and other corrective appliances.
   b. First appointment
      (1) A thorough medical and dental history is taken, and the patient is evaluated clinically, with the patient's motivation toward orthodontics taken into consideration.
      (2) If the patient and/or guardian would like to continue with the process, then the patient's radiographs, photographs, and impression are taken.
         (a) Radiographs include full mouth intraoral series, cephalometric (full cranial), panorex, and occlusal films.
      (3) Study models
         (a) Alginate impressions are poured up in plaster or stone and then polished to a high luster.
      (4) Photographs
         (a) Photographs of the patient's head and neck at several different angles are used to observe facial features and bone growth.
         (b) Mirrors are used to photograph intraoral aspects of the patient's oral cavity.
      (5) Cephalometric tracings
         (a) Cephalometric tracings are used in conjunction with the cephalometric radiograph to determine future bone growth and position of first molars.

Note: Photographs, radiographs, study models, or cephalometric tracings may be performed in the office or in an outside facility.

   c. Second appointment
      (1) The clinical evaluation of the radiographs, tracings, photographs, and study models is discussed with the patient.
      (2) Financial arrangements are made with the patient and/or guardian.
      (3) The patient is referred out for any extractions or restorative work.
      (4) Separators are placed if no referrals are needed.

   d. Third appointment
      (1) Bands and brackets are placed.

(2) A primary coaxial or flexible arch wire is placed and tied with ligature ties.

e. Subsequent appointments
   (1) Reserved for replacement or ligature ties.
   (2) New wires may be placed, or hardware designed to rotate or align malpositioned teeth may be used.
   (3) Checking bands and loose hardware may be done on these appointments.
   (4) Oral hygiene is discussed during these appointments.

f. Final appointment after treatment has been completed
   (1) Bands and brackets are removed.
   (2) Impressions for retainer are done.
   (3) Patient is referred out for radiographs and final study models.
   (4) Prophylaxis appointment is scheduled for patient.

g. Follow-up appointments
   (1) Retainers are delivered and seated.
   (2) Retainer evaluation checkups are done thereafter.

III. BAND AND BRACKET PLACEMENT

A. Successful treatment and correction of malocclusion requires the pushing and pulling forces exerted by extraoral and intraoral software. Tension and strain from ligature ties, wires, springs, and other orthodontic appliances can be used. Bands and brackets must be placed onto the teeth.

B. Band placement
   1. The patient is seated and the procedure is explained. Any separators are removed. Types of separators that may be removed can include TP springs, brass wire, or elastic.
   2. A complete coronal polish is performed using pumice to remove any plaque or debris from the coronal surfaces.
      a. In some states the dental assistant is licensed to perform this function.
   3. The teeth to be banded are determined and the try-in phase is completed. Bands are tried in, contoured, and set aside to be cemented.
   4. After all bands have been tried in and selected, they are set aside in the designated order to be cemented.
   5. Teeth to be banded are dried and isolated.
   6. Upon the dentist's command, the cement is mixed and the bands are lined with permanent cement and handed to the dentist. Bands are usually cemented one quadrant at a time. A new mix for each quadrant is required.
   7. Different instruments such as a band pusher or band seater are handed to the dentist after initial placement of the cement-lined band is seated onto the designated teeth.

C. After all bands have been placed and seated, the patient is instructed to bite down on gauze or cotton rolls until the cement has completely set.

D. After the cement has set, it can then be removed around the occlusal and gingival areas. In some states the registered dental assistant is permitted to perform this function.

E. After oral hygiene is given and care of the bands is discussed, the patient is then dismissed. Usually the parent or guardian is in the operatory at this time.

F. Assistant responsibilities following the banding appointment
   1. Gathers all contaminated materials and takes them to the sterilization area.
   2. After removing the latex treatment gloves, the assistant washes his or her hands and makes an entry into the patient's chart regarding the cementation appointment.
      a. band sizes.
      b. types of cements used.
      c. Any other treatment information that is required by the orthodontist.
   3. The assistant returns to the treatment area, dons utility gloves, and cleans and disinfects the treatment room.

4. All instruments are cleaned and prepared for sterilization in the central sterilization area.

5. The utility gloves are then cleaned and removed, and the assistant washes his or her hands with antimicrobial soap.

G. Armamentarium needed for banding appointment
   1. Basic setup.
   2. Cotton 2 x 2 gauze squares and cotton rolls.
   3. Presized bands with or without bracket and buccal tubes.
   4. Band pusher
      a. Used to apply pressure to the edge of the band while seating.
   5. Band seater
      a. Used to apply force to the band while seating.
   6. Howe pliers
      a. All-around utility pliers.
   7. Contouring pliers
      a. Used to crimp or contour the bands prior to cementation.
   8. Band remover
      a. Used to remove the bands during the try-in phase prior to cementation.
   9. Flexible metal spatula and mixing pad.
   10. Coronal polish setup.
   11. Assorted scalers
      a. Used to remove set cement.
   12. Air-water syringe tip, HVE tip, saliva ejector tip, patient bib and chain.
   13. Other assorted instruments preferred by the orthodontist.

IV. DIRECT BOND BRACKETS

A. Brackets are attached to the facial aspect of the teeth to aid in the support of an arch wire. Many orthodontists prefer brackets rather than full bands because of their esthetic and hygiene pluses.

B. Brackets can be bonded directly onto the tooth with self-cure or light-cure materials.

C. They are easier to keep clean and less traumatic to the tooth and surrounding structures than conventional bands.

D. They come in a variety of material types. Clear plastic and stainless steel are the most popular. Ceramic and resin are also used.

E. Bonding procedure
   1. Patient is seated and the procedure is explained.
   2. A complete coronal polish is performed with pumice to remove any plaque or other debris from the surfaces of the teeth.
   3. The area is then isolated and acid etch is placed on the facial or buccal aspect of the tooth.
      a. Lip retractors or a rubber dam may be placed to isolate and maintain a dry field.
   4. After the etch has been rinsed and dried, the activator is applied.
      a. If the tooth is contaminated with saliva, it will have to be re-etched.
      b. Etching material softens a microscopic layer of enamel and when properly rinsed and dried, it will have a frosty white appearance.
      c. The assistant may don plastic overgloves to keep the individual bonding material containers free from cross-contamination.
   5. After the activator is rinsed and dried, the cement is applied to the back of the bracket and handed to the orthodontist for placement.
      a. The dental assistant, using a disposable brush, also places activator on the back of the bracket.
      b. A conditioner may be used prior to the activator.
   6. The orthodontist is handed a scaler or other instrument of choice to manipulate the bracket into the desired position. The instrument is also used to remove excess cementation material.
   7. If the bonding material is self-cure, then the patient is instructed to remain still until the material is set. If the material is light cure, then the assistant passes the light to the orthodontist and holds the light shield over the curing area. The assistant and the orthodontist during this part of the procedure may wear special glasses.

a. The curing light is placed 2–3 millimeters from the bracket.

b. The bracket cement is activated with the curing light for approximately one to two minutes.

8. After all teeth have been bracketed, the isolation materials are removed and the patient's mouth is rinsed.

9. Oral hygiene instructions and care of the brackets are discussed with the patient and the patient's parent and/or guardian before dismissal.

10. Assisting duties following the placement of direct bond brackets

a. All contaminated materials are removed from the operatory and placed into the central sterilization area for cleaning and sterilization.

b. The assistant removes the latex gloves and washes his or her hands with antimicrobial soap.

c. Information regarding the bracket bonding appointment is recorded into the patient's chart and given to the front office assistant for reappointment.

d. The assistant returns to the operatory and dons the utility gloves for the operatory and instrument cleanup procedure.

e. After the cleanup procedure, the gloves are washed and placed back in their designated place.

Note: The orthodontist may place an arch wire at this appointment.

11. Armamentarium for direct bonding appointment

a. Basic setup.

b. Cotton rolls, 2 x 2 gauze sponges.

c. HVE and saliva ejector tips.

d. Brackets.

e. Bracket placement pliers.

f. Bonding materials.

g. Scaler.

h. Disposable brushes.

V. ARCH WIRE AND LIGATURE PLACEMENT

A. After bands and brackets have been placed, an arch wire, which is a thin, stainless steel wire preformed into a horseshoe shape, is placed within the brackets.

B. The arch wire is ligated and it directs movement of various teeth into their desired positions.

C. The arch wire is tied into place with a ligature tie (stainless steel or elastic) after it has been seated into the bracket.

1. In some states the dental assistant is licensed to ligate an arch wire into place.

VI. ARCH WIRE PLACEMENT AND REMOVAL PROCEDURES

A. The assistant seats the patient and explains the procedure.

1. Armamentarium is set up and the patient is draped.

B. The orthodontist chooses an arch wire using the study model and places the desired loops or crimps using either bird-beak or pesso pliers.

C. The orthodontist places the arch wire and then ties it into place.

1. In some states the assistant performs this function.

D. The patient and the parent or guardian are instructed on oral hygiene and care of the orthodontic appliances.

E. The patient is dismissed and given a subsequent appointment.

F. Assisting duties following the arch wire placement procedure

1. Remove all contaminated materials from the operatory and take them to the central sterilization area.

2. The assistant removes the latex gloves and washes his or her hands with antimicrobial soap.

3. Documentation of the procedure is entered into the chart regarding wire sizes and ligature types.

4. The assistant then dons the utility gloves and disinfects the operatory and cleans and sterilizes the instruments and other armamentarium that was used for the procedure.

5. The utility gloves are then washed and removed and placed in their proper storage area.

G. Armamentarium for arch wire placement
   1. Basic setup.
   2. Preformed arch wire.
   3. Ligature tying pliers.
   4. Howe pliers.
   5. Ligature cutter.
   6. Ligature director.
   7. Hemostats.
   8. Distal end cutters.

H. Arch wire, band, and bracket removal procedure
   1. Seat patient and explain the procedure.
      a. drape patient and set out all needed armamentarium.
   2. The assistant passes the scaler or ligature cutters to the orthodontist so that the ligatures may be removed.
   3. After all ligature ties have been removed, the assistant passes the Howe pliers or hemostats so that the arch wire may be removed.
   4. The assistant then passes the bracket-removing pliers to the orthodontist so that the brackets may be removed.
      a. A small cup may be held under the patient's chin to capture the brackets, bands, and ligature ties.
   5. The orthodontist removes the old cement from the coronal portion of the tooth using an ultrasonic scaler or manual scaler.
      a. In some states the dental assistant is licensed to do this procedure.
      b. The patient may be referred out for a complete prophylaxis.
      c. If a prophylaxis is not needed, a coronal polish may be performed.
   6. Impressions for retention are taken, and after being cleaned up, the patient is dismissed and rescheduled for the next appointment.

7. The assistant follows regular disinfection and sterilization techniques following the procedure.

VII. TYPES OF INTRAORAL APPLIANCES USED IN ORTHODONTICS

A. Hawley retainer
   1. Most commonly used removable retainer following orthodontic treatment.
   2. Worn passively to retain the teeth in their new position.
   3. Constructed of clear acrylic that holds wire clasps on molar teeth.
   4. The plastic portion is placed over the palate.
      a. The plastic can be clear, pink, or multicolored.
   5. On a mandibular retainer, the acrylic part rests on the anterior lingual floor of the mouth.

B. Vacuform custom retainers
   1. Can be fabricated right in the office.
   2. Are custom made for each patient.
   3. Can be constructed out of heavy, clear plastic and are durable.
   4. Are esthetically pleasing.
   5. Are used while the laboratory is constructing a more permanent retainer.

C. Lower fixed 4 x 4
   1. Are banded from cuspid to cuspid and have a lingual bar that travels around the anterior arch of the mandible.
   2. Can be worn for long periods of time with little or no discomfort.
   3. Can provide lower incisor positioning during late growth.

D. Headgear
   1. An orthopedic device used to control growth and tooth movement.
   2. Has two parts
      a. face bow.
      b. traction device.

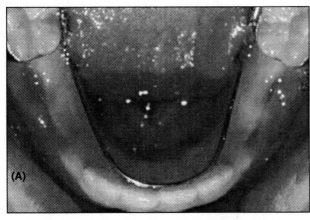

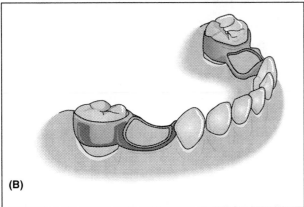

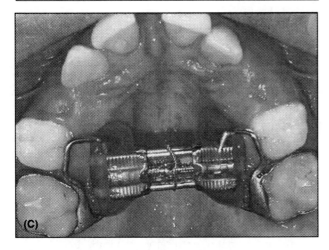

(A) Patient with a lingual arch wire. (B) Space maintainer to hold the space when a tooth is lost prematurely. (C) Palatal separating appliance. *(Courtesy of Rita Johnson, RDH, and Dr. Vincent DeAngelis)*

  E. Space maintainers
    1. Active retainers
      a. Actively move teeth while wearing
    2. Lingual arch
      a. Fixed in the patient's arch and used to hold existing teeth in their place while the permanent teeth erupt.

  F. Rapid palatal expander (RPE)
    1. Used to correct a cross-bite and allow expansion of the maxilla.
    2. Usually cemented onto the first maxillary molars.
    3. Can be activated by the patient using a small key to turn the expander, which widens the palate.

REVIEW QUESTIONS

1. Orthodontic treatment phases include which of the following?
   1. Preventive
   2. Limited
   3. Interceptive
   4. Clinical

   A. 1, 2, 3
   B. 2, 3
   C. 1 only
   D. None of the above

2. Which of the following radiographs are used during orthodontic treatment?
   1. Panorex
   2. Full mouth survey
   3. Occlusal
   4. Cephalometric

   A. 1, 2, 3
   B. 1, 2, 4
   C. 1, 2
   D. 1, 3

3. When cementing bands in place, the assistant should complete which of the following?
   1. Apply cement to all surfaces within the band.
   2. Mix cement thoroughly.
   3. Apply a small amount of cement to the tooth prior to band placement.
   4. Mix enough cement for one quadrant at a time.

   A. 1, 2, 3
   B. 1, 2, 4
   C. 1, 4
   D. 1, 3

Match the following.

_____ 4. Ligature tying pliers

_____ 5. Howe pliers

_____ 6. Distal end cutters

_____ 7. Band pusher

_____ 8. Band seater

_____ 9. Three-pronged pliers

    A. Utility pliers used for general purposes

    B. Instrument used to trim the ends of the arch wire after it has been placed in the brackets and ligated

    C. Pliers used to create loops and bends in the arch wire

    D. Instrument used to apply force when seating the band

    E. Pliers used to ligate stainless steel ties onto the brackets

    F. Instrument that uses the pressure of the patient's bite to seat the bands in place

10. Two common types of measuring devices used to take intraoral measurements are a Boley gauge and a flexible millimeter ruler.
    A. True
    B. False

11. The buccal tube on a posterior band is used to hold the intraoral portion of the headgear in place.
    A. True
    B. False

12. During the preliminary appointment in orthodontic treatment, which of the following may occur?
    1. Clinical examination
    2. Classify malocclusion
    3. Impressions for study models
    4. Complete restoration of teeth

    A. 1, 2, 3
    B. 1, 2, 4
    C. 1, 4
    D. 1, 3

Match the following occlusion with the definition.

_____ 13. The mesiobuccal cusp of the upper first molar occludes with the buccal groove of the lower first molar.

_____ 14. The mesiobuccal cusp of the maxillary first molar is distal to the buccal groove of the mandibular first molar.

_____ 15. The mesiobuccal cusp of the maxillary first molar is mesial to the buccal groove of the mandibular first molar.

_____ 16. Known as mesioclusion

_____ 17. Known as neutroclusion

_____ 18. Known as distoclusion

    A. Class I
    B. Class II
    C. Class III

19. What is the instrument of choice in ligating an arch wire?
    A. Hemostat
    B. Howe pliers
    C. Ligature tying pliers
    D. Utility pliers

20. Loose orthodontic bands may cause
    A. decalcification.
    B. decay under the band.
    C. orthodontic forces to be minimized.
    D. All of the above.

21. Headgear should not be worn during
    A. sports activities.
    B. sleeping.
    C. daytime hours.
    D. school hours.

22. During bracket placement, if the etched enamel is contaminated with saliva, it should be
    A. air dried and isolated.
    B. re-etched.
    C. re-rinsed.
    D. None of the above

23. A/An _____ is when the upper and lower anterior teeth do not occlude, creating an open space when the jaws are closed.
    A. overjet
    B. cross-bite
    C. open bite
    D. closed bite

24. A/An _____ is when one or more of the upper teeth or cusps close inside the lower teeth or cusps during occlusion.
    A. cross-bite
    B. open bite
    C. overjet
    D. None of the above

25. A/An _____ is when the upper teeth overlap the lower teeth too far.
    A. overjet
    B. closed bite
    C. open bite
    D. cross-bite

26. A patient's overjet is measured by
    A. the distance the incisal edges of the maxillary teeth vertically overlap the mandibular teeth.
    B. the horizontal distance the maxillary teeth protrude beyond the mandibular teeth.
    C. the distance between the incisal edge of the maxillary incisors and the gingival edge of the anatomical crown of the mandibular incisors.
    D. having the patient bite in a protruded end to end relationship.

27. When taking impressions for orthodontic study models, which of the following areas should be captured by alginate?
    A. All of the teeth
    B. The entire palate
    C. The retromolar and tuberosity areas
    D. All of the above

28. Ligatures used in orthodontics may include which of the following?
    1. Elastic
    2. Stainless steel
    3. Elastic chains
    4. Floss

    A. 1, 2, 3
    B. 1, 2, 4
    C. 1, 4
    D. 1, 3

29. A Hawley retainer is a type of
    A. removable appliance.
    B. retainer.
    C. retention device.
    D. All of the above

30. Frequent oral hygiene instruction for the orthodontic patient is critical because
    A. intraoral hardware presents more areas for plaque to accumulate.
    B. arch wires cause more tooth decay.
    C. keeping the bands and brackets free from plaque influences overall gum health.
    D. A and C

ANSWERS AND RATIONALES

1. A Preventive: Assessing potential orthodontic problems and treating them before they create a problem.
      Limited: Directing an orthodontic problem to just one area instead of the entire mouth.
      Interceptive: Intervening in a situation and correcting the problem as a whole.

2. B Panorex: Full view of the upper and lower dentition, including the bony facial structures.
      Full mouth survey: Full set of radiographs composed of bitewings and periapical views.
      Cephalometric: Entire view of the cranium, including the first two vertebrae.

3. B When assisting during the cementation of the bands, the assistant should mix only enough cement to seat one quadrant, mixing the cement thoroughly and lining the entire inner surface of the band.

4. E
5. A
6. B
7. D
8. F
9. C
10. A A Boley gauge and a flexible millimeter ruler are used to measure intraoral areas of the mouth. They can be used to measure arch diameter, arch circumference, tooth size, and degree of overjet or overbite.

11. B The buccal tube on the posterior band is used to hold the arch wire. The large tube above the buccal tube is used to hold the headgear.

12. A During the first or second appointment of orthodontic treatment, there will be a clinical examination, impressions for study models will be done, and the orthodontist will classify malocclusion.

13. A
14. C
15. B
16. C
17. A
18. B

19. C The instrument of choice for ligating an arch wire is ligature tying pliers.

20. D When an orthodontic band is loose, decay and decalcification can occur. Also, tooth movement is minimized because there is not adequate force being applied to the anchor tooth.

21. A Because headgear is partially worn outside of the mouth, it is dangerous to wear it during any contact sports. It is customary to wear headgear during sleeping hours and during the daytime.

22. B Saliva will contaminate a newly etched surface. Therefore, it is mandatory that the area be re-etched to guarantee the bonding process of the brackets.

23. C An open bite is characterized by the posterior teeth occluding but not the anterior teeth, leaving the patient's bite "open."

24. D This condition is classified as a Class III malocclusion and the mandible protrudes in front of the maxilla.

25. B A closed bite occurs when the maxillary anterior teeth eclipse the entire crown of the mandibular anteriors. The cause is due to the bite collapsing from inadequate posterior support or abrasion of the posterior teeth.

26. B An overjet is measured by taking a millimeter ruler and measuring the distance in which the maxillary teeth protrude over the mandibular teeth. A horizontal measurement is made by placing the millimeter ruler edge against the facial aspect of the mandibular anteriors and measuring horizontally to the facial aspect of the maxillary anteriors. The distance is recorded as the overjet.

27. D To replicate the dentition adequately, you must get the palate, teeth, vestibule, and retromolar and tuberosities when taking an alginate.

28. A Ligature ties used to ligate an arch wire include elastic, stainless steel, and continuous elastic chains.

29. D A Hawley retainer is a removable appliance constructed out of plastic and wire and is used after orthodontic treatment to retain the dentition in its new place.

30. D Oral hygiene must be stressed during orthodontic treatment. Intraoral appliances cause accumulation of plaque in spaces that are hard to reach unless you have proper instruction and tools. When plaque control is not practiced, gingivitis is likely to occur.

Pharmacology and Pain Control

CHAPTER OVERVIEW

Pain and anxiety control in dentistry is designed to provide patient comfort during routine operative procedures. By using medication such as topical and local anesthetics, the dental office can provide comfort and lessen patient anxiety during dental procedures. Medications are also used following dental procedures that may leave the patient in discomfort or antibiotics are used to prevent infection. This chapter reviews the common drugs and their uses.

KEY TERMS

allergy
analgesics
anaphylaxis
antagonistic
antibiotics
antigen
antiseptic

barbiturates
brand name
Drug Enforcement Agency
generic
germicide
narcotic
pharmacology

prescription
sedative
synergistic
topical anesthetic
tranquilizers
vasoconstrictor

I. DEFINITION

A. Pharmacology is the study of drugs and their effect on the body systems.

B. Drugs defined
   1. A drug can be either found naturally or may be fabricated in a lab with synthetic agents.
   2. Drugs that occur naturally are found in plants, animals, or minerals.
   3. A drug that is classified as synthetic is manufactured from chemicals.
   4. Drugs that are legal have been approved by the Food and Drug Administration (FDA).
   5. Drugs that are sold over the counter (OTC) can be purchased without a prescription.
   6. Drugs that require a prescription from a medical doctor, dentist, or veterinarian can be purchased using a written prescription slip, which is signed by the doctor giving explicit instructions on use.
      a. The prescription must be filled and dispensed by a licensed pharmacist.
      b. Some drugs are kept in the dental office for the benefit of the patient (antibiotics or antianxiety medications).

II. GOVERNMENT LEGISLATION OF DRUGS

A. The Pure Food and Drug Act was passed in 1906.
   1. An attempt by the government to regulate and control the manufacturing, distribution, and sale of drugs.

B. The Harrison Narcotic Act was passed in 1914.
   1. Enabled the FDA to control and regulate the sale of drugs as well as manufacturing and distribution of food and cosmetics.
   2. Required companies to test drugs and render them safe for humans.

C. The comprehensive Drug Abuse Prevention and Control Act was passed in 1970.
   1. Rise of drug abuse spurred this legislation.
   2. The Controlled Substance Act was born.
   3. The Drug Enforcement Agency (DEA) is responsible for the enforcement of this act.
   4. Under this jurisdiction, drugs are divided into five categories.
   5. Controlled substances require the dentist's DEA number and patient's name and address.
   6. This type of prescription cannot be filled more than six months after the prescription has been written.
   7. It cannot be refilled more than five times.

D. Council on Dental Therapeutics
   1. A division of the American Dental Association (ADA).
   2. Evaluates toothbrushes, toothpaste, whiteners, and mouth rinses.
   3. Maintains contact with other research organizations.
   4. ADA approval is granted through this council.
   5. ADA stamp of approval will appear on product label.

E. Generic vs. brand name
   1. Brand name
      a. Drugs that are controlled by business firms and have a registered trademark.
      b. Brand names are always capitalized.
   2. Generic name
      a. Drugs that can belong to any business and are unprotected.
      b. Generic drug names are not capitalized.
      c. Usually furnished using the actual chemical name of the drug.

Parts of a Prescription

1. The dentist's name, address, telephone number, and registration number.

2. The patient's name, address, and the date on which the prescription is written.

3. The *subscription* that includes the symbol Rx ("take thou").

4. The *inscription* that states the names and quantities of ingredients to be included in the medication.

5. The *subscription* that gives directions to the pharmacist for filling the prescription.

6. The *signature* (Sig) that gives the directions for the patient.

7. The dentist's signature blanks. Where signed, indicates if a generic substitute is allowed or if the medication is to be dispensed as written.

8. REPETATUR 0 1 2 3 p.r.n. This is where the dentist indicates whether or not the prescription can be refilled.

9. ☐ LABEL Direction to the pharmacist to label the medication appropriately.

[1]

[2]

[3]

[4]

[5]

[6]

[7]

[8]

[9]

L&K LEWIS & KING, DDS
2501 CENTER STREET
NORTHBOROUGH, OH 12345

Name___Juanita Hansen_____

Address__143 Gregory Lane, Apt. 43__ Date _4/7/--_

Rx

Amoxicillin   500 mg

Disp. #40

Sig   1 cap quid x 10 days

Generic Substitution Allowed __Susan Rice____
                                          D.D.S.
Dispense As Written _____
REPETATUR 0 1 2 3 p.r.n.   D.D.S.
☐ LABEL

Prescription with parts identified.

3. Generic drugs or generic equivalents are sometimes given out instead of their brand name counterpart.
    a. Basically the same as brand but some meet lower standards during testing.
4. Drug information sources
    a. Physicians' Desk Reference
        (1) Published yearly.
        (2) Contains colorful pictures of medication for quick reference and identification.
        (3) Contains an index of pharmaceutical products.
        (4) Each drug has complete listing of most known facts about the drug.
        (5) Indications and use of the drug.
        (6) Contraindications to the use of the drug.
        (7) Warnings and precautions.
        (8) Recommended dosages.
        (9) How the drug is supplied.
    b. United States Pharmacopeia (USP) and National Formulary (NF)
        (1) Contains information specific to the professional dispensing the drug.
5. Drug interactions
    a. Administration of drugs cause many reactions.
        (1) Antagonistic.
            (a) May interact with other foods or drugs to give an undesirable effect.
        (2) Synergistic
            (a) Can interact with other medications to give a more heightened effect than either drug used independently.
6. Drug reactions
    a. Any adverse effect that a drug has on the human body.
    b. Can be mild, moderate, or even life threatening
        (1) Nausea.
        (2) Vomiting.
        (3) Itching, skin rashes, hives.
        (4) Swelling of the eyes, lips, and tongue.
        (5) Wheezing or shortness of breath.
        (6) Loss of consciousness.
    c. Can be life threatening, resulting in anaphylactic shock
        (1) Convulsions.
        (2) Cardiac arrest.
        (3) Cyanosis.
        (4) Very low blood pressure.
7. Commonly used drugs in dentistry
    a. Antibiotics
        (1) Used to combat infection.
        (2) Used as a premedication for heart or joint replacement patients.
    b. Analgesics
        (1) Used to relieve discomfort.
        (2) May be of a narcotic or non-narcotic variety.
    c. Tranquilizers
        (1) Used to reduce anxiety or tension during dental procedures.
    d. Vasoconstrictor
        (1) Used in local anesthetics to constrict the flow of blood.
        (2) Also known as epinephrine.
        (3) Not recommended for patients who are pregnant or have a history of heart disease or hypertension.
    e. Topical anesthetics
        (1) Smeared on the mucosa to produce temporary loss of feeling prior to local anesthetic injections.
        (2) Can be used to control the gag reflex during alginate impressions or radiographs.
        (3) Comes in ointment, spray, or liquid
    f. Topical hemostatic agents
        (1) Used to control bleeding during dental procedures.
    g. General anesthetics
        (1) Administered to render the patient unconscious during dental procedures.
        (2) Can be administered intravenously or by inhalation.
    h. Topical antimicrobial rinses
        (1) Used to reduce the number of microorganisms present in the oral cavity.

8. Dental assistant's role in a drug emergency
   a. Be able to recognize an emergency.
   b. Locate the drug emergency kit.
   c. Be able to prepare the drugs requested by the dentist.
   d. Be ready to prepare any other emergency equipment such as oxygen mask or blood pressure cuff.
   e. Check to ensure that the Emergency Medical Service (EMS) has been notified.
   f. Prevention is the best way to avoid an emergency.
   g. Always check the patient's chart or ask about allergies before the administration of medications.
9. Routes of drug administration
   a. Orally.
   b. By inhalation.
   c. Transdermally.
   d. Subcutaneously.
   e. Intramuscularly.
   f. Intravenously.
   g. Topically.

III. ANESTHETIC SETUP

A. Aspirating syringe
   1. Used to deliver local anesthetic.
   2. Sterilized using an autoclave or chemclave after each use.
   3. Parts of the syringe
      a. Thumb ring.
      b. Finger grip.
      c. Finger bar.
      d. Barrel of syringe.
      e. Piston rod.
      f. Harpoon.
      g. Threaded tip.

IV. LOCAL ANESTHETIC

A. Glass carpule that contains local anesthetic.
B. Has an aluminum diaphragm at one end and a rubber stop at the other.
C. Rubber stops are color coded for easy identification.
D. Strengths of anesthetics
   1. Duration ranges from short acting, intermediate acting, to long acting.

2. Ratios of epinephrine to anesthetic solution range from 1:50,000, 1:100,000, to 1:200,000.
3. Also available without epinephrine.

E. Disinfection of anesthetic carpules
   1. Isopropyl alcohol and a gauze 2 x 2 square.
   2. Provided in blister packs that are already sterilized.

F. Storage of anesthetic carpules
   1. Cool, dry place.
   2. Away from sunlight.
   3. Discard if solution discolors or is outdated.

V. TOPICAL ANESTHETICS

A. Used to temporarily numb the oral mucosa.
B. Provided in an ointment, liquid, or spray.
C. Uses
   1. Prior to local anesthetic injection.
   2. To control the gag reflex.
   3. To relieve symptoms of oral trauma or disease.

VI. DISPOSABLE ANESTHETIC NEEDLES

A. Single-use item.
B. Presterilized.
C. Supplied in different gauges (diameter of the needle)
   1. The higher the gauge number, the thinner the needle.
   2. The lower the gauge number, the thicker the needle.

VII. RECAPPING THE ANESTHETIC NEEDLE

A. One-handed scoop method.
B. Recapping devices.
C. OSHA regulations forbid recapping a needle by holding the cap in one hand and the syringe in the other.

VIII. ADMINISTRATION OF LOCAL ANESTHESIA

A. Maxillary
   1. Infiltration
      a. Anesthetizes only one to two teeth.
      b. Anesthetic is deposited directly at the site of the procedure.

2. Block
   a. Required for most procedures on mandibular teeth.
   b. Mandibular block
      (1) Anesthetic is deposited near the branch of the alveolar nerve.
      (2) Numbness on the half of the jaw where injection was given.
   c. Incisive nerve block
      (1) Inferior alveolar nerve branch at the mental foramen is the site of injection.
      (2) Numbs the anterior and bicuspid teeth.
   d. Periodontal ligament injection
      (1) anesthetic is deposited into the periodontal ligament.
      (2) Used in conjunction with block or infiltration injection.
   e. Other types of injections
      (1) Intraosseous anesthesia injection directly into the spongy portion of the bone.
      (2) Long buccal injection of soft tissues.
      (3) Lingual injection of soft tissue.

IX. NITROUS OXIDE

A. Tanks clearly labeled with specific colors
   1. Blue: Nitrous.
   2. Green: Oxygen.

B. Assistant responsibilities during administration of nitrous oxide sedation
   1. Never leave the patient alone while the patient is on nitrous oxide gas.
   2. Never adjust or start the flow of gases.
   3. Follow the disinfection and sterilization procedures for all equipment.
   4. Check the tanks periodically for supply of gases.
   5. Make sure that all equipment meets safety standards.
      a. Scavenger system.
      b. Proper working condition.
   6. Assistant should use the HVE during procedures in which nitrous oxide is used.
   7. Monitor the patient for any changes in behavior, breathing, or consciousness.

X. IV SEDATION

A. Drugs administered directly into the blood stream.

B. Produces conscious or deep sedation.

C. Assistant's role during IV sedation
   1. Monitor the patient's vitals very closely.
   2. Be prepared to respond to any emergency.
   3. Never leave the patient alone when IV sedation is being used.
   4. Follow infection control procedures when assisting in the administration of IV sedation.
   5. Monitor the patient closely after the effects have worn off.

REVIEW QUESTIONS

Match the definition with the terms.

_____ 1. Injection into the muscle

_____ 2. Injection directly into the vein

_____ 3. Inhaling gases

_____ 4. Taken by mouth

_____ 5. Placed under the tongue

_____ 6. Injection using a hypodermic needle

_____ 7. Injection into the fat layer

_____ 8. Application to the oral mucosa

A. Intravenously
B. Inhalation
C. Topically
D. Intramuscularly
E. Parenterally
F. Sublingually
G. Subcutaneously
H. Orally

9. Brand name drugs have which of the following characteristics?
   1. They are written in triplicate.
   2. The name of the drug is always capitalized.
   3. The drug name is protected by a trademark.
   4. They are stronger than a generic drug.

A. 1, 2, 3
B. 1, 4
C. 2, 3
D. All of the above

10. Which of the following is true regarding antibiotics?
    1. They can irritate the gastrointestinal tract.
    2. They can be taken intravenously.
    3. They are used to treat infection.
    4. They contain flavoring agents.

    A. 1, 2, 3
    B. 2 only
    C. 3, 4
    D. All of the above

11. An anesthetic syringe is made up of which of the following parts?
    1. Barrel
    2. Harpoon
    3. Thumb ring
    4. Aluminum diaphragm

    A. 1, 2, 3
    B. 1, 4
    C. 2 only
    D. All of the above

12. Uses of medicines in dentistry include which of the following?
    A. Help the body overcome infection
    B. Help to control pain
    C. Can be purchased over the counter
    D. All of the above

Choose the appropriate types of injections for the following teeth.

_____ 13. Tooth #3

_____ 14. Tooth #30

_____ 15. Tooth #24

_____ 16. Tooth #14
    A. Mental block
    B. Infiltration
    C. Block

17. Materials you would find on an anesthetic tray would include which of the following?
    1. Topical anesthetic
    2. Cotton-tip applicator
    3. Syringe setup
    4. Mouth mirror

    A. 1, 2, 3
    B. 1, 4
    C. 3 only
    D. All of the above

18. The higher the gauge of the needle, the _____ the diameter of the needle is.
    A. larger
    B. smaller

19. When a patient has a drug allergy, which of the following symptoms may occur?
    1. Nausea
    2. Hives
    3. Fever
    4. Itching

    A. 1, 2, 4
    B. 1, 4
    C. 2 only
    D. All of the above

20. Drug information may be obtained from which of the following?
    1. Physicians' Desk Reference
    2. Label on the back of the bottle
    3. Pharmacist
    4. National Formulary

    A. 1, 2, 3
    B. 1, 4
    C. 3 only
    D. All of the above

21. Drugs that are legal to dispense
    A. are available by prescription only.
    B. must be dispensed by a licensed pharmacist.
    C. are approved by the Food and Drug Administration.
    D. are never kept in a dental office.

22. Premedication for mitral valve prolapse prevents the patient from
    A. fainting.
    B. acquiring a bacterial infection that may affect the valves of the heart.
    C. having a heart attack.
    D. having an allergic reaction to pain medication.

23. The ADA approves which of the following products for use?
    1. Antibiotics for use in the dental field
    2. Professional tooth whitening bleach
    3. Toothbrushes
    4. Dentifrices

    A. 1, 2, 3
    B. 2, 3, 4
    C. 1 only
    D. All of the above

24. Which of the following is true regarding generic drugs?
    A. They have a registered trademark.
    B. They are unprotected and can be distributed by any company.
    C. They meet higher standards during testing than brand name drugs.
    D. Their name is always capitalized.

25. As you are loading an anesthetic syringe, you notice that the solution in the anesthetic carpule is cloudy. This could be caused by
    A. anesthetic that has been contaminated.
    B. anesthetic that has expired.
    C. anesthetic that has been frozen and then thawed.
    D. anesthetic that has been exposed to light.

26. Antagonistic refers to a drug that interacts with another to create a heightened or desirable effect.
    A. True
    B. False

27. Synergistic refers to a drug that has an adverse effect when combined with another drug.
    A. True
    B. False

28. A drug reaction is any adverse effect that a drug has on the human body.
    A. True
    B. False

29. A potentially life-threatening allergic reaction is called anaphylactic shock.
    A. True
    B. False

30. Responsibilities delegated to the dental assistant during the administration of nitrous oxide sedation include which of the following?
    1. Never leave the patient alone while under nitrous oxide sedation.
    2. Never start the flow of gases.
    3. Keep equipment in good working order and have it checked regularly by a licensed professional.
    4. Follow sterilization procedures after the sedation procedure has been completed.

    A. 1, 2, 3
    B. 2, 3, 4
    C. 1 only
    D. All of the above

ANSWERS AND RATIONALES

1. D
2. A
3. B
4. G
5. F
6. E
7. H
8. C
9. C Brand name drugs always have the name of the drug capitalized. The company that the drug belongs to has financed the research and marketing that goes into selling the drug on the market. It is protected by that company's trademark.
10. A Antibiotics destroy good bacteria as well as bad bacteria. This can lead to gastrointestinal upset and may cause diarrhea or nausea. They are used to treat infection and can be taken orally or may be administered intravenously. Oral administration is most common in the dental office.
11. A The anatomy of an anesthetic syringe includes the barrel, which is where the carpule is secured; the thumb ring, which is where the operator places the thumb and uses pressure to inject the medication; and the harpoon, which is the sharp tip connected to the piston rod that is lodged into the rubber stopper of the anesthetic carpule, which forces the anesthetic into the needle.
12. D Several types of medications are used in dentistry. Antibiotics are used to help the body overcome infection, and analgesics are used to help control pain. A dentist may elect to prescribe a pain reliever that does not require a prescription but may be purchased over the counter at a local drug store.
13. B
14. C
15. A
16. B
17. D When setting up an anesthetic tray, the following items should be present: topical anesthetic and a cotton-tip applicator for placement, a mouth mirror, and a syringe setup (carpule, needle, and syringe).
18. A The higher the gauge of a needle (25, 27, and 30 are most commonly used in dentistry), the larger or more rigid the needle is.

19. A When a patient is having a reaction to the administration of a drug, severe nausea, hives, and itching may occur. A fever is the body's response to infection, not allergy.

20. D Information regarding the administration, side effects, and dosage rates may be obtained from the pharmacist at the time of dispensing or from the label on the bottle. The Physicians' Desk Reference or National Formulary is available for more technical information regarding drugs.

21. C Any medication that is legal to dispense, either over the counter or through the pharmacist, has been approved by the Food and Drug Administration. Any medication or drug that has not been approved by the FDA is either illegal or has not met the federal safety standards and could be dangerous.

22. B Mitral valve prolapse is a condition in which the left valve of the heart does not close tightly after blood has entered the heart. If a dental procedure is performed in which bacteria can be introduced into the bloodstream, there is a potential for it to settle around the valve and cause a bacterial infection known as bacteremia endocarditis. A prophylactic of antibiotics is taken to prevent this from occurring.

23. B Some of the items that are approved by the American Dental Association include toothbrushes, toothpastes and other dentifrices, and professional whitening or bleaching solutions.

24. B Generic drugs do not belong to any company; therefore, they do not have to have a trademark name. Generic drugs are referred to by their chemical name.

25. A Anesthetic carpules that contain cloudy solution have been contaminated in some way, either by bacterial growth or by leakage of cold sterile solution into the carpule. They should be discarded immediately.

26. B Antagonistic refers to a drug that does not interact well with another specific drug and causes an adverse or life-threatening reaction.

27. B Synergistic refers to the action of a drug when it works well with other drugs. Drugs that have a synergistic effect will achieve a more desirable effect than they would if one was used alone.

28. A A drug reaction is any adverse effect that a drug has on the human body.

29. A A potentially life-threatening allergic reaction is called anaphylactic shock and can result in death if emergency care is not delivered.

30. D During the nitrous oxide sedation procedure, the dental assistant's role is to monitor patient responses by staying in the room with the patient at all times. She should never start the flow of any gases. And equipment should be maintained by following all sterilization procedures and regular maintenance of tanks, hoses, masks, and scavenger systems.

CHAPTER 15

Medical and Dental Emergencies

CHAPTER OVERVIEW

Medical and dental emergencies are those emergencies that are classified as situations that require immediate attention. A variety of medical and dental emergencies may occur in the dental office. An emergency can happen not only to a patient but also to a fellow employee. This chapter reviews some of the common medical and dental emergencies and the proper method of treatment and includes a brief review of cardiopulmonary resuscitation.

KEY TERMS

anaphylactic shock
avulsed
cardiac arrest
chemical injury

CPR
diabetic emergency
epilepsy

first aid
syncope
vital signs

I. DIAGNOSTIC VITAL SIGNS

A. Serve as an indicator of what kind of health a patient is in
   1. Pulse rate
      a. Radial pulse: Wrist.
      b. Carotid pulse: Neck.
      c. Brachial pulse: Inside of arm near the bicep muscle.
      d. Taken for one minute.
   2. Respiration rate
      a. Breaths per minute.
      b. Taken for one minute.
      c. Normal respiration for an adult is 10–20 breaths per minute.
   3. Blood pressure
      a. Systolic: The highest pressure exerted by the cardiovascular system.
      b. Diastolic: The lowest pressure of the cardiovascular system.
      c. Read with a stethoscope and sphygmomanometer.
      d. Can be taken manually or with an electronic blood pressure cuff.
   4. Temperature
      a. Taken by placing thermometer under the tongue.
      b. Optimal time is two minutes.
      c. Normal reading is 98.6°F.
      d. Standard mercury thermometer or digital thermometer.

II. CARDIOPULMONARY RESUSCITATION

A. Can be performed if the patient has stopped breathing and has no heartbeat. Careful assessment of the victim should be done before CPR is started.
   1. Check for unresponsiveness.
   2. Alert Emergency Medical Service (EMS).
   3. Roll adult victim onto back and make sure victim is on a firm surface.
   4. Open airway.
   5. Check for breathing.
   6. If not breathing, give two slow breaths.
   7. Can reposition head and try two breaths if first breaths were unsuccessful.
   8. Check for pulse (carotid).
   9. If there is no pulse and no breathing, begin cardiopulmonary resuscitation.

B. Cardiopulmonary resuscitation techniques
   1. Adult
      a. Fifteen compressions.
      b. Two breaths.
      c. After four cycles of 15 to 2, check your victim's pulse and breathing.
      d. Continue CPR until you are exhausted, help arrives, or your patient regains breathing and heartbeat function.
      e. Compression depths are 1½ to 2 inches.
   2. Child
      a. Follow steps 1 through 9.
      b. Five compressions.
      c. Two breaths.
      d. Use the palm of one hand to deliver compressions.
      e. Compression depths are 1 to 1½ inches.
   3. Infant
      a. Follow steps 1 through 7.
      b. Give a puff of air instead of a full breath.
      c. Pulse is checked in the brachial artery.
      d. Five compressions are delivered using the middle and ring finger of one hand between the nipple line.
      e. Compression depths are ½ to 1 inch.
   4. Rescue breathing
      a. Used in the event that a victim has a pulse but no respiration.
      b. Drowning or electrical shock would temporarily stop respiration.
      c. Procedure
         (1) Head tilt, chin lift, and attempt to open airway.
         (2) Sweep the mouth for any airway blockage.
         (3) Deliver two full breaths.
         (4) Maintain five breaths per minute.
         (5) If blockage is due to a foreign object, attempt the Heimlich maneuver.
   5. Rescue breathing for a child or infant
      a. Head tilt, chin lift.
      b. Check for any foreign objects.
      c. Do not do a blind finger sweep on an infant (may lodge object farther into infant's throat).
      d. Deliver two breaths (less pressure than for an adult).
      e. If blockage is due to a foreign object, attempt the Heimlich maneuver by back blows alternating with chest thrusts for an infant and arms around the victim's waist and fist under rib cage for a child.

III. MEDICAL EMERGENCIES

A. Shock
   1. Life-threatening injuries must be addressed first.
   2. Prevent loss of body heat by covering with a blanket.
   3. Elevate the victim's legs 8–12 inches if possible.
   4. Do not give the victim anything to eat or drink.
   5. If victim is having difficulty breathing, place in a supine position.
   6. If victim is vomiting or unconscious, place victim on side.

B. Syncope (fainting)
   1. Lay victim down and elevate the legs 8–12 inches (in the dental chair, recline chair back until legs are above victim's chest).
   2. Loosen tight clothing.

3. Moisten a washcloth with cool water and place on victim's face.

4. Do not use smelling salts or ammonia inhalants.

5. Do not give victim anything to eat or drink until victim has fully recovered.

C. Chemical injuries
1. Flood the eye with warm water immediately.
2. Use the eyewash station if available.
3. Rinse area at least 15 minutes.
4. Cover eye loosely with bandage and seek medical attention.

D. Foreign body in eye
1. Do not rub the eye.
2. Lift lower eyelid over upper eyelid and allow eyelashes to brush particle out.
3. Attempt to flush particle out with warm water for at least 15 minutes.
4. Seek medical attention if you cannot dislodge particle safely.

E. Heart attack
1. Victim may feel pressure, fullness, squeezing, or pain in the center of the chest lasting two minutes or longer.
2. Pain may spread to either shoulder, the neck, the lower jaw, or either arm.
3. Victim may feel nausea, dizziness, sweating, or shortness of breath.
4. Contact EMS and make victim as comfortable as possible.

F. Stroke
1. Victim will feel sudden weakness or numbness of the face, arm, and leg on one side of the body.
2. Loss of speech, trouble talking or understanding conversation.
3. Dimness or loss of vision.
4. Sudden severe headache.
5. Victim should be kept calm and EMS should be contacted immediately.

G. Diabetic emergencies
1. Insulin shock victims should be given sugar (candy, fruit juice).
2. Keep victim as calm as possible.
3. Insulin-dependent victim should be given insulin injection as soon as possible.
4. Seek medical attention for victim.

H. Epilepsy
1. Epilepsy is not a medical emergency.
2. Move anything out of the way that could cause harm to the patient during the seizure.
3. Cushion the victim's head with something soft.
4. Do not restrain the victim in any way.
5. Loosen any tight clothing.
6. Turn the victim onto side.
7. Call EMS if the victim has never had a seizure. A second seizure or difficulty breathing afterward may occur.

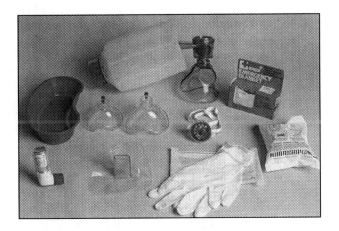

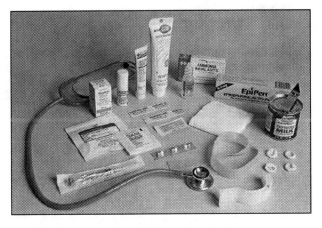

Example of a dental office emergency kit.

IV. DENTAL INJURIES

A. Objects wedged between teeth
1. Attempt to remove with dental floss.
2. Attempt to remove with a toothpick or other oral hygiene aid.
3. If unsuccessful, call dentist.

B. Trauma to lip or tongue
1. Apply pressure with sterile gauze to area.
2. If swelling occurs, apply a cold pack.
3. If bleeding does not subside, call dentist.

C. Avulsed teeth
1. Rinse tooth off; do not scrub.
2. Do not touch the root of the tooth.
3. Place tooth in a cup of whole milk.
4. Call dentist for an appointment to reimplant and stabilize.

D. Partially avulsed tooth
1. Gently push the tooth back into place without rinsing tooth.
2. Make an appointment with dentist to stabilize.

E. Fractured tooth
1. Clean any dirt, blood, and debris from the injured area.
2. Apply a cold compress on the face next to the injured tooth.
3. For jaw fractures, immobilize the jaw with a scarf over and under the chin and tie both ends together on top of the head.
4. Make an appointment with dentist to stabilize or refer out to oral surgeon for treatment.

REVIEW QUESTIONS

1. Normal respiration for an adult is _____ breaths per minute.
   A. 12–18
   B. 10–12
   C. 18–20
   D. 10–20

2. The expansion and contraction of an artery, which can be felt with the tips of your fingers, is known as
   A. systolic pressure.
   B. pulse.
   C. heart rhythm.
   D. defibrillation.

3. The artery in the neck where the pulse can be felt is called the _____ artery.
   A. femoral
   B. brachial
   C. carotid
   D. radial

4. The ABCs of basic life support stand for airway, breathing, and compressions.
   A. True
   B. False

5. Which of the following are common medical emergencies that may occur in the dental office?
   1. Heart murmur
   2. Cardiac arrest
   3. Anaphylactic shock
   4. Syncope

   A. 1, 2, 3
   B. 1, 4
   C. 2, 3, 4
   D. All of the above

6. The ratio for compressions to ventilation on an adult is _____.
   A. 15:1
   B. 15:4
   C. 15:2
   D. 15:6

7. Syncope is another word for fainting.
   A. True
   B. False

8. What is the optimal time to leave a thermometer in a patient's mouth?
   A. Two minutes
   B. Three minutes
   C. Four minutes
   D. Five minutes

9. When a patient experiences an epileptic seizure, the dental personnel should respond by
   1. not restraining the patient in any way.
   2. standing back and letting the patient have the seizure.
   3. moving chairs and tables out of the patient's way.
   4. placing a wooden pencil or pen between the patient's teeth so that the patient does not bite the tongue.

   A. 1, 2, 3
   B. 2, 3, 4
   C. 1, 4
   D. All of the above

10. The normal temperature for a healthy adult is
    A. 99.4°F.
    B. 98.6°F.
    C. 96.5°F.
    D. 97.6°F.

11. A patient is in the dental chair and complains of sudden weakness, numbness of the face, and dizziness. It is possible they may be suffering from
    A. a fainting episode.
    B. anaphylactic shock.
    C. a heart attack.
    D. a stroke.

12. If the airway of a victim seems obstructed after the first attempt to give rescue breaths, the rescuer should
    A. check the victim's pulse.
    B. reposition the head and attempt to ventilate again.
    C. begin chest compressions.
    D. check for foreign body obstruction.

List in order, starting with A, the steps in delivering cardiopulmonary resuscitation to an adult victim.

13. _____

14. _____

15. _____

16. _____

17. _____

18. _____

19. _____

20. _____
    A. Activate EMS.
    B. Give two slow breaths.
    C. Begin chest compressions if there is no pulse.
    D. Roll the victim onto the back.
    E. Check for breathing.
    F. Check for pulse.
    G. Check victim for unresponsiveness.
    H. Open the airway.

21. EMS stands for
    A. emergency monitoring sequence.
    B. emergency medical stands.
    C. emergency medical service.
    D. emergency medication substances.

22. A frantic mother calls to say that her son has fallen and "knocked his tooth completely out." As the dental assistant who took the call, you would respond by telling her to
    A. place the tooth in a clean cloth, control bleeding, and come right in.
    B. scrub all of the debris off the tooth, place it in a bag of ice, and come right in.
    C. place the tooth in a glass of milk, apply pressure to the area to control bleeding, and come right in.
    D. None of the above

23. Symptoms of a heart attack
    A. include pain that radiates to the jaw.
    B. could be mistaken for indigestion.
    C. could be mild and ignored.
    D. All of the above

24. In a medical emergency situation, the dental assistant should
    1. activate EMS.
    2. know where the oxygen tank is kept and how to set it up for the delivery of oxygen.
    3. know where the emergency kit is.
    4. be prepared to administer injectable medication for an allergic reaction.

    A. 2, 3, 4
    B. 1, 2, 3
    C. 2, 4
    D. All of the above

Match which factors can be changed and which cannot be changed to increase your chances of not having a heart attack.

25. _____Heredity

26. _____Sex

27. _____High blood pressure

28. _____Age

29. _____High cholesterol
    A. Can be changed
    B. Cannot be changed

30. Prudent heart living includes which of the following?
    A. A diet low in fat
    B. Regular exercise program
    C. Reduction in stress
    D. All of the above

ANSWERS AND RATIONALES

1. A   The normal respiration for an adult is 12–18 breaths per minute. Respiration is the inhalation and expiration of air.

2. B   A patient's pulse is the expansion and contraction of the elastic arterial walls as blood rushes through on its way away from the heart. A pulse cannot be felt in a vein.

3. C   The depression in the patient's neck between the trachea and the sternocleidomastoid muscle is where the carotid artery can be felt.

4. B   The ABCs of life support stand for airway, breathing, and circulation. These are the first three responses that you check when assessing for the administration of cardiopulmonary resuscitation.

5. C   Common medical emergencies that may occur in the dental field include a heart attack, a severe allergic reaction to local anesthetic, or fainting.

6. C   Compressions to ventilations for an adult are 15:2 (fifteen compressions for every two breaths of air). After four cycles of compressions to ventilations, the rescuer should reassess the victim.

7. A   The word syncope means fainting.

8. B   The optimal time to wait before recording the temperature on a standard mercury thermometer is three minutes. Two minutes is adequate, but three is optimal.

9. A   An epileptic seizure is not considered a medical emergency. It is an emergency only if the victim does not have a history of seizure disorders or is pregnant. The dental personnel should remove all furniture that the patient may hurt themselves on and stand back and let the patient have the seizure. Never place anything in the mouth while the patient is having a seizure.

10. B   The temperature for an adult who has not just smoked a cigarette or consumed a hot or cold beverage and is not ill should read 98.6°F.

11. D   Numbness of the face, weakness, and dizziness are all signs of a stroke.

12. B   Repositioning the patient's head for a second time rules out the possibility of the rescuer not maintaining an adequate airway for the first time.

13. G
14. A
15. D
16. H
17. E
18. B
19. F
20. C

21. C   EMS stands for emergency medical service. In some states, one number summons the police, fire department, and ambulance. In other states, each of these agencies has to be called separately.

22. C   When a tooth has been avulsed (torn completely from the socket), it must be placed in a cup of whole milk and bleeding should be controlled. An immediate visit to the dentist is recommended because the sooner the tooth is reimplanted, the greater the chance for survival and reattachment. Never recommend cleaning the tooth. Periodontal ligaments and other fibers responsible for attachment could be lost, diminishing the chances of reattachment.

23. D   A patient who may be experiencing a heart attack in your office may deny that anything is wrong, tell you that it feels like indigestion, or complain of pain radiating to the jaw and begin to perspire.

24. B   The dental assistant should be ready for any and all medical and dental emergencies. Responding to an emergency can mean life or death for your patient. Knowing how to activate your EMS and the location of the emergency kit and oxygen tank should be common knowledge.

25. B
26. B
27. A
28. B
29. A
30. D   According to the American Heart Association, prudent heart living starts with consuming a diet low in saturated fats, getting on a regular exercise program, and reducing stress.

Oral Evacuation and Instrument Transfer

CHAPTER OVERVIEW

While assisting during restorative and surgical procedures, the dental assistant must keep a dry field and maintain visibility for the operator. By using a high volume evacuator, saliva ejector, and cotton rolls, the assistant is able to keep the field clear and dry. This chapter reviews some of the methods used to maintain a clear field and examines some of the techniques for achieving this.

KEY TERMS

classifications of motion	palm grasp	surgical suction tip
clock positions	pen grasp	svedopter
dental dam	saliva ejector	three-way syringe
high volume evacuator tip		

I. ORAL EVACUATION

A. Oral evacuation is the removal of debris and saliva from the oral cavity during operative procedures.
   1. Using an oral evacuator aids in patient comfort by keeping the oral cavity free of saliva and eliminating the need to expectorate or swallow.
   2. Improves operator visibility.
   3. Reduces aerosol spatter and splashing of saliva or other infectious pathogens.

B. Types of evacuators
   1. High volume evacuator (HVE)
      a. Can remove large amounts of fluids and debris.
      b. Should be changed between each patient and lines should be flushed with a commercial evacuation product or bleach and water mixed at a ratio of 10 parts water to 1 part bleach.
   2. Saliva ejector
      a. Referred to as a low volume evacuator.
      b. Can be used by patient during procedures when the operator works alone (i.e., prophylaxis or coronal polish) or evacuation is not needed on a constant basis.

3. Svedopter
   a. A long thin retraction/suction device that comes in several different sizes and is attached to the saliva ejector hose.
   b. Can be slipped under the tongue while the patient is wearing a rubber dam and is used to remove pooled saliva that collects in the floor of the mouth.
   c. Should be discarded after each use and suction lines should be flushed with water and bleach at a ratio of 10:1.
   d. Cannot pick up solid pieces of debris.
4. Surgical suction tip
   a. Used in oral surgery to remove blood and saliva from the oral cavity during surgical procedures.
   b. Comes in disposable single use or stainless steel, which can be cleaned and sterilized using an autoclave or chemclave.
   c. Lines should be flushed with a mixture of water and bleach at a ratio of 10:1 after each patient use.

C. Using the HVE oral evacuation tip
   1. Can be held using a reverse palm-thumb or modified pen grasp.
   2. Should be held securely to avoid dropping.
   3. Engage the suction tip securely into the suction hands before using.
   4. When using the HVE, use the beveled tip toward the hard tissues.
   5. Always use a commercial evacuation solution or water and bleach mix at a ratio of 10:1 after each patient.

D. Using the saliva ejector
   1. Can be manipulated to fit into patient's mouth.
   2. Keep soft tissue away from saliva ejector so that suction will not be impeded.
   3. Discard after each use.

E. Using the surgical suction tip
   1. Used in a wiping motion.
   2. Keep tip clear by keeping a container of water nearby so that the tip may be cleared frequently to prevent clogging.

3. The suction tip may be left on during surgery and occluded with a cotton gauze sponge when not in immediate use.

F. Three-way or air-water syringe
   1. Used in conjunction with the HVE and saliva ejector.
   2. Aids in keeping the oral cavity clean and free of liquids during treatment procedures.
   3. Creates an air, water, or combination spray.
   4. Limits the need for patient to rinse and expectorate.
   5. Aids in retracting soft tissue during operative procedures.

G. Maintaining the oral evacuation system
   1. Lines should be flushed after each patient.
   2. HVE tips can be cleaned with soap and water and then placed in a glutaraldehyde solution for 10 or more hours to sterilize.
   3. Routine maintenance of the main suction should be performed on a regular basis.
   4. Hoses and lines should be checked for wear and replaced when needed.
   5. Changing the main trap and smaller traps on a regular schedule keeps the suction system running efficiently.

II. ISOLATION TECHNIQUES

A. Keeping a dry field and improving visibility for the doctor is one of the most important functions of the dental assistant. Using cotton rolls, saliva ejectors, and high volume evacuation tips can help you accomplish this task.
   1. Indications for isolation
      a. Aids in the management of the patient.
      b. Maintains a clear and dry field.
      c. Keeping aerosol spatter and fluids out of the oral cavity aids in the infection control process.
      d. Cotton rolls alone and cotton roll holders provide retraction of soft tissues while keeping the area dry.
      e. Increases patient comfort.

2. Types of isolation materials
   a. Cotton rolls.
   b. 2 x 2 cotton gauze sponges.
   c. Dental dam.
   d. Dry angles.
   e. Svedopters.
   f. Saliva ejector.
   g. Absorbent paper discs.
3. Cotton roll isolation
   a. Can be placed in the vestibule or under the tongue to absorb excess saliva.
   b. Are disposable and easy to manipulate.
4. Cotton 2 x 2 gauze squares
   a. Can be folded into fourths and used to blot surgical sites.
   b. Can be placed in the back of the patient's mouth during oral surgery procedures to prevent patient from aspirating materials or fluids.
5. Saliva ejectors and svedopters
   a. Can be bent or manipulated to fit operative area.
   b. Are disposable and easy to assemble.
6. Dental dam
   a. Used to isolate one or more teeth.
   b. Improves visibility for operator and assistant.
   c. Aids in patient management.
   d. Retracts soft tissue (tongue and gingival tissues).

III. CLOCK POSITIONS

A. Clock positions are used to situate the operator and the assistant around the patient for easier visibility and access to the patient's oral cavity. When referring to the clock positions, we use a standard numeric clock to orient ourselves around the treatment area, using the patient's nose as the center of the clock.
   1. Operating zone
      a. Right-handed operator: 7 to 12 o'clock
      b. Left-handed operator: 12 to 5 o'clock
   2. Assisting zone
      a. Right-handed operator: 2 to 4 o'clock
      b. Left-handed operator: 8 to 10 o'clock

3. Static zone
   a. Right-handed operator: 12 to 2 o'clock
   b. Left-handed operator: 10 to 12 o'clock
   c. Rear delivery carts are located in the static zone.
4. Transfer zone
   a. The area below the patient's nose where instruments are exchanged.
   b. Right-handed operator: 4 to 7 o'clock
   c. Left-handed operator: 5 to 8 o'clock

IV. CLASSES OF MOTION

A. There are five classifications of motion, which state the range of motion that the dental team uses.
   1. Class I
      a. Involves only finger movements.
   2. Class II
      a. Involves movements of the fingers and wrist.
   3. Class III
      a. Involves finger, wrist, and elbow movements.
   4. Class IV
      a. Involves movement of the entire arm and shoulder.
   5. Class V
      a. Involves movements of the arm and twisting of the body.

V. INSTRUMENT TRANSFER

A. Key rules
   1. Place working end of instrument in the proper position so that it faces the arch being treated.
   2. The assistant holds the instrument at the top when passing it, allowing the operator to grasp it at the bottom.
   3. Pick up the instrument at the end of the tray that is closest to the assistant.
   4. Grasp the instrument between the index finger and thumb, supporting the handle with the middle finger.
   5. Keep instruments in order of use.

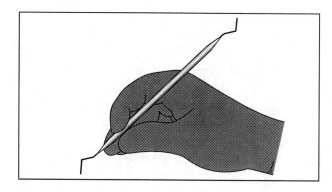

Pen grasp.

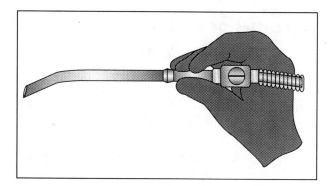

Modified pen grasp.

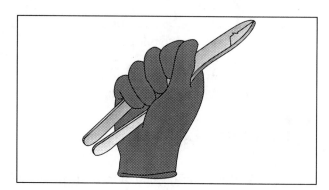

Palm grasp.

B. One-handed transfer
1. Leaves one hand free to suction.
2. Assistant picks up one instrument, makes the transfer, and is able to place the previous instrument back on the tray using only one hand.

C. Two-handed transfer
1. Assistant uses both hands to pass and retrieve instruments.
2. Used for bulky items.
3. Used for passing surgical instruments.

REVIEW QUESTIONS

1. The auxiliary uses the three-way syringe in which of the following ways to cool the tooth and keep the field clear while the dentist performs operative procedures using a high-speed handpiece?
   A. Air
   B. Water
   C. A mist of air and water
   D. All of the above

2. When utilizing the assistant's chair, which of the following techniques may be used?
   A. The chair may be adjusted at least four to five inches higher than the operator's chair.
   B. The assistant may use the circular ring at the base of the chair to rest the feet on.
   C. The padded extension arm may be placed in front of the assistant's torso for more support.
   D. All of the above

3. When delivering an instrument to the operator, the instrument should be positioned _____ the instrument being returned.
   A. below
   B. parallel to
   C. above
   D. behind

4. When assisting a right-handed operator, the assistant delivers and retrieves instruments with
   A. the left hand.
   B. the right hand.
   C. both hands.

5. When assisting a left-handed operator, the auxiliary is seated in the _____ position.
   A. 12 to 2 o'clock
   B. 8 to 10 o'clock
   C. 2 to 3 o'clock
   D. 4 to 8 o'clock

6. When using a high volume evacuator tip in the posterior region, the auxiliary places the suction tip
   A. at the gingival third of the tooth being prepared.
   B. on the occlusal surface of the tooth being prepared.
   C. parallel to the buccal or lingual surfaces of the tooth being prepared.
   D. A and C

7. The most common movements of the dental auxiliary during four-handed dentistry include
   A. movements of the fingers only.
   B. movements of fingers and wrist only.
   C. movements of fingers, wrist, and elbow.
   D. All of the above

8. When the operator is seated in the 10 o'clock position, the auxiliary is most efficient seated in the _____ position.
   A. 1 to 3 o'clock
   B. 2 to 3 o'clock
   C. 1 to 4 o'clock
   D. 2 to 4 o'clock

9. Which of the following is true regarding oral evacuation?
   1. Aids in patient comfort
   2. Improves operator visibility
   3. Can remove large amounts of debris and saliva from the oral cavity
   4. Cools the tooth during operative procedures

   A. 1, 2, 3
   B. 1, 4
   C. 3 only
   D. All of the above

10. Which of the following is a type of oral evacuator tip?
    1. Saliva ejector
    2. Svedopter
    3. High volume evacuator
    4. Surgical suction

    A. 1, 2, 3
    B. 1, 4
    C. 3 only
    D. All of the above

11. After using the oral evacuation system on a patient, it should be flushed with
    1. hot, soapy water.
    2. commercial evacuation system cleaner.
    3. water and bleach ratio at 10:1.
    4. cold sterile solution.

    A. 1, 2, 3
    B. 2, 3
    C. 1 only
    D. All of the above

12. A surgical suction tip is utilized
    A. in a dabbing motion.
    B. by placing it stationary to the surgical site.
    C. with a light, sweeping motion.
    D. All of the above

13. When using the high volume evacuator, the bevel should be placed
    A. on the occlusion.
    B. parallel to the hard tissues or tooth being treated.
    C. next to the tongue.
    D. behind the retromolar area.

Match the following clock positions for a right-handed operator.

_____ 14. 7:00 to 12:00 o'clock position

_____ 15. 4:00 to 7:00 o'clock position

_____ 16. 2:00 to 4:00 o'clock position

_____ 17. 12:00 to 2:00 o'clock position

    A. transfer zone
    B. operator's zone
    C. static zone
    D. assistant's zone

Match the following transfer techniques with the instrument to be transferred.

_____ 18. High-speed handpiece

_____ 19. Burnisher

_____ 20. Cowhorn extraction forceps

_____ 21. Air-water syringe

_____ 22. Scalpel

_____ 23. Cleoid-discoid carver

_____ 24. Extraction elevator

    A. One-handed transfer method
    B. Two-handed transfer method

25. Instruments are arranged in order of use on the bracket tray, with the instrument used first farthest from the operator.
    A. True
    B. False

26. A svedopter may be used to retract the tongue and remove saliva without the aid of an auxiliary when placed in the patient's mouth.
    A. True
    B. False

27. Keeping a dry field is not as important as passing instruments on time and in order.
    A. True
    B. False

28. Which of the following are reasons why you would isolate an area during operative procedures?

    1. Maintains a dry field
    2. Helps the patient to be more comfortable by eliminating the need to expectorate
    3. Keeps aerosol spatter down for infection control purposes
    4. Aids in retraction of tissues

    A. 1, 2, 3
    B. 3, 4
    C. 1 only
    D. All of the above

29. Which of the following grasps is used for the high volume evacuator tip?
    1. Modified pen grasp
    2. Pen grasp
    3. Reverse palm-thumb grasp
    4. Underhand grip

    A. 1, 2, 3
    B. 1, 3
    C. 3 only
    D. All of the above

30. The saliva ejector tip is designed to be cleaned and sterilized after each patient use.
    A. True
    B. False

ANSWERS AND RATIONALES

1. D   The three-way syringe is used with water, air, or a combination of spray to cool and clean the tooth periodically throughout the procedure.

2. D   The assistant's chair is designed to seat the auxiliary comfortably during dental procedures. The extension arm is used to support the assistant's torso, and the foot bar is designed to give support to the feet and legs. The assistant should be positioned at least four to five inches above the operator for maximum visibility.

3. B   During the delivery of an instrument, the instrument being delivered is even and parallel with the instrument being returned. This places the instrument in the position it is intended to be used.

4. B   The auxiliary uses her left hand to retrieve and deliver instruments. The right hand is too far away and not convenient when assisting the right-handed operator.

5. B   The 8 to 10 o'clock position places the auxiliary at the patient's right while the operator is seated at the patient's left.

6. D   Placing the bevel of the evacuator tip parallel and at the gingival third gives the operator room to maneuver and the auxiliary access to clear the field as needed.

7. D   When utilizing four-handed dentistry, all of the classifications of movement are used. Limited movements involving moving the entire torso or twisting are avoided.

8. B   The 2 to 3 o'clock position gives the dental auxiliary the best visibility and access to instrumentation.

9. A   An oral evacuator is a suction device that removes debris and saliva to improve visibility and aid in patient comfort. An air-water syringe is used to cool the tooth during operative procedures.

10. D   Saliva ejector, svedopter, high volume evacuator, and surgical suction are used to remove saliva, blood, and debris from the patient's oral cavity.

11. B   Commercial evacuation solutions or bleach and water are acceptable evacuation solutions to clean and disinfect the evacuation lines. A cold sterile solution is not economically sound, and soapy water does not disinfect at the level needed.

12. C   When using a surgical suction tip, it is best utilized when moving in a sweeping and wiping motion over the immediate area.

13. B   To avoid suctioning the soft tissues and tongue, the bevel is placed facing the tooth or hard tissues.

14. B

15. A

16. D

17. C

18. A

19. A

20. B

21. B

22. B

23. A

24. B

25. A   Instruments are easier to manage when they are arranged in order of use.

26. A   The curly shape of the svedopter is designed to attach to the patient's cheek and retract the tongue while evacuating saliva.

27. B   Keeping a clear field is more important than passing instruments to the dentist. The dentist can retrieve instruments if you are occupied with clearing the field.

28. D   Keeping an area isolated during the operative procedure keeps aerosol spatter to a minimum, helps to retract tissues for operator efficiency, and improves patient comfort.

29. B   The modified pen grasp and the reverse palm-thumb grasp are the safest and most effective ways to hold the high volume evacuator tip.

30. B   Because of the diameter of saliva ejectors, they are difficult to clean. They are packaged and priced as a single-use item.

CHAPTER 17

Law and Ethics in the Dental Field

CHAPTER OVERVIEW

In the delivery of dental care to patients, we are constantly faced with legal and ethical issues. In today's society, the dental office is held up to the highest professional standards. Legal regulations and laws govern the way we practice dentistry; therefore, the members of the dental health team must be committed both legally and ethically. This chapter reviews some of the key concepts and ideas regarding legal and ethical behavior in the dental workplace.

KEY TERMS

act of commission	ethics	malpractice
act of omission	jurisprudence	written consent
Board of Dental Examiners	lawsuit	
Dental Practice Act	litigation	

I. RESPONSIBILITIES

A. Responsibilities of the dental assistant to the dentist
   1. Always treat your dentist with loyalty and respect.
   2. Support your dentist in whatever decisions he or she makes for your patients.
   3. Any information learned about the dentist or the patient must be held in the strictest of confidences.
   4. Perform only those functions that are delegated to you by law.
   5. Follow the instructions of the dentist and do the task assigned to the best of your ability.
   6. Conduct yourself in a professional manner that will reflect favorably upon you, the dentist, and the office.

B. Responsibilities of the dental assistant to the patients
   1. Perform all tasks to the best of your ability.
   2. Accept all patients and hold their dental health concerns in the highest regard.
   3. Learn to meet different patient needs and be willing to help all patients achieve their dental goals.
   4. Update skills and knowledge on a regular basis.
   5. Strive to improve yourself.

6. Dress appropriately and have proper grooming skills.
7. Strive to educate and motivate patients toward better oral health.
8. Your attitude should always reflect positively toward the field of dentistry.

C. Responsibilities to other dental health team members
  1. Treat all team members with respect and strive to work harmoniously and as a team.
  2. Demonstrate the desire to help other team members when the need arises.
  3. Arrive at your work site on time and be prepared to stay late if treatment on a patient goes over the normal office hours.
  4. Handle any grievances in a timely manner and through the proper channels.
  5. Refrain from accepting gratuities from patients.

II. ETHICS

A. Ethics deals with moral conduct or duty as it applies to the dental field. It is not a formal written law but a personal belief when dealing with issues of right and wrong in the delivery of dental care. It is a standard followed by all dental health-care workers and should be adhered to at all times.

B. American Dental Assistants Association Principles of Ethics
  1. Any individual involved in the practice of dentistry must strive to maintain and enrich the profession.
  2. Each individual must observe the Gold Rule and treat each patient based on individual need.
  3. Each individual must strive to maintain confidentiality and respect for the dentist.
  4. Each individual must update and expand his or her technical expertise on a regular basis for the benefit of the patient and the employer.
  5. Each individual must seek to sustain and improve the American Dental Assistants Association at all levels.

Note: The format but not the content has been altered slightly for review purposes.

III. JURISPRUDENCE

A. Dental jurisprudence deals with the law as it pertains to the practice of dentistry.
  1. May include statutes regulating dentistry.
  2. Professional liability.
  3. Professional incorporation.

B. Dental Practice Act
  1. Developed within your own state.
  2. Outlines the legal practices of dentistry as well as the scope in which they may be practiced.
  3. Developed through legislation.
  4. Defines conditions under which an auxiliary may practice.
  5. Defines the type of supervision under which a dental auxiliary may perform a function or task
    a. Direct: The dentist is in the office at the time that the function is being performed. The dentist has previously given the auxiliary a direct order and is available for assistance, guidance, and evaluation.
    b. General: The dentist is not in the office during the procedure. However, the dentist is aware that the procedure is being performed and takes full responsibility.

C. State Dental Board of Examiners
  1. Individual state boards are responsible for administering licensing examinations and maintaining all records regarding the dental team and the license under which dental team members are practicing.
  2. Most states require continuing education courses when renewing licensure.
  3. The State Board of Dental Examiners requires a record of these courses before renewing any license.
  4. The Board of Dental Examiners also keeps a record of all applicants and pass and fail rates and accreditates dental schools and dental hygiene and dental assisting programs.
  5. Investigates infractions of the Dental Practice Act within own state.

D. Common negligent acts in the dental office
   1. Mistaken identity
      a. Treating one patient using another patient record.
   2. Material spills
      a. May injure or debilitate the patient.
   3. Abandonment
      a. Deciding not to complete treatment started on a patient without just cause.
   4. Medication errors
      a. Administering a medication that may have allergic or other detrimental effects for the patient.
   5. Disease transmission
      a. Inadvertent transmission of communicable disease such as hepatitis or HIV.
   6. Treating a patient without proper consent
      a. Treating the pediatric patient without written consent from the caregiver.
      b. Treating a pediatric patient without the caregiver in the room or on the premises.
      c. Not obtaining written consent when performing any dental procedure on a patient.
   7. Loss or damage of patient's personal property
      a. Jewelry, wallet, or handbag.
      b. Materials spilled onto patient clothing, resulting in permanent damage.
   8. Inadvertent bodily injury to patient
      a. Accidental laceration with scalpels or high-speed burs.
      b. Accident through faulty or malfunctioning equipment.

REVIEW QUESTIONS

1. When working as an assistant, you have certain responsibilities to your dentist. These responsibilities include which of the following?
   1. Treat your dentist with respect.
   2. Support your dentist in any decision made for the patient.
   3. Perform only those tasks that are delegated to you by law.
   4. Conduct yourself professionally in the dental office.

   A. 1 only
   B. 1, 3, 4
   C. 1, 4
   D. All of the above

2. Patient perception is one of the most important concepts in the delivery of patient care. Methods that convey a positive image include which of the following?
   1. Accept all patients without regard to their ethnic background, socioeconomic situation, or financial position.
   2. Keep all information regarding patient care confidential.
   3. Maintain a positive attitude toward your dentist and the office.
   4. Keep an upbeat attitude toward your coworkers.

   A. 1, 2, 4
   B. 3 only
   C. 2, 4
   D. All of the above

3. The best way to avoid malpractice is through
   1. communication and prevention.
   2. documentation of all treatment.
   3. following the "silence is golden" rule.
   4. obtaining written consent for all treatment.

   A. 1, 2, 4
   B. 1, 3
   C. 4 only
   D. All of the above

4. You cannot be dismissed from your position for refusing to perform an illegal function ordered by your supervisory dentist.
   A. True
   B. False

5. The dentist technically owns all records of treatment and radiographs. However, the patient has the right to access and retrieve copies of all records.
   A. True
   B. False

6. Ethics is the part of philosophy that deals with moral conduct, duty, and judgment.
   A. True
   B. False

7. _____ supervision means that the dentist is in the office or treatment facility and personally authorizes treatment to be performed.
   A. Direct
   B. Indirect
   C. Local
   D. Personal

8. Malpractice is
   A. a misdemeanor.
   B. performing an act that a "reasonable and prudent man would perform."
   C. unethical conduct.
   D. professional negligence.

9. When a patient breaks an appointment, this may be interpreted as
   A. abandonment.
   B. contributory negligence.
   C. forgetfulness.
   D. malpractice.

10. _____ is the science dealing with the law as it applies to dentistry.
    A. Dental jurisprudence
    B. Ethics
    C. Malpractice
    D. Respondeat superior

11. The principle of "reasonable skill, care, and judgment" applies to
    A. the dentist.
    B. the dental auxiliaries.
    C. the licensed dental personnel.
    D. all dental team members.

12. In each state, the _____ contains the legal restrictions and controls that govern the practice of dentistry.
    A. ADA Code of Ethics
    B. Federal Principles of Ethics
    C. State Board of Dentistry
    D. state Dental Practice Act

13. Failure to comply with the Dental Practice Act or any other laws governing the practice of dentistry could result in
    A. a fine.
    B. license revocation.
    C. A and B
    D. None of the above.

Match the following.

_____ 14. Act of commission

_____ 15. Jurisprudence

_____ 16. Malpractice

_____ 17. Due care

_____ 18. Consent

_____ 19. Act of omission

_____ 20. Ethics

_____ 21. Direct supervision

_____ 22. Duty of care

_____ 23. General supervision

A. Given when a patient enters the dental office and gives permission for treatment.
B. The dentist remains in the office while the auxiliary performs a task.
C. The dentist has a legal obligation to deliver just and proper care to the patient.
D. Addresses the law as it applies to dentistry.
E. An act that a reasonable individual would not perform.
F. The patient expects the dentist to be licensed and use reasonable skills and up-to-date medications and materials.
G. Also known as professional negligence.
H. The dentist remains responsible even though he or she is not in the treatment facility.
I. Failure to perform an act that a reasonable individual would.
J. Moral conduct and judgment.

24. When there is an entry in the patient's chart that is an error, it should be crossed out once with a pen, initialed, and the correct entry written below it.
    A. True
    B. False

25. Respondeat superior is Latin for
    A. "respond to your superior."
    B. "let the assistant respond."
    C. "respond in care."
    D. "let the master answer."

ANSWERS AND RATIONALES

1. D The dentist is the authority figure in the office. Respect toward the dentist and the dentist's decisions is key.
2. D Patient perception during the delivery of care makes the difference between patient acceptance and rejection of the office, staff, and treatment plan. Acceptance of all patients and conveying a positive approach to the delivery of treatment is fundamental in improving patient perception.
3. D Malpractice can be avoided if you follow some basic concepts. Document all treatment and do not make critical remarks about another dentist or the treatment rendered by the dentist. Obtaining a signed consent for treatment can diminish your chances for a malpractice lawsuit.
4. A It is illegal to practice any dental assisting duties that are not delegated to you by law. You can be charged and held liable if you are convicted of practicing illegal functions.
5. A The dentist owns all records of treatment and radiographs. However, the patient has the right to access and retrieve copies of all records.
6. A Ethics is concerned with standards for judging whether actions are right or wrong.
7. A Direct supervision is when the dentist is in the facility and is authorizing treatment to be performed. The dentist is available to evaluate any duties performed by the auxiliary.

8. D Professional negligence is considered the same as malpractice in that the welfare and well-being of the patient were compromised during the delivery of dental treatment.
9. B Contributory negligence is based on the philosophy that the patient should be involved in the overall delivery of dental treatment. By scheduling and attending the appointment, the patient is actively participating in the delivery of care. When a patient breaks an appointment, the patient is contributing to the breakdown of delivering care.
10. A Dental jurisprudence is the term used to include statutes regulating the legal aspects of the practice of dentistry.
11. D All dental team members are responsible for using good judgment and reasonable skills when treating or managing the dental patient.
12. D Each state has its own compilation of legal restrictions and laws that govern the personnel in the dental office.
13. C When you fail to comply with the law as it is written, you may be fined or have your license revoked.
14. E
15. D
16. G
17. C
18. A
19. I
20. J
21. B
22. F
23. H
24. A Never erase or white out an entry in a patient chart. Patient charts are legal documents and may have to be used in a court of law.
25. D Respondeat superior is Latin for "let the master answer," which means the dentist is held responsible for the actions of employees.

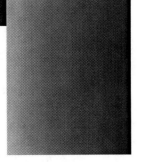

CHAPTER 18

Dental Office Management

CHAPTER OVERVIEW

This chapter reviews the basic front office duties and aspects of dental office management. Claim forms, job duties, and insurance information are covered. Aspects of patient management and marketing are also covered.

KEY TERMS

accounts payable
accounts receivable
communication
dental claim forms

dental insurance
external marketing
inventory and supplies

nonverbal cues
patient management
recall systems

I. THE FRONT OFFICE

A. Office manager
   1. Responsible for delegation and follow-through of duties in the dental office.
   2. Handles all aspects of running the dental practice.
   3. Maintains patient relations
      a. Schedules appointments.
      b. Greets patients.
      c. Obtains health history forms.
      d. Prepares consultation materials.
      e. Explains office policies.
      f. Discusses financial arrangements.
      g. Implements marketing strategies.
   4. Maintains dental staff relations
      a. Conducts staff meetings.
      b. Helps to resolve conflicts within the staff.
      c. Provides support to the staff.
      d. Interviews, hires, and trains all new staff members.
      e. Places job advertisements.
      f. Assigns workloads.
      g. Arranges for risk management and OSHA seminars.
   5. Should be able to operate and troubleshoot electronic office equipment
      a. Fax machine.
      b. Calculators.
      c. Computers.
      d. Time-card clock.
      e. Copy machine.
      f. Postage equipment.
      g. Telephones.
      h. Intercom or paging system.

6. Should be able to manage all records in the office
    a. Prepares clinical charts.
    b. Prepares insurance forms.
    c. Prepares laboratory requisitions.
    d. Maintains employee records.
    e. Appoints an OSHA coordinator to maintain material safety data sheets and other safety-related data.
    f. Writes checks.
    g. Reconciles bank statements.
    h. Handles petty cash and change funds.
    i. Prepares monthly statements.
    j. Prepares state and federal tax documents (quarterly basis).
7. Should be able to manage any correspondence within the office
    a. Opens and classifies mail.
    b. Weighs mail and computes postage.
    c. Prepares special handling for mail (UPS, FedEx, USPS).

B. There may be more than one front office person and the duties can be divided.
    1. Receptionist
        a. Greets patients.
        b. Makes appointments.
        c. Confirms appointments.
        d. Gives out all necessary forms to new and existing patients.
        e. Keeps the reception area neat and tidy.
        f. Answers phones.
        g. Fields all calls and takes messages when appropriate.
        h. Takes patient payments.
    2. Insurance or billing receptionist
        a. Handles all correspondence with insurance companies.
        b. Fills out all necessary insurance forms and submits them to the carrier.
        c. Takes all necessary insurance information from the patient.
        d. Posts all payments for treatment to patient accounts.
        e. Handles all monthly billing procedures.
        f. Fields all questions regarding patient billing.
        g. Handles all collection procedures.
        h. Handles accounts payable and receivable.
        i. Prepares the daily deposit.

II. PATIENT MANAGEMENT

A. Patients have special needs.
    1. Recognizing nonverbal cues
        a. Nervousness.
        b. Clenching hands together.
        c. Crossing arms.
        d. Locking ankles together.
        e. Defensiveness
            (1) Crossed arms and clenched fists.
            (2) Hands on hips.
            (3) Standing at a farther-than-normal distance
        f. Openness
            (1) Sit in front of the patient with no barrier when communicating.
            (2) Do not cross arms.
            (3) Smile and use gestures that exhibit friendliness.
        g. Touching
            (1) Touch the patient's shoulder to reassure a patient showing signs of nervousness.
            (2) An arm around a senior citizen's shoulder indicates warmth and caring.
            (3) A light touch on a pediatric patient's arm may be comforting.
        h. Embarrassment
            (1) Patients who cover their mouth may be hiding an embarrassing smile.
            (2) Tightening the upper lip to hide a smile.
    2. Recognizing the patient who has a disability
        a. Physical disability
            (1) Blind or deaf.
            (2) Stroke victim.
            (3) Missing limbs.
        b. Patient with a walker or in a wheelchair.
        c. Mentally disabled.
            (1) Alzheimer's disease.
            (2) Cerebral palsy.

3. Giving extra care to the patient with disabilities
   a. Clearing a path for the patient to maneuver in.
   b. Adjusting the dental chair so that the patient may enter and exit freely.
   c. Having an extra assistant help during procedures.
   d. Taking extra time and effort to make the patient with the disability comfortable.
4. Financial arrangements for the disabled patient
   a. If patients do not have all of their mental faculties, arrange with family ahead of time for payment of services.
   b. Be prepared before the patient arrives to have all necessary fees for service documented and be ready to discuss arrangements with patient or family member.
   c. Treat all patients the same; if they are regular patients, bill them as you would any other patient.

III. MARKETING FOR THE DENTAL PRACTICE

A. In a competitive, consumer-oriented society, dentists around the country have come to realize that marketing their dental practice is an integral part to staying in business.

B. Marketing increases practice loads, spreads goodwill, and can increase the knowledge of certain dental services out into the community that otherwise may have gone unknown.
   1. Two types of marketing
      a. Internal: What an office does to maintain the patients who are already in the practice
         (1) Newsletters.
         (2) Gifts to patients for referrals.
         (3) Greeting cards (Christmas, birthday, or grief).
         (4) Special promotions for existing patients.
         (5) Managing the office staff to improve customer relations, efficiency, and goodwill.
         (6) Attending seminars that center around delivering total patient care.
         (7) Clean and attractive office with quality care delivered.
      b. External: Determining prospective patients and then centering activities toward bringing those patients in
         (1) Special coupons or promotions.
         (2) Open house.
         (3) Telephone book.
         (4) Referral services.
         (5) Extended office hours to accommodate individuals who cannot leave the office.
         (6) Newspaper announcements of services or grand opening of office.
         (7) Special seminars for the public (temporomandibular disorders, bleaching techniques).
   2. Complex media advertising
      a. Commercials
      b. Weekly newspaper columns
      c. Identifying local organizations and offering specials centered around their needs.

IV. INVENTORY AND SUPPLY ORDERING FOR THE DENTAL OFFICE

A. Inventory ordering
   1. Types of supplies
      a. Consumable supplies
         (1) Items that are consumed upon each use
             (a) Dental cements
             (b) Radiographic film
             (c) Local anesthetics
             (d) Stationery
      b. Nonconsumable supplies
         (1) Items that are reusable and that are of relatively low cost
             (a) Dental instruments
             (b) Radiographic intraoral film holders
      c. Capital items
         (1) Large, costly items that are seldom replaced
             (a) Sterilizer.
             (b) Handpieces.
             (c) Computer.
             (d) Dental units.

V. CHOOSING SUPPLIES

A. Dental supply house
   1. Provides all basic dental supplies.
   2. Carries brand name and generic items.
   3. Provides quick service and special rates on many items.
   4. Usually has a toll free number to order from and can set up an account for you.
   5. May send a representative to the office on a regular basis.

B. Purchasing medications
   1. Can be bought from a local pharmacy.
   2. Can usually be delivered by the pharmacy.
   3. Can be called in by the dentist.
   4. Local pharmacy may set up an account for the dentist.

C. Purchasing office supplies
   1. Local stationery stores carry most products needed by office.
   2. Local stationery stores usually deliver.
   3. Large local wholesale warehouses carry bulk items for less.
   4. Most stationery stores or warehouses can carry an account for the dentist.
   5. Discount warehouses may also carry cleaning supplies and other items routinely needed by the office.

VI. SETTING UP AN INVENTORY SYSTEM

A. All offices must have some type of inventory control system.
   1. Capital equipment
      a. Must have a detailed card made out for each item listing the manufacturer, the manufacturer's phone number, the phone number for the repair center, and maintenance data.
      b. Schedule all preventive maintenance when the doctor is out of the office.
   2. Expendable and nonexpendable items
      a. Never keep a large stock on hand.
      b. Always keep enough materials to give you an adequate lead time when ordering.
      c. Rotate stock when needed.
      d. Take advantage of quantity discount purchases when ordering.

   e. Special computer software packages are available for keeping track of stock and ordering.
   f. Keep a direct line of communication with the back office so that you can order in a timely manner.
   g. Set up a manual card system.
   3. Receiving orders
      a. Open the box and remove the packing slip.
      b. Check the quantity and types of items in the box against the packing slip.
      c. Make a note of any items that are missing or backordered.
      d. Put materials away in a timely manner.
      e. Place the packing slip or invoice where it can be referred to at the end of the month for payment.
      f. Remove any material safety data sheets and place in the MSDS binder.
      g. Send back any items that were not ordered or should be returned making a note for future reference.

VII. DENTAL INSURANCE

A. Dental insurance is designed to financially assist in the expense of treatment and care of the dental patient. In the early 1900s, dental insurance was not heard of. However, by 1965, 1.9 million people were covered by dental insurance, and by 1985, 95 million Americans were covered by some form of dental insurance.
   1. Insurance involves four parties
      a. Patient.
      b. Insured or subscriber
         (1) Could be a spouse or dependent child.
      c. Organized group that is participating in the plan
         (1) Any company or business that has negotiated benefits with a particular insurance company.
      d. Dentist
         (1) The provider of services for the insured.

B. Carrier
  1. The insurance company that distributes money to the dentist or provider for services rendered.
  2. Types of prepaid dental programs
    a. Usual, customary, and reasonable fee.
    b. Fees that are charged by a provider
      (1) Usual: Provider's usual fee that is charged for a service.
      (2) Customary: Provider's fee that is charged in a similar limited geographic area and with the same training as those providers in that area.
      (3) Reasonable: Those fees that are charged by a provider when the provider lives in the same limited geographic area and those fees are reasonable for the specific procedure performed.
    c. Fixed fee
      (1) An established fee set down by the office for a particular service.
      (2) Usually federally supported.
      (3) The provider must follow a set fee schedule and cannot charge the patient any more for the service than what is listed on that set schedule.
  3. Table of allowance
    a. A specified amount that will be paid toward the cost of dental services.
    b. The patient has to pay the difference between what is covered and what is not.
C. Other dental delivery systems
  1. Capitation plans
    a. The dentist is paid a fixed amount for delivering services to a group of insured subscribers per month.
    b. Regardless of the number of patients seen or services rendered, the provider receives the same amount of reimbursement.
    c. The provider is not paid for individual services; instead, the provider is paid for performing as many services as are needed per month.

  2. Health maintenance organizations
    a. A legal entity that will accept all financial risk for providing dental benefits and services.
    b. Specified services are provided to a population at a specific time for a specific cost.
    c. Designated providers must be used while on this plan.
    d. Subscribers are charged a specific premium and are required to remain on the plan for a designated amount of time.
  3. Preferred provider organizations
    a. Individual practitioner, partnership, or clinic may contract to provide dental services at a lower-than-normal cost.
    b. The purchaser of benefits then tells that group of insured that the provider is available and at a lower-than-advertised cost.
    c. The provider then has the opportunity to acquire additional patients to the practice.
  4. Franchise dentistry
    a. Usually marketed under a trade name.
    b. Dentists in the corporation are hired as employees.
    c. Dentists who are part of the franchise enjoy the benefits of larger advertising budgets and bigger markets.
    d. If dentists do not become employees, they may become investors in the company as well as practice within the company.

VIII. PREPARING DENTAL CLAIM FORMS

A. Accuracy
  1. Claim forms must be filled out with accurate information regarding the insured's name and Social Security number as well as the subscriber's information.
  2. Information regarding procedures and correct codes must appear on the claim form.
  3. Claim forms should contain up-to-date information.

4. Information regarding deductibles and maximum should be observed when filling out claim forms.

B. Appropriate signatures
   1. The provider's (dentist's) signature must appear on the bottom of the claim form.
   2. The patient's or insured's signature must appear on the claim form or "signature on file" should appear on the patient or parent line.

C. Parts of an ADA claim form
   1. Patient information
      a. Information about the patient is contained in this area.
         (1) Name, relationship to the insured, sex, birthdate, Social Security number.
         (2) Information about coverage on another plan.
      b. Information about the subscriber is contained in this area.
         (1) Name, address, Social Security number, employer, and birth date.
   2. Billing dentist
      a. Information about the dentist is contained in this area.
         (1) Dentist's name, address, and phone number.
         (2) Social Security number and license number.
   3. Treatment record
      a. Information regarding treatment
         (1) Tooth numbers, surfaces, type of procedure, coding numbers, and cost.
         (2) Dentist signature.
   4. Carrier information
      a. Located in the upper right-hand corner
         (1) Carrier name and address.
   5. Additional information
      a. Patient's signature or parent's signature if patient is a minor.
      b. Dentist's signature.
      c. Information regarding nature of treatment.

IX. FINANCIAL RECORDS IN DENTAL OFFICE MANAGEMENT

A. Accounts receivable
   1. A system used to maintain data regarding charges, payments, and credits to the patient's individual or family accounts.
   2. Also can be called a ledger card.
   3. Patient has a constant running balance on the ledger card or on the accounts receivable record.
   4. The data is used for tracking income generated by the practice and also for tax purposes.
   5. All pertinent information must be recorded when managing accounts receivable.
      a. Endorse all checks with a restrictive endorsement upon receiving.
      b. Record all payments in patient ledger card.
      c. Prepare deposit slip and deposit into the bank.

B. Accounts payable
   1. A system used to maintain data regarding all monies being paid by the dentist.
      a. Fixed overhead.
      b. Variable overhead.
   2. Checks may be written by the office manager and signed by the dentist.
   3. The data is also used to reconcile bank statements and for budgeting analysis.
   4. All pertinent information must be recorded when issuing a check.
      a. Payee.
      b. Amount of check.
      c. Check number.
      d. Purpose of the check.
      e. New balance in account.

C. Other reports used in the dental office
   1. Walkout statement
      a. Given to patient after treatment and contains treatment performed, any payments that were received, and patient's running balance.
   2. Daily journal sheet
      a. A listing of all activity for that day.
      b. Payments received.
      c. All treatment performed.

3. Charge slip
   a. Given to the front office indicating what procedures were performed on a particular patient.
   b. Used by the front office for billing purposes.
4. Deposit slip
   a. Contains all cash, checks, and charges for the day.
   b. Divides all forms of payment into separate categories.
   c. Checks are listed by routing numbers followed by totals.
   d. Charge card slips have verification numbers listed and totals.
   e. Cash is separated by currency and coin.
   f. Complete total is listed at the bottom of the deposit slip.
   g. Must contain the dentist's name, address, and bank account number.

X. OTHER FORMS OF BOOKKEEPING SYSTEMS

A. Pegboard
   1. A one-write system.
   2. Manual style of bookkeeping.

B. Computerized
   1. More efficient.
   2. Provides ease in entering payments and posting treatment.

C. Both systems contain the same categories but are in different formats.

XI. TYPES OF WRITTEN COMMUNICATION

A. Business letters
   1. Types of business letters that are generated in the dental office
      a. Welcome letters.
      b. Collection letters.
      c. Referrals to other dentists (specialists).
      d. Birthday or congratulatory.
      e. Thank you.
   2. Guidelines to follow when creating a business letter
      a. Remember that the letter is a reflection on the dental office.
      b. Use language that the reader can understand. Stay away from technical terms that the reader may not be able to interpret.
      c. Use correct grammar and always check spelling.
      d. Always maintain patient confidentiality.
      e. Be sure all information is accurate and correct.
      f. Send clean copies free of ink smudges.

B. Office procedure manual
   1. An office procedure manual outlines the policies and practices of the office.
   2. This manual must be clear and concise and easy to understand. The office manager is responsible for distributing the manual to new and existing employees.
   3. The manual is a description of policies and step-by-step practices related to the day-to-day running of the dental office.
   4. It can be used as a training manual for all new employees.
   5. It is designed only for the office staff, not the patients.
   6. It can be used as a reference source for the office.

C. Written office policy
   1. A written office policy is designed for the patient. It outlines the procedures and policies as they relate to managing the patient. An office policy can be handed out to the patient in the form of a pamphlet, or it can be posted near the front desk. It should be in plain view for the patient to see.
      a. Can be sent to the patient in the welcome letter.
      b. Usually outlines policies, procedures, and the overall office philosophy.
      c. It helps the patient to understand both patient and office expectations.

D. MSDS binder
   1. The MSDS binder is used to store all of the material safety data sheets that are included in every hazardous material that is sent to the office. These sheets must be maintained in a binder and made available to all staff members.
   2. The MSDS sheets are provided by OSHA.

3. The sheets contain information such as manufacturer's name, address, emergency numbers, ingredients, and what to do if an exposure occurs.

E. OSHA compliance manual
   1. An Occupational Safety and Health Administration manual must be set up for the office staff. This manual is maintained by the office assistant or office manager. This manual contains information on all OSHA regulations.
   2. Information contained in the OSHA Compliance Manual can be used as a reference guide.
   3. Information on all regulations regarding infection control, hazard communication, training procedures, and medical waste disposal is discussed.
   4. The OSHA Compliance Manual is designed to protect the dental health-care worker.

F. Recall systems
   1. A recall system is designed to put patients on a regular appointment schedule. Patients are entered into the system and then when the designated appointment arrives, the patient is then notified. Recall appointments can be for prophylaxis, examinations, denture checks, retainer checks, orthodontic maintenance, or periodontal evaluations.
      a. Types of recall systems
         (1) Recall by mail: Notices are sent out at the appropriate intervals to patients, reminding them to contact the office for their appointment.
         (2) Recall by telephone: Patients are called to schedule an appointment around the designated recall time.
         (3) Advanced booking: Patients make an appointment for the designated recall appointment in the future at the time of their current recall appointment. A reminder card is usually mailed to patients a week before the appointment to remind them.

REVIEW QUESTIONS

1. What are the two types of bookkeeping systems using in the dental office?
   1. Computerized
   2. One-write
   3. Ledger card
   4. Numeric

   A. 1, 4
   B. 2, 3
   C. 4 only
   D. 1, 2

Match the following terms with the correct definition.

_____ 2. Insured

_____ 3. Spouse

_____ 4. Customary

_____ 5. Reasonable

_____ 6. Covered service

_____ 7. Medicaid

_____ 8. Capitation program

_____ 9. Pretreatment

_____ 10. Dual coverage

_____ 11. Co-payment

A. Dental coverage under more than one plan
B. Predetermination for treatment
C. The beneficiary's share of the fees after the insurance company has paid
D. Subscriber
E. Within the range of usual fees charged by the dentist in the same area
F. Services for which payment is provided under the terms of the insurance contract
G. Husband or wife of the insured
H. Government-sponsored program
I. Fee that is justified under special circumstances
J. Program in which payment for services is based on an agreed fee, which is distributed on a per-capita basis

12. An exclusion is a benefit that is not covered by an insurance company under a particular dental plan.
    A. True
    B. False

13. A buffer period is time set aside for special patients to come in for extractions.
    A. True
    B. False

14. A unit of time is considered a block of time that is reserved for restorative treatment.
    A. True
    B. False

15. All of the following are key items needed for an entry in an appointment book EXCEPT
    A. patient's age.
    B. patient's name.
    C. procedure.
    D. contact phone number.

16. All appointment book entries are written in
    A. ink.
    B. pencil.

17. A system that enables the front office to find materials under an alphabetic filing system is referred to as a/an
    A. numeric filing system.
    B. alpha filing system.
    C. chronologic filing system.
    D. cross-reference filing system.

18. _____ ensure the practice has a constant supply of materials and eliminate the need to store an abundance of one item.
    A. Automatic shipments
    B. Bulk ordering
    C. Purchase quantity
    D. Limited ordering

19. Accounts payable are
    A. money that is leaving the practice.
    B. supplies purchased for the office.
    C. fixed overhead expenses.
    D. insurance payments.

20. After receiving the bank statement, it should be reconciled with the
    A. general ledger.
    B. day sheet.
    C. check register.
    D. expense records.

21. _____ is not a federal payroll deduction.
    A. FICA
    B. FUTA
    C. Additional federal withholdings
    D. Worker's compensation

22. The _____ is the maximum amount of a product that is to be ordered at one time.
    A. order amount
    B. reorder point
    C. reorder quantity
    D. maximum quantity discount

23. Types of on-hold messages include
    A. on-hold music.
    B. professional announcements of products or services.
    C. silence with intermittent messages thanking the caller for holding.
    D. All of the above

24. Which of the following are considered to be accounts receivable?
    1. Personal checks from patients
    2. Payments made by an insurance company
    3. Payment of utilities
    4. Payment for supplies

    A. 1, 2, 3
    B. 1, 2
    C. 4 only
    D. All of the above

Match the following terms with the correct definition.

_____ 25. EOB

_____ 26. Payment plan

_____ 27. Small claims court

_____ 28. Collection letter

_____ 29. Electronic claim

_____ 30. ROA

A. Legal action taken to regain money that has not been paid to the practice by the patient

B. Written correspondence indicating a demand for payment

C. Sending information via modem to an insurance company for processing

D. A sheet sent along with payment explaining benefits that were paid by that insurance

E. Money that is received and posted to the patient account

F. A contract that outlines method and frequency of payment to an account

ANSWERS AND RATIONALES

1. **D** Computerized and one-write systems are used for bookkeeping purposes in the dental office.
2. **D**
3. **G**
4. **E**
5. **I**
6. **F**
7. **H**
8. **J**
9. **B**
10. **A**
11. **C**
12. **A** An exclusion is a benefit that is not covered. Examples would include any cosmetic dentistry such as vital bleaching or orthodontic treatment for esthetic purposes.
13. **B** A buffer period is time that is set aside for emergencies.
14. **B** A unit of time is an increment of time determined by the office. It can be in 10- or 15-minute increments. These increments are grouped together depending on the length of time needed for the procedure being performed.
15. **A** Name, phone number, and procedure are listed in the appointment book entry. The patient's age is not required unless the patient is a child.
16. **B** All appointment book entries are written in pencil due to the constant changes that are taking place throughout the scheduling process.
17. **B** Alpha filing systems arrange patient files in alphabetical order using the last name first and the first name last. Color coding the first letter of the first and last name is a common practice to provide easy identification during filing and retrieving.
18. **A** Automatic shipments are sent on a regular basis according to the rate at which the office uses the specific supply. It ensures a regular supply without creating a storage problem.
19. **A** An account payable is considered all money that is leaving the practice (for example, all fixed and variable overhead that is paid on a regular basis).
20. **C** A check register lists all checks that have been written for the practice. The bank statement should be reconciled with the check register as soon as it is received.
21. **D** Worker's compensation is a fund that is paid into by the employer on a state level.
22. **C** Reorder quantity is the amount of a supply that is to be reordered without creating an overabundance of one item.
23. **D** The most common types of on-hold systems include a recording discussing services or products that are provided by the office, easy listening music, or a reminder that the caller is still on hold and has not been disconnected.
24. **B** Accounts receivable are considered money that is coming into the practice via patient payments or insurance payments.
25. **D**
26. **F**
27. **A**
28. **B**
29. **C**
30. **E**

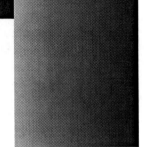

Comprehensive Practice Exam

The following questions are examples of test questions and formats that may or may not appear on the DANB exam. These questions are for review purposes only and are not to be construed as a replication of exam test questions found on the DANB exam. Please mark your answers on the answer sheet that has been provided.

1. Movements of the fingers and wrist are classified as
   A. Class I.
   B. Class II.
   C. Class III.
   D. Class IV.

2. When the operator is seated at the 2 o'clock position, the assistant is most efficient at the _____ position.
   A. 8 to 10 o'clock
   B. 9 to 10 o'clock
   C. 9 to 11 o'clock
   D. 11 to 12 o'clock

3. The basic setup includes
   A. mouth mirror.
   B. explorer.
   C. cotton pliers.
   D. All of the above

4. A circulating assistant is utilized during _____ dentistry.
   A. four-handed
   B. six-handed
   C. recall
   D. stand up

5. When setting up a procedure tray, the assistant should place instruments on the tray
   A. in reverse order of use.
   B. in order of use.
   C. in a random order.
   D. in order of largest to smallest.

6. A dental assistant's hands should be _____.
   A. manicured with unchipped nail polish.
   B. short and clean with clear nail polish.
   C. groomed at the assistant's discretion because gloves are generally worn.
   D. well groomed with short, clean fingernails.

7. During dental treatment, if assistants need to retrieve an instrument out of a drawer, they can _____.
   A. use their gloved hand as long as they use a paper towel to open the drawer to retrieve the instrument.
   B. use an overglove.
   C. use the blue nitrile or heavy latex glove to retrieve the instrument.
   D. use their gloved hand as long as they wash it before opening the drawer to retrieve the instrument.

8. When an assistant and operator sit down to perform a procedure and all necessary instruments and materials are not present, this causes
   A. the operator to become frustrated.
   B. the assistant to break the chain of asepsis to retrieve needed items.
   C. increased chair time for the patient.
   D. All of the above

9. The utilization of four-handed dentistry promotes which of the following?
   A. Decrease in operator attention turned away from restorative site
   B. Increased speed in utilization of materials
   C. Increased efficiency for the dental team
   D. A and C
   E. B and C

10. When assisting a right-handed operator, the assistant delivers and retrieves the instruments using
    A. the right hand.
    B. the left hand.
    C. either hand.
    D. the hand that the assistant uses to write with.

11. During assisting, the assistant is seated _____ inches higher than the operator.
    A. one to two
    B. two to three
    C. three to four
    D. four to five

12. During operative procedures, the best method of cooling the tooth and keeping the field clear is by using
    A. a three-way syringe and a saliva ejector.
    B. air and an HVE tip.
    C. a mist of air and water and the HVE tip.
    D. a stream of water and a surgical suction tip.

13. During four-handed dentistry, the instrument is retrieved with the _____ and passed with the _____.
    A. ring finger, thumb and middle finger
    B. little finger, thumb and forefinger
    C. the palm, thumb and forefinger
    D. None of the above

14. Generally, the light should be positioned at least _____ inches from the patient's mouth.
    A. 6
    B. 12
    C. 18
    D. 24

15. If the operator is restoring tooth #3, the bevel of the HVE tip should be positioned on the
    A. lingual of tooth #3.
    B. buccal of tooth #3.
    C. buccal of tooth #30.
    D. lingual of tooth #30.

Using the clock concept for a right-handed operator, match the following zones.

_____ 16. Operating zone

_____ 17. Transfer zone

_____ 18. Static zone

_____ 19. Assisting zone

   A. Between 4 and 8 o'clock
   B. Between 2 and 4 o'clock
   C. Between 6 and 11 o'clock
   D. Between 11 and 12 o'clock

20. The air compressor is used to provide which of the following?
    1. Air for the three-way air-water syringe
    2. The oral evacuation system
    3. To drive the slow- and high-speed handpiece
    4. To operate the dental chair

    A. 1, 2, 3
    B. 1, 3
    C. 1, 3, 4
    D. 1 only

21. In four-handed dentistry, the transfer zone is located
    A. over the patient's eyes.
    B. under the patient's chin.
    C. over the patient's chest.
    D. under the patient's nose.

22. Cells that are responsible for the formation of enamel are referred to as
    A. enamelblasts.
    B. ameloblasts.
    C. odontoblasts.
    D. dentinoblasts.

23. A _____ forms when two developmental centers join together.
    A. groove
    B. fissure
    C. pit
    D. fossa

24. The enamel cuticle is also referred to as
    A. Hertwig's epithelium.
    B. Sharpey's fibers.
    C. Nasmyth's membrane.
    D. Angle's classifications.

25. The process by which a tooth breaks through the gingiva and moves into a functional space is referred to as
    A. exfoliation.
    B. apposition.
    C. eruption.
    D. proliferation.

26. The process by which deposits of calcium are laid down and the cusps and the various surfaces are formed is referred to as
    A. calcification.
    B. osteoblastosis.
    C. dentinogenesis.
    D. cementoblastosis.

27. Supernumerary teeth are characterized as teeth that are in excess of the permanent 32 teeth.
    A. True
    B. False

28. When two or more teeth grow together during the developmental stage, _____ is the result.
    A. conjunction
    B. fusion
    C. hypoplasia
    D. hypercalcification

29. The anatomic portion of the crown includes
    A. the part of the crown that extends from the top third of the crown to the bottom third.
    B. the portion that extends from the occlusal surface to the cementoenamel junction.
    C. the part of the crown that is covered with enamel and extends to 1 mm above the free gingiva.
    D. None of the above

30. Like dentin, enamel is capable of regenerating itself.
    A. True
    B. False

31. When a tooth has a furcation, it can be said that it has more than one root.
    A. True
    B. False

32. Functions of the cementum include
    1. attachment.
    2. compensation.
    3. growth.
    4. nutritive.

    A. 1, 2, 4
    B. 1, 2, 3
    C. 1, 3
    D. 4 only

33. Masticatory mucosa
    1. is part of the gingival unit.
    2. is designed to withstand forces from chewing.
    3. covers the hard palate.
    4. is freely movable and can tear or injure easily.

    A. 1, 2, 3
    B. 1, 2, 4
    C. 2, 3
    D. All of the above

34. Healthy gingival tissue is
    A. pink, spongy, and porous.
    B. taut and pink, with little bleeding.
    C. pink and stippled, with 1–3 mm sulcus depth.
    D. glossy, pigmented, and bulbous.

35. What charting system uses two digit numbers, the first digit indicating the quadrant where the tooth is located and the second number indicating the tooth?
    A. Palmer notation
    B. ADA system
    C. Fédération Dentaire
    D. Universal charting method

36. The imaginary line that travels through the center of the tooth is referred to as the
    A. proximal angle.
    B. apical line.
    C. axial surface.
    D. distal line angle.

37. The surface of a tooth that dips inward is referred to as
    A. concave.
    B. convex.
    C. reverted.
    D. retruded.

38. When a closed stable contact is made and the maxillary and mandibular arches are evenly distributed with force, this is referred to as
    A. malocclusion.
    B. centric occlusion.
    C. distocclusion.
    D. mesiocclusion.

Match the following terms with the anatomical landmarks.

_____ 39. Fossa

_____ 40. Cusp of Carabelli

_____ 41. Cingulum

_____ 42. Mamelon

_____ 43. Fissure

    A. Also known as the fifth cusp; appears on the first maxillary molars
    B. A depression on the occlusal surface of a posterior tooth
    C. The line that occurs along a developmental groove
    D. The lobes found on a newly erupted incisal ridge
    E. A prominence found on the lingual surface of the cuspids

44. The _____ length radiograph is used to establish the length of the canal during debridement.
    A. periapical
    B. working
    C. obturating
    D. All of the above

45. Material used to obturate or fill a canal following root canal therapy is called _____.
    A. silver points.
    B. gutta-percha.
    C. glass ionomer.
    D. polycarboxylate cement.

46. An endodontic explorer is _____ a traditional explorer.
    A. longer than
    B. shorter than
    C. the same length as
    D. thinner than

47. A/An _____ is used to place canal sealer into the canal of the tooth prior to filling.
    A. endodontic broach
    B. Lentulo spiral
    C. Peeso reamer
    D. K-type file

48. A finger plugger is used
    A. to condense gutta-percha into the canal.
    B. to place canal sealer into the canals.
    C. to enlarge the canal.
    D. in the debridement process.

49. An endodontic broach is used to
    A. remove old gutta-percha from the canals.
    B. remove large amounts of pulpal tissue.
    C. shape and enlarge the canals.
    D. enlarge the opening of the apex.

50. A glass bead sterilizer is used for
    A. heating obturating instruments.
    B. sterilizing paper points and gutta-percha at chairside.
    C. sterilizing files, reamers, and other hand instruments at chairside.
    D. heating sodium hypochlorite to irrigate the canals.

51. When establishing the vitality of a tooth, which of the following methods may be used?
    1. Percussion
    2. Vitalometer
    3. Transillumination
    4. Cold testing

    A. 1, 2, 4
    B. 1, 4
    C. 3 only
    D. All of the above

52. Paper points are used to
    A. measure the length of a canal.
    B. dry the canal.
    C. obtain a sample for a culture.
    D. B and C

53. The ideal temperature for incubating an endodontic culture is
    A. 98.5°F
    B. 97.6°F.
    C. 98.6°F.
    D. 100°F.

54. A pulpotomy is the
    A. partial removal of the pulp.
    B. complete removal of the pulp.
    C. removal of necrotic tissue.
    D. A and C

55. Indications for endodontic therapy include
    1. dead or dying pulp.
    2. trauma to the pulp, causing irreversible damage.
    3. deep, carious lesions that extend to the pulp horns.
    4. in anticipation for a post and buildup.

    A. 1, 2, 3
    B. 1, 4
    C. 1, 2, 4
    D. All of the above

56. A/An _____ handpiece is used in conjunction with a Gates-Glidden to enlarge the pulp canals.
    A. high-speed contra-angle
    B. slow-speed latch-type
    C. ultrasonic unit
    D. A and C

Match the following.

_____ 57. Barbed broach

_____ 58. Lentulo spiral

_____ 59. K-type file

_____ 60. Hedström file

_____ 61. Gates-Glidden

_____ 62. Peeso reamer

_____ 63. Finger plugger

_____ 64. Irrigating syringe

    A. Used to condense gutta-percha into the canal
    B. Used to administer irrigants into the canal
    C. Used to enlarge and plane the walls of the canal
    D. Used to deliver canal sealer into the canal prior to obturating
    E. Used to remove large amounts of pulpal tissue
    F. A drill used exclusively to enlarge the canal
    G. Manufactured with sharp cutting edges to plane the walls of the canal
    H. Used to enlarge canal and is attached to a latch-type contra-angle

65. A size 30 file is _____ than a size 60 file.
    A. smaller
    B. larger

66. Removing organic and inorganic material from the canals is called
    A. palpation.
    B. debridement.
    C. condensation.
    D. aspiration.

67. An apicoectomy is
    A. the partial removal of the pulpal tissues.
    B. the complete removal of the root of the tooth.
    C. the removal of the apex only through overlying bone and gingival tissues.
    D. also called a retrograde.

List in the correct sequence below the events that take place during the use of a pulp vitalometer, beginning with A and ending with F.

_____ 68. A small amount of toothpaste is applied to the buccal or facial aspect of the tooth.

_____ 69. Isolate the tooth or teeth to be tested.

_____ 70. Place the vitality probe on the tooth to be tested.

_____ 71. Start at zero and increase the setting gradually until a tingle is felt by the patient.

_____ 72. Record your findings.

_____ 73. Explain to the patient the procedure and ask for cooperation in signaling you when a sensation is felt.

74. The _____ test requires the application of a light source to the tooth to determine small fractures in the crown of the tooth.
    A. percussion
    B. transillumination
    C. fiber-optic
    D. heat

75. Which of the following would not be found on the tray for the obturating appointment?
    A. Lentulo spiral
    B. Gutta-percha
    C. Canal sealer
    D. Barbed broach

76. When irrigating a canal during the debridement process, the irrigant of choice is
    A. alcohol.
    B. saline solution.
    C. sodium hypochlorite.
    D. non-epinephrine anesthetic.

77. A K-type file has a smooth-edged spiral shape as opposed to the Hedström, which has a sharp, spiral cutting edge.
    A. True
    B. False

78. When a canal is not accurately measured, this may lead to the overfilling or underfilling of the canal when obturating.
    A. True
    B. False

79. The master cone is also called accessory points.
    A. True
    B. False

80. The glass bead sterilizer may be filled with glass beads or table salt.
    A. True
    B. False

81. To chelate means to
    A. fill the canal with canal sealer.
    B. dry the canal until no moisture is present.
    C. debride the canal by chemical means.
    D. measure the canal for the master cone.

82. Plaque forms in the mouth every _____ hours.
    A. 8
    B. 24
    C. 36
    D. 72

83. Vitamin _____ promotes healing of gingival tissues and maintains overall soft tissue health.
    A. A
    B. D
    C. E
    D. C

84. Topical application of acidulated phosphate fluoride is generally _____ minutes.
    A. 2
    B. 4
    C. 6
    D. 12

85. Systemic fluoride can be found in
    A. topical fluoride.
    B. fluoride rinses.
    C. fluoridated water.
    D. disclosing tablets.

86. The vitamin that aids in the clotting of blood is vitamin
    A. A.
    B. D.
    C. E.
    D. K.

87. Which of the following are the four major signs of inflammation?
    1. Redness
    2. Edema
    3. Bleeding
    4. Heat
    5. Pain

    A. 1, 2, 3, 5
    B. 2, 3, 5
    C. 1, 2, 4, 5
    D. 3 only

88. Sealants are applied to the _____ of primary teeth.
    A. grooves and buccal area
    B. pits and fissures
    C. lingual area and pits
    D. occlusal and lingual area

Match the following as either A *for a key nutrient or* B *for a food group.*

_____ 89. Water

_____ 90. Carbohydrates

_____ 91. Breads and cereals

_____ 92. Milk or dairy

_____ 93. Vitamins

_____ 94. Minerals

_____ 95. Fats

_____ 96. Proteins

_____ 97. Vegetables and fruits

98. The _____ brushing technique is performed by placing the toothbrush at a 45° angle and cleaning the sulcus as well as the entire tooth structure.
    A. modified Stillman
    B. Bass
    C. press and roll
    D. Fones

99. The simplest form of sugar that is utilized by the body is called
    A. a disaccharide.
    B. a polysaccharide.
    C. nucleotides.
    D. glucose.

100. To manufacture tissue proteins, all _____ amino acids must be present.
    A. 22
    B. 24
    C. 26
    D. 32

101. Plaque is composed of which of the following?
    1. Bacteria
    2. Saliva
    3. Cellular debris
    4. Epithelial tissue

    A. 1, 2, 3
    B. 1, 3, 4
    C. 1, 2
    D. All of the above

102. The cement most commonly used for temporary crowns and restorations is
    A. glass ionomer.
    B. zinc oxide eugenol.
    C. polycarboxylate.
    D. zinc phosphate cement.

103. The tooth that replaces the missing tooth on a three-unit bridge is called a/an
    A. abutment.
    B. pontic.
    C. veneer.
    D. PFM.

104. Bite registration material is used to record the relationship of the upper and lower bite when preparing a tooth for a crown.
    A. True
    B. False

105. When fabricating a custom temporary crown, a/an _____ impression is taken.
    A. hydrocolloid
    B. polyvinylsiloxane
    C. alginate
    D. polyether

106. Tooth #3 has a porcelain-fused-to-metal crown and tooth #30 has to be restored with full coverage. What type of crown would be indicated?
    A. A porcelain-fused-to-metal
    B. full gold
    C. acrylic
    D. resin

107. When mixing polyvinylsiloxane impression material, a base and a catalyst are mixed simultaneously until a homogenous mix is attained.
    A. True
    B. False

108. Which of the following instruments would appear on a crown preparation tray?
    1. Retraction cord
    2. Retraction cord instrument
    3. Basic setup
    4. A diamond bur

    A. 1, 2, 3
    B. 1, 2, 4
    C. 3 only
    D. All of the above

109. Retraction cord that contains epinephrine is used to
    A. control bleeding after the impression is taken.
    B. control bleeding while the impression is being taken.
    C. decrease inflammation after the impression is taken.
    D. decrease bleeding prior to the impression being taken.

110. When there is advanced periodontitis involved in the area where a fixed crown or bridge is needed, the fixed crown or bridge is usually
    A. indicated.
    B. contraindicated.
    C. constructed with the knowledge that it is temporary.
    D. constructed out of composite.

111. When placing a core buildup, what materials are most commonly used?
    1. Composite
    2. ZOE
    3. Amalgam
    4. Resin buildup material

    A. 1, 2, 3
    B. 1, 3
    C. 1, 3, 4
    D. All of the above

112. Latex gloves may retard the setting of putty impression material. _____ may be used to mix the material.
    1. Heavy latex gloves
    2. Plastic overgloves
    3. Vinyl gloves
    4. Non-powdered latex gloves

    A. 1, 2, 3
    B. 1, 2
    C. 2, 3
    D. All of the above

113. A veneer covers the _____ aspect of the tooth.
    A. buccal
    B. lingual
    C. facial
    D. distal

114. When cementing a crown, the cement should _____ inside of the crown.
    A. line the
    B. fill the
    C. partially set
    D. A or C

115. A mechanical means of retracting the gingiva prior to taking the final impression would be to place a temporary that extends beyond the margin and into the gingiva.
    A. True
    B. False

116. Which of the following items would appear on a seating tray?
    1. Prophy setup with pumice
    2. Bite stick
    3. Permanent cement
    4. Retraction cord packing device

    A. 1, 2, 3
    B. 1, 3
    C. 1, 2, 4
    D. All of the above

117. The following are part of a partial denture EXCEPT
    A. saddle.
    B. framework.
    C. occlusal rim.
    D. clasp.

118. A custom tray is
    A. fabricated to be used only on the patient it was fitted for.
    B. fabricated to extend over the tuberosities.
    C. shaped to relieve the labial frenum attachments.
    D. All of the above

119. An immediate denture is placed _____ following extractions.
    A. 24 hours
    B. 48 hours
    C. 72 hours
    D. on the same appointment

120. A chairside reline is
    A. designed to restore a snug fit of the denture.
    B. designed to adhere the denture to the alveolar ridge.
    C. designed as a temporary measure.
    D. required at each adjustment appointment.

121. When polishing a removable prosthesis, _____ is used.
    1. a sterilized rag wheel
    2. a sander
    3. a dremel tool
    4. pumice

    A. 1, 2, 3
    B. 1, 4
    C. 3 only
    D. All of the above

122. After impressions for a custom tray are taken, the assistant should _____ before sending to the lab.
    1. spray with hot water
    2. spray with an EPA-approved disinfectant
    3. place in a bag with a biohazard label on it
    4. spray with alcohol

    A. 1, 3
    B. 2, 3
    C. 1, 4
    D. 3 only

123. When choosing the shade for a complete denture, the assistant should
    A. try to make it as white as possible without looking unnatural.
    B. try to match the patient's skin tone and coloring with the teeth.
    C. let the patient choose the shade.
    D. not show the patient any shades to avoid confusion.

124. When sending out a denture for a laboratory reline, the assistant should set up an impression for
    A. the patient without dentures in place.
    B. the patient's dentures.
    C. the patient's bite.
    D. the patient's dentures while in the mouth.

Place the full denture construction procedure in order, beginning with the letter A and ending with the letter E.

_____ 125. Wax setup

_____ 126. Baseplates and bite rim try-in

_____ 127. Impression for a custom tray

_____ 128. Adjustment appointment

_____ 129. Final try-in or delivery

130. Elastic separators
    1. are used to separate the anterior teeth prior to bracket placement.
    2. are placed directly into the contact of the posterior teeth.
    3. are placed prior to banding the posterior teeth.
    4. are seated using a scaler.

    A. 1, 2, 3
    B. 1, 3
    C. 2, 3
    D. All of the above

131. A Hawley retainer is a type of _____ appliance.
    A. fixed
    B. removable

132. Angle's Class III malocclusion is also called
    A. mesioclusion.
    B. disoclusion.
    C. linguoversion.
    D. neutroclusion.

133. A Boley gauge is used in the placement of direct bond brackets.
    A. True
    B. False

134. Part of the clinical examination for an orthodontic workup includes which of the following?
    1. Radiographs
    2. Study models
    3. Medical and dental history
    4. Arch measurements

    A. 1, 2, 3
    B. 1, 2, 4
    C. 2, 3
    D. All of the above

135. An arch wire may be ligated with all of the following EXCEPT
    A. elastic chain.
    B. individual elastic rings.
    C. stainless steel ligatures.
    D. elastic separator.

Match the following with the correct letter.

_____ 136. Correcting bad oral habits

_____ 137. Referral for extractions

_____ 138. Construction of a palatal expander

_____ 139. Construction of a space maintainer

_____ 140. Caries control

_____ 141. Orthognathic surgery

    A. Preventive
    B. Interceptive
    C. Corrective

142. A buccal tube is designed to
    A. receive the end of the headgear apparatus.
    B. receive the end of the arch wire.
    C. anchor the Class II elastics.
    D. aid in the seating of the band.

143. Which of the following instruments would not appear on the banding appointment tray?
    1. Basic setup
    2. Presized bands
    3. Handpiece with prophy cup and pumice
    4. Scaler

    A. 1, 2, 3
    B. 1, 2, 4
    C. 2, 4
    D. All would appear on the tray.

144. Which types of radiographs are required in orthodontic treatment?
    1. Full mouth survey
    2. Cephalometric radiograph
    3. Occlusal film
    4. Panorex

    A. 1, 2, 3
    B. 1, 2
    C. 1, 2, 4
    D. All of the above

145. Which instruments would appear on the arch wire and ligature placement tray?
    1. Preformed arch wire
    2. Ligature wires
    3. Howe pliers
    4. Bracket placement cement

    A. 1, 2, 4
    B. 1, 2, 3
    C. 1, 2
    D. 3, 4

146. A patient who was in for a retie the day before calls in to report that two brackets have come off. The assistant would
    A. instruct the patient to wait until the next appointment and the office will recement them in place.
    B. tell the patient to come in immediately.
    C. tell the patient that it is alright and schedule an appointment later in the month.
    D. reprimand the patient for being careless about home care and schedule the patient for the next available appointment.

147. Retainers that are worn after orthodontic treatment are designed
    A. to keep teeth aligned and be worn indefinitely.
    B. to keep teeth in their new place while the bone becomes calcified.
    C. for splinting purposes.
    D. for the comfort of the patient.

148. An overjet is measured with a
    A. millimeter ruler.
    B. Boley gauge.
    C. standard ruler.
    D. small measuring tape.

149. Maintaining good oral hygiene during orthodontic treatment is critical because
    1. when plaque accumulates under bands, the teeth become susceptible to a plaque acid attack.
    2. maintaining adequate oral hygiene during orthodontic treatment aids in the overall health of the gingiva.
    3. high cariogenic foods adhere to teeth and can contribute to tooth decay.
    4. periodontal disease leads to bone loss, which can compromise the outcome of orthodontic treatment.

    A. 1, 2, 3
    B. 1, 2, 4
    C. 1, 3
    D. All of the above

150. Upon entering the practice for the first time that day, the office assistant should perform which of the following functions?
    1. Turn on lights and computer.
    2. Check messages.
    3. Confirm the day's appointments.
    4. Adjust the heating or air conditioning settings.

    A. 1, 2, 3
    B. 1, 2, 4
    C. 1, 3
    D. All of the above

151. Sorting mail is a task that is delegated to the dentist because it is his or her practice. The front office assistant should forward all mail to the dentist as it comes in.
    A. True
    B. False

152. Each time an insurance claim form is prepared, it is acceptable for the front office assistant to
    A. sign the dentist's name.
    B. use a rubber stamp with the dentist's signature on it.
    C. ask the dentist to sign the claim form with a black pen.
    D. sign your name since you were the one who prepared it.

153. If patients enter the office and have an outstanding balance, it is appropriate for the front office assistant to
    A. mention to them after they have taken a seat that they have a balance.
    B. take them outside to talk about their outstanding balance in private.
    C. run a current summary of treatment and payments and talk to them in the dentist's office or consultation area about their outstanding balance.
    D. wait until they are back in the operatory and then talk to them about the outstanding balance.

154. A call group is utilized when
    A. the dentist will be out of the office and not available to take patient emergencies.
    B. the answering service does not know where the dentist is.
    C. the dentist's answering machine gives his or her beeper number for emergency situations.
    D. the dentist has a meeting and will be returning to the office before the end of the workday.

155. Accounts payable are
    A. fees owed by the patients.
    B. fees owed by the practice.
    C. fees owed by the suppliers.
    D. monies dispersed by suppliers.

156. Fixed overhead is regarded as
    1. property rental.
    2. equipment rental.
    3. utility payments.
    4. salaries.

    A. 1, 2, 3
    B. 1, 2, 4
    C. 3 only
    D. All of the above

157. A pretreatment estimate is
    A. used to give patients an idea of what they will be spending on treatment.
    B. an estimate of treatment that will be done, which is sent to the insurance company for prior approval.
    C. an estimate that the dentist uses to follow the required treatment that needs to be done.
    D. a listing of services given by the dentist that explains the procedure to the patient.

158. For insurance purposes, an exclusion is when the insurance company will not pay for the insured's spouse.
    A. True
    B. False

159. A release of information is confidential information about the patient's treatment and may be released only with the patient's written authorization.
    A. True
    B. False

160. Signature on file refers to
    A. the dentist's signature on the insurance form prior to sending it out for processing.
    B. the patient's signature on a blank insurance form prior to sending it out for processing.
    C. the insurance company's signature on the claim form after it has been processed.
    D. None of the above

161. A recall system is used for
    A. returning patients who have restorative work pending.
    B. patients who have insurance claims pending.
    C. patients who return on a regular basis for cleanings.
    D. a patient who can come in on short notice.

162. A prophy brush is used to
    A. clean the interproximal surfaces of the teeth.
    B. clean the occlusal surfaces of the posterior teeth.
    C. clean the incisal surfaces of the anterior teeth.
    D. All of the above

163. Care is taken not to apply too much pressure to the tooth during coronal polish because
    A. too much pressure may wear the enamel off.
    B. too much frictional heat may cause damage to the pulp.
    C. too much pressure may create trauma to the gingiva.
    D. a light stroke removes stain as efficiently as a heavy stroke.

164. A fulcrum is used during coronal polish because
    A. a fulcrum creates more pressure than not using a fulcrum.
    B. a fulcrum is not necessary when coronal polishing.
    C. a fulcrum will steady the hand to avoid slipping and traumatizing the soft tissues.
    D. a fulcrum is used to control the amount of prophy paste that is distributed onto the tooth.

165. Fluoride can be applied using which of the following?
    1. Gauze sponge
    2. Toothbrush
    3. Cotton rolls
    4. Trays

    A. 1, 2, 3
    B. 1, 2, 4
    C. 2, 3, 4
    D. All of the above

166. General duties performed by the dental assistant during periodontal treatment include which of the following?
    1. Seating and preparing the patient
    2. Maintaining a clear field during surgery
    3. Measuring periodontal pockets
    4. Preparing preset trays and the operatory before surgery

    A. 1, 2, 3
    B. 1, 2, 4
    C. 1, 4
    D. All of the above

Match the following.

_____ 167. Hoe scaler

_____ 168. File scaler

_____ 169. Chisel scaler

_____ 170. Jaquette scaler

_____ 171. Sickle scaler

_____ 172. Ultrasonic scaler

    A. A universal instrument used to remove gross amounts of supragingival calculus
    B. Provided in pairs and used for the right or left sides of the mouth; used to remove facial or lingual calculus from the posterior teeth
    C. Has a single straight cutting edge; is turned 100° to the shank at the end of the working edge
    D. Has a single straight cutting edge and the blade is straight but the end is beveled at a 45° angle
    E. Scaler containing a serrated edge on a rounded or rectangular base
    F. Instrument that vibrates at the tip using sound waves, removing calculus supragingivally as well as subgingivally

173. Which instruments would appear on a periodontal surgery tray?
    1. Basic setup
    2. Scalpel handle
    3. Periodontal knives
    4. Scalers
    5. 1157 carbide bur

    A. 1, 2, 3, 4
    B. 1, 2, 3, 5
    C. 1, 3, 4, 5
    D. All of the above

174. Which of the following are included in the initial examination of the periodontal patient?
    1. Medical and dental history
    2. Radiographs
    3. Oral examination, including probe depths
    4. Postoperative instructions

    A. 1, 2, 3
    B. 2, 3, 4
    C. 1, 4
    D. All of the above

175. Root planing and scaling usually require the patient to be anesthetized.
    A. True
    B. False

176. A periodontal pocket marker is used to make perforations that indicate pocket depth.
    A. True
    B. False

177. Before the patient is dismissed following the periodontal examination, it is the responsibility of the assistant to ensure that
    1. the patient has been given a prescription for antibiotics.
    2. a review of oral hygiene instruction has been given.
    3. all charting notations have been entered.
    4. if appropriate, the nature of the next visit has been discussed.

    A. 1, 2, 3
    B. 1, 3, 4
    C. 2, 3, 4
    D. All of the above

178. Immediately following the placement of sealants, articulating paper is used to
    A. check the contacts.
    B. check the occlusion for high spots.
    C. ensure that a sealant was placed.
    D. check for occlusal wear.

179. Sealants can either be self-curing or will require the use of a curing light to complete the setting process.
    A. True
    B. False

180. When charting periodontal pockets, a reading of 3 mm indicates
    A. normal gingiva.
    B. mild periodontitis.
    C. moderate periodontitis.
    D. advanced periodontitis.

181. A grafting procedure removes tissue from one area and replaces it in another area to stop recession.
    A. True
    B. False

182. Removing necrotic tissue from a periodontal pocket is called
    A. scaling.
    B. root planing.
    C. curettage.
    D. polishing.

183. The organization responsible for developing and enforcing standards for workplace safety and health is known as
    A. EPA.
    B. OSHA.
    C. FDA.
    D. ADA.

184. Some dental health-care workers are at special risk for
    1. HIV.
    2. HBV.
    3. DPT.
    4. MMR.

    A. 1, 3
    B. 1, 4
    C. 1, 2
    D. All of the above

185. In the United States, approximately _____ people each year are infected with HBV.
    A. 30,000
    B. 300,000
    C. 4,000
    D. 40,000

186. Because dental health-care workers come into contact with _____, _____, and _____, their chances of contracting HIV are increased if precautions are not taken.
    A. saliva, blood, tears
    B. saliva, blood, mucus
    C. blood, lymph, saliva
    D. saliva, blood, sulcular fluids

187. Universal precautions include which of the following?
    1. Gloves
    2. Masks
    3. Goggles
    4. Shoe covers

    A. 1, 2, 3
    B. 1, 2, 4
    C. 1, 2
    D. All of the above

188. Although protective gloves may be worn as a barrier against saliva and blood, they cannot protect you from
    A. acid etch solution.
    B. puncture wounds.
    C. radiography chemicals.
    D. harsh cleaning products.

189. Protective clothing should be worn when
    A. splashes or spills are likely to happen.
    B. there are housekeeping duties that must be performed.
    C. you work with large amounts of blood, saliva, or gingival fluids.
    D. All of the above.

190. The agency responsible for tracking the spread of disease is known as
    A. ADA.
    B. CDA.
    C. CDE.
    D. CDC.

Match the following terms with their definitions.

_____ 191. Body fluids

_____ 192. Carrier

_____ 193. Germicide

_____ 194. HBV

_____ 195. HIV

_____ 196. Hyperimmune globulin

_____ 197. Infectious

_____ 198. PPE

_____ 199. Sharps

_____ 200. Universal precautions

    A. Hepatitis B virus
    B. Needles, blades, and orthodontic wires
    C. Injection that helps the body fight off HBV infection
    D. Blood, saliva, and gingival fluid
    E. Capable of killing germs
    F. Human immunodeficiency virus
    G. Guidelines for the prevention of spreading HIV or HBV at work
    H. Capable of spreading infection
    I. Gloves, masks, goggles, and gowns
    J. A person who can spread HBV or HIV

201. When handling sharps, it is approved by OSHA to
    A. bend the needle before disposing to eliminate the possibility of being punctured.
    B. break the needle in half to prevent an exposure incident.
    C. do nothing to the needle but remove it and place it in the sharps container for disposal.
    D. discard the needle by placing it in a bag that is clearly labeled biohazard.

202. Monitoring sterilization equipment is performed by using
    A. a dipstick for cold sterile solution.
    B. biological monitoring strips.
    C. a dosimeter badge.
    D. heat indicator tape.

List in order the steps for cleaning and sterilizing instruments beginning with A *and ending with* E.

_____ 203. Wrap or bag instruments and place in chemclave or autoclave.

_____ 204. Place instruments in the ultrasonic basket and place the basket in a holding solution.

_____ 205. Don nitrile or latex housekeeping gloves.

_____ 206. Place ultrasonic basket into the ultrasonic cleaner.

_____ 207. Thoroughly rinse and dry instruments.

208. A steam sterilizer is effective at
    A. a temperature of 210°F and 15 psi for 20 minutes.
    B. a temperature of 250°F and 11 psi for 30 minutes.
    C. a temperature of 280°F and 10 psi for 20 minutes.
    D. a temperature of 250°F and 15 psi for 30 minutes.

209. When instruments are loaded into a steam or chemical sterilizer, the instruments are
    A. loaded largest to smallest.
    B. loaded vertically.
    C. loaded horizontally with the largest instruments on top.
    D. loaded horizontally with the smallest instruments on top.

210. Steam and chemical sterilizers should be spore tested
    1. once a week.
    2. once a month.
    3. when a new type of packaging is used.
    4. when a patient with a communicable disease is treated in the office.

    A. 1, 2, 3
    B. 1, 3
    C. 2, 4
    D. All of the above

211. Biofilm in dental unit waterlines is best defined as a collection of microorganisms that affix to surfaces that are exposed to any type of moisture.
    A. True
    B. False

212. Which of the following are methods to minimize the spread of pathogenic organisms in the dental field?
    1. Use of a dental dam
    2. Use of disposable or single-use items
    3. Use of an HVE tip
    4. Use of an antimicrobial mouth rinse prior to starting the procedure

    A. 1, 2, 3
    B. 1, 2, 4
    C. 1, 3
    D. All of the above

213. The degree of blackness on a dental film is referred to as
    A. contrast.
    B. density.
    C. opaqueness.
    D. sharpness.

214. The difference in the degree of blackness on a radiographic film is referred to as
    A. density.
    B. radiolucency.
    C. contrast.
    D. detail.

215. Film fog is caused by
    A. scatter radiation.
    B. the primary beam not being centered.
    C. too much time in the fixer.
    D. too little time in the developer.

216. Intraoral film packets with a size of No. 0 can be used for
    A. occlusal radiographs.
    B. adult bitewings.
    C. a radiograph for a child.
    D. an adult periapical.

217. When mounting films, the dot convex
    A. gives you a lingual view of the dentition
    B. gives you a labial view of the dentition
    C. does not make a difference in viewing
    D. is used only when taking bitewings

218. Tissues that are the most sensitive to ionizing radiation include
    1. reproductive tissues.
    2. blood forming tissues.
    3. thyroid tissues.
    4. skin and muscle tissues.

    A. 1, 2, 3
    B. 1, 2, 4
    C. 1, 4
    D. All of the above

219. The thickness of a lead apron should be at least
    A. 0.10 mm.
    B. 0.25 mm.
    C. 10 mm.
    D. 20 mm.

220. A blurred image may be caused by
    A. incorrect exposure time.
    B. patient movement during exposure.
    C. weak fixer.
    D. mA settings that are too high.

221. Using the same film packet twice can create
    A. a light image.
    B. a blurred image.
    C. two images on one film.
    D. darkened film.

222. The technique of choice for periapical film exposure is the
    A. bisecting angle technique.
    B. paralleling technique.
    C. Both
    D. Neither

223. When taking an edentulous survey, the exposure times are reduced by a factor of
    A. one-half.
    B. one-third.
    C. one-fourth.
    D. one-sixteenth.

224. A panorex or panelipse film reveals which of the following?
    1. Entire maxilla and mandible
    2. Orbital sockets of the eyes
    3. Retained roots
    4. Impacted third molars

    A. 1, 2, 3
    B. 1, 2, 4
    C. 1, 3, 4
    D. All of the above

225. Exposed dental film contains a latent image and should be processed as soon as possible.
    A. True
    B. False

226. The main reason why a stop bath is used is to rinse fixer from the film and stop the film development process.
    A. True
    B. False

227. Rapid processing of dental film can be accomplished by
    1. higher solution temperatures.
    2. concentrated solutions.
    3. constant agitation of the film.
    4. limiting the fixer bath to 10 seconds.

    A. 1, 2, 3
    B. 1, 2, 4
    C. 1, 4
    D. All of the above

228. The dip tanks should be covered when not in use to keep the chemicals from becoming oxidized and weakening.
    A. True
    B. False

229. Lighting for the dental darkroom should include a/an
    A. safelight.
    B. overhead white light.
    C. outside warning light.
    D. viewing safelight.
    E. All of the above

230. The main source of electrons in the x-ray tube comes from the
    A. position indicator device.
    B. tungsten filament.
    C. aluminum filter.
    D. milliamperage control.

231. The quality or penetrating power of an x-ray is controlled by the
    A. kilovoltage.
    B. milliamperage.
    C. tungsten filament.
    D. film position.

232. The quantity of x-rays that is produced is determined by the
    A. milliampere dial.
    B. kilovoltage.
    C. density.
    D. thickness of the aluminum filter.

233. A bur that fits into a straight handpiece is referred to as
    A. friction grip.
    B. latch type.
    C. long shank.
    D. snap type.

234. Round burs are numbered
    A. ½ to 11.
    B. 556 to 563.
    C. 699 to 703.
    D. 55½ to 62.

235. A _____ is used to mount a polishing disc to the latch-type contra-angle.
    A. bur chuck
    B. mandrel
    C. latch
    D. friction attachment

236. A spoon is used to
    A. remove undermined enamel.
    B. plane the walls of the preparation.
    C. remove soft decay.
    D. carve detailed anatomy after placing an amalgam.

237. After using an anesthetic syringe, recapping the needle can be accomplished by
    1. using a recapping device.
    2. using the one-handed scoop method.
    3. handing it to the operator for recapping.
    4. placing the needle cap in one hand and the syringe in the other and then recapping the needle.

    A. 1, 2, 3
    B. 1, 3
    C. 1, 2
    D. Any of the above methods are acceptable.

238. The harpoon of the anesthetic syringe makes it possible to aspirate during the administration of anesthetic.
    A. True
    B. False

239. A wooden wedge and matrix band are used to replace the missing wall of a Class II restoration.
    A. True
    B. False

240. Which of the following instruments would appear on an amalgam restoration tray?
    A. Amalgam carrier
    B. Condenser
    C. Carver
    D. Burnisher
    E. All of the above

Match the following instruments with their definitions.

_____ 241. Chisel

_____ 242. Cleoid-discoid

_____ 243. Gingival margin trimmers

_____ 244. Hollenback carver

_____ 245. Amalgam well

_____ 246. Amalgamator

_____ 247. Acorn burnisher

    A. Used to carve the interproximal surfaces of an amalgam restoration
    B. Used to smooth and seal the occlusal surfaces of an amalgam restoration
    C. Used to store the amalgam while it is being condensed into the carrier
    D. Used to triturate amalgam
    E. Used to trim the mesial and distal margins of a preparation prior to amalgam placement
    F. Used to carve the occlusal surfaces of the amalgam restoration
    G. Used to cut undermined tooth structure during the preparation of a cavity

248. A Class V restoration involves the
    A. interproximal surfaces on the posterior teeth.
    B. the interproximal surfaces on the anterior teeth.
    C. the smooth surfaces on all teeth.
    D. the occlusal surfaces on posterior teeth.

249. Contraindications for the use of zinc oxide eugenol include which of the following?
    1. It cannot be used under acrylic or resin materials.
    2. It is not used for a final base under an amalgam restoration.
    3. It cannot be used as a temporary filling because of its solubility.
    4. It is generally used to cement aluminum crowns.

    A. 1, 2, 3
    B. 1, 2, 4
    C. 1, 3
    D. None of the above are contraindications.

List in the correct sequence beginning with A and ending with D the use of materials on an amalgam preparation.

_____ 250. Varnish

_____ 251. Insulating base

_____ 252. Liner

_____ 253. Amalgam restoration

254. Calcium hydroxide when used as a liner
    A. aids in the adhering of amalgam to the tooth.
    B. stimulates the formation of reparative dentin.
    C. aids in the sealing of dentin tubules.
    D. can act as a bonding agent for resin materials.

255. Class II restorations require the use of
    1. amalgam.
    2. resin.
    3. acid etch.
    4. cleoid-discoid.

    A. 1, 2, 3
    B. 1, 2, 4
    C. 1, 3
    D. 2, 3

256. The smoothing and adaptation of the marginal ridge after applying restorative material to the tooth structures is called margination.
    A. True
    B. False

257. An inlay is designed to restore
    1. one to three surfaces of a tooth.
    2. the mesial, distal, or buccal surfaces of a tooth.
    3. the mesial, distal, or occlusal surfaces of a tooth.
    4. the mesial, distal, or facial surfaces of a tooth.

    A. 1, 2, 3
    B. 1, 2, 4
    C. 1, 3
    D. All of the above

258. Before non-cohesive gold can be used for gold foil restorations, it must be
    A. melted.
    B. annealed.
    C. triturated.
    D. flattened into thin pieces.

259. When administering a block injection, anesthetizing tooth #30, a _____ needle is used.
    A. short
    B. long
    C. 40 gauge
    D. extra short

260. A dental dam, when used in restorative dentistry, can do which of the following?
    1. Aid in patient comfort
    2. Aid in moisture control
    3. Aid in infection control
    4. Prevent dental materials from coming into contact with the patient's soft tissues

    A. 1, 2, 3
    B. 1, 4
    C. All of the above
    D. None of the above

261. When mixing zinc phosphate, it is advisable to use a _____ to slow the setting time.
    A. parchment pad
    B. cool, dry glass slab
    C. a regular paper pad
    D. a dappen dish

262. An abrasive agent is generally used to polish
    A. amalgam.
    B. enamel.
    C. composite.
    D. full gold crowns.

263. Minimizing an unfavorable reaction to topical or local anesthetics can be increased by
    1. using an aspirating syringe to establish whether or not you have infiltrated a vein.
    2. reviewing the medical and dental history for any allergies.
    3. using the smallest concentration possible at the lowest dosage.
    4. observing the patient for any reactions immediately following the application.

    A. 1, 2, 3
    B. 1, 2, 4
    C. 1, 3
    D. All of the above

264. A short acting anesthetic lasts less than
    A. 20 minutes.
    B. 30 minutes.
    C. 45 minutes.
    D. one hour.

265. The main cause of fainting in the dental office is due to
    1. the dental visit becoming a stressful event.
    2. the lack of blood flow to the brain.
    3. being seated in a supine position for extended periods of time.
    4. respiratory difficulties.

    A. 1, 4
    B. 1, 3
    C. 1, 2
    D. 2, 4

266. A patient who is experiencing a stroke in the dental office may
    1. become confused about his or her surroundings.
    2. have acetone breath.
    3. lose consciousness.
    4. be unable to communicate by talking.

    A. 1, 2
    B. 1, 4
    C. 1, 3, 4
    D. All of the above

Match the following.

_____ 267. Astringent

_____ 268. Vasoconstrictor

_____ 269. Coagulant

     A. Agent that is used topically to control bleeding

     B. Agent that is used to control minor bleeding of the gingiva

     C. Agent that promotes blood clotting

270. The legality of a dental assistant performing a scaling would be discussed under
    A. ethics.
    B. jurisprudence.
    C. duty of care.
    D. direct supervision.

271. Legal restrictions that control the actions of the dentist and staff would be found in
    A. a JADA journal.
    B. an ADA journal.
    C. the state Dental Practice Act.
    D. on an "implied consent" form.

272. Malpractice is the same as
    A. professional negligence.
    B. failure to exercise due care.
    C. an act of commission.
    D. All of the above.

273. Practices that would decrease the potential for litigation would include
    1. maintaining proper documentation.
    2. keeping a good rapport with your patients.
    3. avoiding any unpleasant discussions regarding consequences from treatment.
    4. obtaining written and implied consent for all treatment.

    A. 1, 2, 3
    B. 1, 2, 4
    C. 1, 3
    D. All of the above

274. If a patient refuses radiographs during the course of treatment, the best reaction from the dental assistant would be to
    A. insist on radiographs or the patient may have to seek treatment elsewhere.
    B. document the conversation in the chart and have the patient sign below it.
    C. explain that radiographs are necessary and the dentist cannot continue without them.
    D. Any of the above responses could be used.

275. A space maintainer is designed to
    A. splint two or more teeth.
    B. protect the area where a tooth has been prematurely lost.
    C. maintain the area where a tooth has been prematurely lost.
    D. be placed instead of an obturator.

276. Trimming a cementing stainless steel crown is not delegated to the dental assistant because
    A. it requires extensive knowledge of the tooth anatomy.
    B. it is not legal for the dental assistant to fabricate a stainless steel crown.
    C. the assistant is busy doing other functions.
    D. it is legal for the dental assistant to fabricate a stainless steel crown.

277. During an indirect pulp cap, the material of choice to place over the near pulpal exposure is
    A. polycarbonate cement.
    B. calcium hydroxide.
    C. glass ionomer.
    D. zinc oxide eugenol.

278. If a Class III fracture of a primary tooth is present,
    1. the dentist may smooth any sharp edges and reappoint the patient in six months.
    2. the dentist may perform an extraction and place a space maintainer.
    3. the dentist may perform a pulpotomy or pulpectomy depending on the extent of the injury.
    4. the dentist may remove all decay and place a stainless steel crown.

    A. 1, 2, 3
    B. 1, 3
    C. 3, 4
    D. None of the above

279. Extrusion is displacement outward.
    A. True
    B. False

280. If the dentist plans to perform an uncomplicated extraction, the assistant would take which of the following radiographs?
    A. Bitewing
    B. Periapical
    C. Panorex
    D. Cephalometric

281. Postoperative instructions are given
    1. in writing.
    2. orally.
    3. to the driver.
    4. before surgery.

    A. 1, 2, 3
    B. 1, 2, 4
    C. 1, 3
    D. All of the above

282. A holding solution is
    1. used to soak instruments prior to putting them in the chemclave.
    2. used to soak instruments prior to putting them in the ultrasonic.
    3. used to prevent blood from drying on the instruments.
    4. used to prevent rusting of instruments.

    A. 1, 2, 3
    B. 1, 2, 4
    C. 1, 3
    D. 2, 3

283. An anti-inflammatory drug that may be prescribed by the dentist to control pain and inflammation may be
    A. Tylenol #3
    B. Dilaudid
    C. Darvocet
    D. Motrin

284. Part of the dental assistant's duties during oral surgery include
    1. keeping the field clear.
    2. maintaining the chain of asepsis.
    3. holding the patient's head and mandible.
    4. passing and receiving instruments.

    A. 1, 2, 3
    B. 1, 2, 4
    C. 1, 4
    D. All of the above

285. Which of the following are methods to control bleeding?
    1. Ice pack following surgery
    2. Heat pack following surgery
    3. Pressure using gauze
    4. Ibuprofen

    A. 1, 2, 3
    B. 2, 3, 4
    C. 1, 3, 4
    D. All of the above

280. Rongeurs are used to
    A. smooth bone.
    B. reduce a large amount of bone structure.
    C. trim bone.
    D. remove small root tips.

287. When removing sutures
    A. the suture is clipped on the loop farthest from the knot and then it is gently pulled out.
    B. the suture is clipped on the lingual side close to the knot and then gently pulled through.
    C. the suture is clipped in the interproximal and then pulled through.
    D. Any of the above methods can be used.

288. Smoothing or contouring the alveolar bone is called
    A. alveolectomy.
    B. osteoplasty.
    C. alveoplasty.
    D. Any of the above.

289. Which of the following instruments would not appear on a soft tissue impaction surgical tray setup?
    A. Cowhorn forceps
    B. Surgical bur
    C. Straight elevator
    D. Surgical curette

290. All of the following are types of suture material EXCEPT
    A. gut.
    B. silk.
    C. polyester.
    D. latex.

291. Which of the following are considered facial bones?
    A. Mandible
    B. Vomer
    C. Sphenoid
    D. Lacrimal bones

292. Which of the following are functions of the sinuses?
    1. Lighten the weight of the skull
    2. Create resonance when you speak
    3. Warm air as it enters the body
    4. Act as a filter to prevent dust from entering the body

    A. 1, 2, 3
    B. 1, 2, 4
    C. 1, 3
    D. 1, 4

293. The two types of mucosa that line the oral cavity are referred to as the lining and masticatory mucosa.
    A. True
    B. False

294. The largest salivary gland is called the
    A. submandibular.
    B. parotid.
    C. sublingual.
    D. accessory parotid.

295. The product in saliva responsible for breaking down starches is called
    A. ptylin.
    B. mucin.
    C. amylase.
    D. serous fluid.

296. The gingiva consists of two types of gingiva called attached and free gingiva.
    A. True
    B. False

297. The teeth that replace the primary teeth are referred to as _____ teeth.
    A. deciduous
    B. succedaneous
    C. natal
    D. None of the above

298. Which of the following items would appear on an endodontic tray?
    1. Broach
    2. Irrigating syringe
    3. Lentulo spiral
    4. Curette
    5. Gutta-percha

    A. 1, 2, 3, 4
    B. 1, 2, 3, 5
    C. 1, 2
    D. All of the above

299. Following oral surgery, which of the following can slow the rate of healing?
    1. Physical stress
    2. Smoking tobacco
    3. Overingestion of vitamin C
    4. Lack of adequate nutrition

    A. 1, 2, 3
    B. 1, 2, 4
    C. 1, 5
    D. All of the above

300. If an employee has a gross wage total of $560 and that wage is taxed at $125, the employee's income will have
    A. an increase of $125 in the net total.
    B. a decrease of $125 in the gross total.
    C. a total net wage of $685.
    D. a total net wage of $560.

Answer Sheet for Comprehensive Practice Exam

Name _____ Date _____
             Last   First   Middle

Directions:

1. Using pencil, fill in only one circle representing your answer for each question.
2. Keeping your marks inside the circle, blacken the circle completely.
3. Completely erase any answer you wish to change, and make no stray marks.

Correct: Ⓐ ● Ⓒ Ⓓ Ⓔ Ⓕ Ⓖ Ⓗ Ⓘ Ⓙ   Wrong: ⊗ ⓑ ○ ☑ ⊘ Ⓕ Ⓖ Ⓗ Ⓘ Ⓙ

1. Ⓐ Ⓑ Ⓒ Ⓓ Ⓔ	27. Ⓐ Ⓑ Ⓒ Ⓓ Ⓔ	53. Ⓐ Ⓑ Ⓒ Ⓓ Ⓔ	79. Ⓐ Ⓑ Ⓒ Ⓓ Ⓔ
2. Ⓐ Ⓑ Ⓒ Ⓓ Ⓔ	28. Ⓐ Ⓑ Ⓒ Ⓓ Ⓔ	54. Ⓐ Ⓑ Ⓒ Ⓓ Ⓔ	80. Ⓐ Ⓑ Ⓒ Ⓓ Ⓔ
3. Ⓐ Ⓑ Ⓒ Ⓓ Ⓔ	29. Ⓐ Ⓑ Ⓒ Ⓓ Ⓔ	55. Ⓐ Ⓑ Ⓒ Ⓓ Ⓔ	81. Ⓐ Ⓑ Ⓒ Ⓓ Ⓔ
4. Ⓐ Ⓑ Ⓒ Ⓓ Ⓔ	30. Ⓐ Ⓑ Ⓒ Ⓓ Ⓔ	56. Ⓐ Ⓑ Ⓒ Ⓓ Ⓔ	82. Ⓐ Ⓑ Ⓒ Ⓓ Ⓔ
5. Ⓐ Ⓑ Ⓒ Ⓓ Ⓔ	31. Ⓐ Ⓑ Ⓒ Ⓓ Ⓔ	57. Ⓐ Ⓑ Ⓒ Ⓓ Ⓔ Ⓕ Ⓖ Ⓗ	83. Ⓐ Ⓑ Ⓒ Ⓓ Ⓔ
6. Ⓐ Ⓑ Ⓒ Ⓓ Ⓔ	32. Ⓐ Ⓑ Ⓒ Ⓓ Ⓔ	58. Ⓐ Ⓑ Ⓒ Ⓓ Ⓔ Ⓕ Ⓖ Ⓗ	84. Ⓐ Ⓑ Ⓒ Ⓓ Ⓔ
7. Ⓐ Ⓑ Ⓒ Ⓓ Ⓔ	33. Ⓐ Ⓑ Ⓒ Ⓓ Ⓔ	59. Ⓐ Ⓑ Ⓒ Ⓓ Ⓔ Ⓕ Ⓖ Ⓗ	85. Ⓐ Ⓑ Ⓒ Ⓓ Ⓔ
8. Ⓐ Ⓑ Ⓒ Ⓓ Ⓔ	34. Ⓐ Ⓑ Ⓒ Ⓓ Ⓔ	60. Ⓐ Ⓑ Ⓒ Ⓓ Ⓔ Ⓕ Ⓖ Ⓗ	86. Ⓐ Ⓑ Ⓒ Ⓓ Ⓔ
9. Ⓐ Ⓑ Ⓒ Ⓓ Ⓔ	35. Ⓐ Ⓑ Ⓒ Ⓓ Ⓔ	61. Ⓐ Ⓑ Ⓒ Ⓓ Ⓔ Ⓕ Ⓖ Ⓗ	87. Ⓐ Ⓑ Ⓒ Ⓓ Ⓔ
10. Ⓐ Ⓑ Ⓒ Ⓓ Ⓔ	36. Ⓐ Ⓑ Ⓒ Ⓓ Ⓔ	62. Ⓐ Ⓑ Ⓒ Ⓓ Ⓔ Ⓕ Ⓖ Ⓗ	88. Ⓐ Ⓑ Ⓒ Ⓓ Ⓔ
11. Ⓐ Ⓑ Ⓒ Ⓓ Ⓔ	37. Ⓐ Ⓑ Ⓒ Ⓓ Ⓔ	63. Ⓐ Ⓑ Ⓒ Ⓓ Ⓔ Ⓕ Ⓖ Ⓗ	89. Ⓐ Ⓑ Ⓒ Ⓓ Ⓔ
12. Ⓐ Ⓑ Ⓒ Ⓓ Ⓔ	38. Ⓐ Ⓑ Ⓒ Ⓓ Ⓔ	64. Ⓐ Ⓑ Ⓒ Ⓓ Ⓔ Ⓕ Ⓖ Ⓗ	90. Ⓐ Ⓑ Ⓒ Ⓓ Ⓔ
13. Ⓐ Ⓑ Ⓒ Ⓓ Ⓔ	39. Ⓐ Ⓑ Ⓒ Ⓓ Ⓔ	65. Ⓐ Ⓑ Ⓒ Ⓓ Ⓔ	91. Ⓐ Ⓑ Ⓒ Ⓓ Ⓔ
14. Ⓐ Ⓑ Ⓒ Ⓓ Ⓔ	40. Ⓐ Ⓑ Ⓒ Ⓓ Ⓔ	66. Ⓐ Ⓑ Ⓒ Ⓓ Ⓔ	92. Ⓐ Ⓑ Ⓒ Ⓓ Ⓔ
15. Ⓐ Ⓑ Ⓒ Ⓓ Ⓔ	41. Ⓐ Ⓑ Ⓒ Ⓓ Ⓔ	67. Ⓐ Ⓑ Ⓒ Ⓓ Ⓔ	93. Ⓐ Ⓑ Ⓒ Ⓓ Ⓔ
16. Ⓐ Ⓑ Ⓒ Ⓓ Ⓔ	42. Ⓐ Ⓑ Ⓒ Ⓓ Ⓔ	68. Ⓐ Ⓑ Ⓒ Ⓓ Ⓔ Ⓕ	94. Ⓐ Ⓑ Ⓒ Ⓓ Ⓔ
17. Ⓐ Ⓑ Ⓒ Ⓓ Ⓔ	43. Ⓐ Ⓑ Ⓒ Ⓓ Ⓔ	69. Ⓐ Ⓑ Ⓒ Ⓓ Ⓔ Ⓕ	95. Ⓐ Ⓑ Ⓒ Ⓓ Ⓔ
18. Ⓐ Ⓑ Ⓒ Ⓓ Ⓔ	44. Ⓐ Ⓑ Ⓒ Ⓓ Ⓔ	70. Ⓐ Ⓑ Ⓒ Ⓓ Ⓔ Ⓕ	96. Ⓐ Ⓑ Ⓒ Ⓓ Ⓔ
19. Ⓐ Ⓑ Ⓒ Ⓓ Ⓔ	45. Ⓐ Ⓑ Ⓒ Ⓓ Ⓔ	71. Ⓐ Ⓑ Ⓒ Ⓓ Ⓔ Ⓕ	97. Ⓐ Ⓑ Ⓒ Ⓓ Ⓔ
20. Ⓐ Ⓑ Ⓒ Ⓓ Ⓔ	46. Ⓐ Ⓑ Ⓒ Ⓓ Ⓔ	72. Ⓐ Ⓑ Ⓒ Ⓓ Ⓔ Ⓕ	98. Ⓐ Ⓑ Ⓒ Ⓓ Ⓔ
21. Ⓐ Ⓑ Ⓒ Ⓓ Ⓔ	47. Ⓐ Ⓑ Ⓒ Ⓓ Ⓔ	73. Ⓐ Ⓑ Ⓒ Ⓓ Ⓔ Ⓕ	99. Ⓐ Ⓑ Ⓒ Ⓓ Ⓔ
22. Ⓐ Ⓑ Ⓒ Ⓓ Ⓔ	48. Ⓐ Ⓑ Ⓒ Ⓓ Ⓔ	74. Ⓐ Ⓑ Ⓒ Ⓓ Ⓔ	100. Ⓐ Ⓑ Ⓒ Ⓓ Ⓔ
23. Ⓐ Ⓑ Ⓒ Ⓓ Ⓔ	49. Ⓐ Ⓑ Ⓒ Ⓓ Ⓔ	75. Ⓐ Ⓑ Ⓒ Ⓓ Ⓔ	101. Ⓐ Ⓑ Ⓒ Ⓓ Ⓔ
24. Ⓐ Ⓑ Ⓒ Ⓓ Ⓔ	50. Ⓐ Ⓑ Ⓒ Ⓓ Ⓔ	76. Ⓐ Ⓑ Ⓒ Ⓓ Ⓔ	102. Ⓐ Ⓑ Ⓒ Ⓓ Ⓔ
25. Ⓐ Ⓑ Ⓒ Ⓓ Ⓔ	51. Ⓐ Ⓑ Ⓒ Ⓓ Ⓔ	77. Ⓐ Ⓑ Ⓒ Ⓓ Ⓔ	103. Ⓐ Ⓑ Ⓒ Ⓓ Ⓔ
26. Ⓐ Ⓑ Ⓒ Ⓓ Ⓔ	52. Ⓐ Ⓑ Ⓒ Ⓓ Ⓔ	78. Ⓐ Ⓑ Ⓒ Ⓓ Ⓔ	104. Ⓐ Ⓑ Ⓒ Ⓓ Ⓔ

105. Ⓐ Ⓑ Ⓒ Ⓓ Ⓔ	154. Ⓐ Ⓑ Ⓒ Ⓓ Ⓔ	203. Ⓐ Ⓑ Ⓒ Ⓓ Ⓔ	252. Ⓐ Ⓑ Ⓒ Ⓓ Ⓔ
106. Ⓐ Ⓑ Ⓒ Ⓓ Ⓔ	155. Ⓐ Ⓑ Ⓒ Ⓓ Ⓔ	204. Ⓐ Ⓑ Ⓒ Ⓓ Ⓔ	253. Ⓐ Ⓑ Ⓒ Ⓓ Ⓔ
107. Ⓐ Ⓑ Ⓒ Ⓓ Ⓔ	156. Ⓐ Ⓑ Ⓒ Ⓓ Ⓔ	205. Ⓐ Ⓑ Ⓒ Ⓓ Ⓔ	254. Ⓐ Ⓑ Ⓒ Ⓓ Ⓔ
108. Ⓐ Ⓑ Ⓒ Ⓓ Ⓔ	157. Ⓐ Ⓑ Ⓒ Ⓓ Ⓔ	206. Ⓐ Ⓑ Ⓒ Ⓓ Ⓔ	255. Ⓐ Ⓑ Ⓒ Ⓓ Ⓔ
109. Ⓐ Ⓑ Ⓒ Ⓓ Ⓔ	158. Ⓐ Ⓑ Ⓒ Ⓓ Ⓔ	207. Ⓐ Ⓑ Ⓒ Ⓓ Ⓔ	256. Ⓐ Ⓑ Ⓒ Ⓓ Ⓔ
110. Ⓐ Ⓑ Ⓒ Ⓓ Ⓔ	159. Ⓐ Ⓑ Ⓒ Ⓓ Ⓔ	208. Ⓐ Ⓑ Ⓒ Ⓓ Ⓔ	257. Ⓐ Ⓑ Ⓒ Ⓓ Ⓔ
111. Ⓐ Ⓑ Ⓒ Ⓓ Ⓔ	160. Ⓐ Ⓑ Ⓒ Ⓓ Ⓔ	209. Ⓐ Ⓑ Ⓒ Ⓓ Ⓔ	258. Ⓐ Ⓑ Ⓒ Ⓓ Ⓔ
112. Ⓐ Ⓑ Ⓒ Ⓓ Ⓔ	161. Ⓐ Ⓑ Ⓒ Ⓓ Ⓔ	210. Ⓐ Ⓑ Ⓒ Ⓓ Ⓔ	259. Ⓐ Ⓑ Ⓒ Ⓓ Ⓔ
113. Ⓐ Ⓑ Ⓒ Ⓓ Ⓔ	162. Ⓐ Ⓑ Ⓒ Ⓓ Ⓔ	211. Ⓐ Ⓑ Ⓒ Ⓓ Ⓔ	260. Ⓐ Ⓑ Ⓒ Ⓓ Ⓔ
114. Ⓐ Ⓑ Ⓒ Ⓓ Ⓔ	163. Ⓐ Ⓑ Ⓒ Ⓓ Ⓔ	212. Ⓐ Ⓑ Ⓒ Ⓓ Ⓔ	261. Ⓐ Ⓑ Ⓒ Ⓓ Ⓔ
115. Ⓐ Ⓑ Ⓒ Ⓓ Ⓔ	164. Ⓐ Ⓑ Ⓒ Ⓓ Ⓔ	213. Ⓐ Ⓑ Ⓒ Ⓓ Ⓔ	262. Ⓐ Ⓑ Ⓒ Ⓓ Ⓔ
116. Ⓐ Ⓑ Ⓒ Ⓓ Ⓔ	165. Ⓐ Ⓑ Ⓒ Ⓓ Ⓔ	214. Ⓐ Ⓑ Ⓒ Ⓓ Ⓔ	263. Ⓐ Ⓑ Ⓒ Ⓓ Ⓔ
117. Ⓐ Ⓑ Ⓒ Ⓓ Ⓔ	166. Ⓐ Ⓑ Ⓒ Ⓓ Ⓔ	215. Ⓐ Ⓑ Ⓒ Ⓓ Ⓔ	264. Ⓐ Ⓑ Ⓒ Ⓓ Ⓔ
118. Ⓐ Ⓑ Ⓒ Ⓓ Ⓔ	167. Ⓐ Ⓑ Ⓒ Ⓓ Ⓔ Ⓕ	216. Ⓐ Ⓑ Ⓒ Ⓓ Ⓔ	265. Ⓐ Ⓑ Ⓒ Ⓓ Ⓔ
119. Ⓐ Ⓑ Ⓒ Ⓓ Ⓔ	168. Ⓐ Ⓑ Ⓒ Ⓓ Ⓔ Ⓕ	217. Ⓐ Ⓑ Ⓒ Ⓓ Ⓔ	266. Ⓐ Ⓑ Ⓒ Ⓓ Ⓔ
120. Ⓐ Ⓑ Ⓒ Ⓓ Ⓔ	169. Ⓐ Ⓑ Ⓒ Ⓓ Ⓔ Ⓕ	218. Ⓐ Ⓑ Ⓒ Ⓓ Ⓔ	267. Ⓐ Ⓑ Ⓒ Ⓓ Ⓔ
121. Ⓐ Ⓑ Ⓒ Ⓓ Ⓔ	170. Ⓐ Ⓑ Ⓒ Ⓓ Ⓔ Ⓕ	219. Ⓐ Ⓑ Ⓒ Ⓓ Ⓔ	268. Ⓐ Ⓑ Ⓒ Ⓓ Ⓔ
122. Ⓐ Ⓑ Ⓒ Ⓓ Ⓔ	171. Ⓐ Ⓑ Ⓒ Ⓓ Ⓔ Ⓕ	220. Ⓐ Ⓑ Ⓒ Ⓓ Ⓔ	269. Ⓐ Ⓑ Ⓒ Ⓓ Ⓔ
123. Ⓐ Ⓑ Ⓒ Ⓓ Ⓔ	172. Ⓐ Ⓑ Ⓒ Ⓓ Ⓔ Ⓕ	221. Ⓐ Ⓑ Ⓒ Ⓓ Ⓔ	270. Ⓐ Ⓑ Ⓒ Ⓓ Ⓔ
124. Ⓐ Ⓑ Ⓒ Ⓓ Ⓔ	173. Ⓐ Ⓑ Ⓒ Ⓓ Ⓔ	222. Ⓐ Ⓑ Ⓒ Ⓓ Ⓔ	271. Ⓐ Ⓑ Ⓒ Ⓓ Ⓔ
125. Ⓐ Ⓑ Ⓒ Ⓓ Ⓔ	174. Ⓐ Ⓑ Ⓒ Ⓓ Ⓔ	223. Ⓐ Ⓑ Ⓒ Ⓓ Ⓔ	272. Ⓐ Ⓑ Ⓒ Ⓓ Ⓔ
126. Ⓐ Ⓑ Ⓒ Ⓓ Ⓔ	175. Ⓐ Ⓑ Ⓒ Ⓓ Ⓔ	224. Ⓐ Ⓑ Ⓒ Ⓓ Ⓔ	273. Ⓐ Ⓑ Ⓒ Ⓓ Ⓔ
127. Ⓐ Ⓑ Ⓒ Ⓓ Ⓔ	176. Ⓐ Ⓑ Ⓒ Ⓓ Ⓔ	225. Ⓐ Ⓑ Ⓒ Ⓓ Ⓔ	274. Ⓐ Ⓑ Ⓒ Ⓓ Ⓔ
128. Ⓐ Ⓑ Ⓒ Ⓓ Ⓔ	177. Ⓐ Ⓑ Ⓒ Ⓓ Ⓔ	226. Ⓐ Ⓑ Ⓒ Ⓓ Ⓔ	275. Ⓐ Ⓑ Ⓒ Ⓓ Ⓔ
129. Ⓐ Ⓑ Ⓒ Ⓓ Ⓔ	178. Ⓐ Ⓑ Ⓒ Ⓓ Ⓔ	227. Ⓐ Ⓑ Ⓒ Ⓓ Ⓔ	276. Ⓐ Ⓑ Ⓒ Ⓓ Ⓔ
130. Ⓐ Ⓑ Ⓒ Ⓓ Ⓔ	179. Ⓐ Ⓑ Ⓒ Ⓓ Ⓔ	228. Ⓐ Ⓑ Ⓒ Ⓓ Ⓔ	277. Ⓐ Ⓑ Ⓒ Ⓓ Ⓔ
131. Ⓐ Ⓑ Ⓒ Ⓓ Ⓔ	180. Ⓐ Ⓑ Ⓒ Ⓓ Ⓔ	229. Ⓐ Ⓑ Ⓒ Ⓓ Ⓔ	278. Ⓐ Ⓑ Ⓒ Ⓓ Ⓔ
132. Ⓐ Ⓑ Ⓒ Ⓓ Ⓔ	181. Ⓐ Ⓑ Ⓒ Ⓓ Ⓔ	230. Ⓐ Ⓑ Ⓒ Ⓓ Ⓔ	279. Ⓐ Ⓑ Ⓒ Ⓓ Ⓔ
133. Ⓐ Ⓑ Ⓒ Ⓓ Ⓔ	182. Ⓐ Ⓑ Ⓒ Ⓓ Ⓔ	231. Ⓐ Ⓑ Ⓒ Ⓓ Ⓔ	280. Ⓐ Ⓑ Ⓒ Ⓓ Ⓔ
134. Ⓐ Ⓑ Ⓒ Ⓓ Ⓔ	183. Ⓐ Ⓑ Ⓒ Ⓓ Ⓔ	232. Ⓐ Ⓑ Ⓒ Ⓓ Ⓔ	281. Ⓐ Ⓑ Ⓒ Ⓓ Ⓔ
135. Ⓐ Ⓑ Ⓒ Ⓓ Ⓔ	184. Ⓐ Ⓑ Ⓒ Ⓓ Ⓔ	233. Ⓐ Ⓑ Ⓒ Ⓓ Ⓔ	282. Ⓐ Ⓑ Ⓒ Ⓓ Ⓔ
136. Ⓐ Ⓑ Ⓒ Ⓓ Ⓔ	185. Ⓐ Ⓑ Ⓒ Ⓓ Ⓔ	234. Ⓐ Ⓑ Ⓒ Ⓓ Ⓔ	283. Ⓐ Ⓑ Ⓒ Ⓓ Ⓔ
137. Ⓐ Ⓑ Ⓒ Ⓓ Ⓔ	186. Ⓐ Ⓑ Ⓒ Ⓓ Ⓔ	235. Ⓐ Ⓑ Ⓒ Ⓓ Ⓔ	284. Ⓐ Ⓑ Ⓒ Ⓓ Ⓔ
138. Ⓐ Ⓑ Ⓒ Ⓓ Ⓔ	187. Ⓐ Ⓑ Ⓒ Ⓓ Ⓔ	236. Ⓐ Ⓑ Ⓒ Ⓓ Ⓔ	285. Ⓐ Ⓑ Ⓒ Ⓓ Ⓔ
139. Ⓐ Ⓑ Ⓒ Ⓓ Ⓔ	188. Ⓐ Ⓑ Ⓒ Ⓓ Ⓔ	237. Ⓐ Ⓑ Ⓒ Ⓓ Ⓔ	286. Ⓐ Ⓑ Ⓒ Ⓓ Ⓔ
140. Ⓐ Ⓑ Ⓒ Ⓓ Ⓔ	189. Ⓐ Ⓑ Ⓒ Ⓓ Ⓔ	238. Ⓐ Ⓑ Ⓒ Ⓓ Ⓔ	287. Ⓐ Ⓑ Ⓒ Ⓓ Ⓔ
141. Ⓐ Ⓑ Ⓒ Ⓓ Ⓔ	190. Ⓐ Ⓑ Ⓒ Ⓓ Ⓔ	239. Ⓐ Ⓑ Ⓒ Ⓓ Ⓔ	288. Ⓐ Ⓑ Ⓒ Ⓓ Ⓔ
142. Ⓐ Ⓑ Ⓒ Ⓓ Ⓔ	191. Ⓐ Ⓑ Ⓒ Ⓓ Ⓔ Ⓕ Ⓖ Ⓗ Ⓘ Ⓙ	240. Ⓐ Ⓑ Ⓒ Ⓓ Ⓔ	289. Ⓐ Ⓑ Ⓒ Ⓓ Ⓔ
143. Ⓐ Ⓑ Ⓒ Ⓓ Ⓔ	192. Ⓐ Ⓑ Ⓒ Ⓓ Ⓔ Ⓕ Ⓖ Ⓗ Ⓘ Ⓙ	241. Ⓐ Ⓑ Ⓒ Ⓓ Ⓔ Ⓕ Ⓖ	290. Ⓐ Ⓑ Ⓒ Ⓓ Ⓔ
144. Ⓐ Ⓑ Ⓒ Ⓓ Ⓔ	193. Ⓐ Ⓑ Ⓒ Ⓓ Ⓔ Ⓕ Ⓖ Ⓗ Ⓘ Ⓙ	242. Ⓐ Ⓑ Ⓒ Ⓓ Ⓔ Ⓕ Ⓖ	291. Ⓐ Ⓑ Ⓒ Ⓓ Ⓔ
145. Ⓐ Ⓑ Ⓒ Ⓓ Ⓔ	194. Ⓐ Ⓑ Ⓒ Ⓓ Ⓔ Ⓕ Ⓖ Ⓗ Ⓘ Ⓙ	243. Ⓐ Ⓑ Ⓒ Ⓓ Ⓔ Ⓕ Ⓖ	292. Ⓐ Ⓑ Ⓒ Ⓓ Ⓔ
146. Ⓐ Ⓑ Ⓒ Ⓓ Ⓔ	195. Ⓐ Ⓑ Ⓒ Ⓓ Ⓔ Ⓕ Ⓖ Ⓗ Ⓘ Ⓙ	244. Ⓐ Ⓑ Ⓒ Ⓓ Ⓔ Ⓕ Ⓖ	293. Ⓐ Ⓑ Ⓒ Ⓓ Ⓔ
147. Ⓐ Ⓑ Ⓒ Ⓓ Ⓔ	196. Ⓐ Ⓑ Ⓒ Ⓓ Ⓔ Ⓕ Ⓖ Ⓗ Ⓘ Ⓙ	245. Ⓐ Ⓑ Ⓒ Ⓓ Ⓔ Ⓕ Ⓖ	294. Ⓐ Ⓑ Ⓒ Ⓓ Ⓔ
148. Ⓐ Ⓑ Ⓒ Ⓓ Ⓔ	197. Ⓐ Ⓑ Ⓒ Ⓓ Ⓔ Ⓕ Ⓖ Ⓗ Ⓘ Ⓙ	246. Ⓐ Ⓑ Ⓒ Ⓓ Ⓔ Ⓕ Ⓖ	295. Ⓐ Ⓑ Ⓒ Ⓓ Ⓔ
149. Ⓐ Ⓑ Ⓒ Ⓓ Ⓔ	198. Ⓐ Ⓑ Ⓒ Ⓓ Ⓔ Ⓕ Ⓖ Ⓗ Ⓘ Ⓙ	247. Ⓐ Ⓑ Ⓒ Ⓓ Ⓔ Ⓕ Ⓖ	296. Ⓐ Ⓑ Ⓒ Ⓓ Ⓔ
150. Ⓐ Ⓑ Ⓒ Ⓓ Ⓔ	199. Ⓐ Ⓑ Ⓒ Ⓓ Ⓔ Ⓕ Ⓖ Ⓗ Ⓘ Ⓙ	248. Ⓐ Ⓑ Ⓒ Ⓓ Ⓔ	297. Ⓐ Ⓑ Ⓒ Ⓓ Ⓔ
151. Ⓐ Ⓑ Ⓒ Ⓓ Ⓔ	200. Ⓐ Ⓑ Ⓒ Ⓓ Ⓔ Ⓕ Ⓖ Ⓗ Ⓘ Ⓙ	249. Ⓐ Ⓑ Ⓒ Ⓓ Ⓔ	298. Ⓐ Ⓑ Ⓒ Ⓓ Ⓔ
152. Ⓐ Ⓑ Ⓒ Ⓓ Ⓔ	201. Ⓐ Ⓑ Ⓒ Ⓓ Ⓔ	250. Ⓐ Ⓑ Ⓒ Ⓓ Ⓔ	299. Ⓐ Ⓑ Ⓒ Ⓓ Ⓔ
153. Ⓐ Ⓑ Ⓒ Ⓓ Ⓔ	202. Ⓐ Ⓑ Ⓒ Ⓓ Ⓔ	251. Ⓐ Ⓑ Ⓒ Ⓓ Ⓔ	300. Ⓐ Ⓑ Ⓒ Ⓓ Ⓔ

Answer Sheet for Comprehensive Practice Exam

Name _____ Date _____
         Last   First   Middle

Directions:

1. Using pencil, fill in only one circle representing your answer for each question.
2. Keeping your marks inside the circle, blacken the circle completely.
3. Completely erase any answer you wish to change, and make no stray marks.

Correct: Ⓐ ● Ⓒ Ⓓ Ⓔ Ⓕ Ⓖ Ⓗ Ⓘ Ⓙ   Wrong: Ⓧ Ⓑ ○ Ⓓ Ⓔ Ⓕ Ⓖ Ⓗ Ⓘ Ⓙ

1. Ⓐ Ⓑ Ⓒ Ⓓ Ⓔ	27. Ⓐ Ⓑ Ⓒ Ⓓ Ⓔ	53. Ⓐ Ⓑ Ⓒ Ⓓ Ⓔ	79. Ⓐ Ⓑ Ⓒ Ⓓ Ⓔ
2. Ⓐ Ⓑ Ⓒ Ⓓ Ⓔ	28. Ⓐ Ⓑ Ⓒ Ⓓ Ⓔ	54. Ⓐ Ⓑ Ⓒ Ⓓ Ⓔ	80. Ⓐ Ⓑ Ⓒ Ⓓ Ⓔ
3. Ⓐ Ⓑ Ⓒ Ⓓ Ⓔ	29. Ⓐ Ⓑ Ⓒ Ⓓ Ⓔ	55. Ⓐ Ⓑ Ⓒ Ⓓ Ⓔ	81. Ⓐ Ⓑ Ⓒ Ⓓ Ⓔ
4. Ⓐ Ⓑ Ⓒ Ⓓ Ⓔ	30. Ⓐ Ⓑ Ⓒ Ⓓ Ⓔ	56. Ⓐ Ⓑ Ⓒ Ⓓ Ⓔ	82. Ⓐ Ⓑ Ⓒ Ⓓ Ⓔ
5. Ⓐ Ⓑ Ⓒ Ⓓ Ⓔ	31. Ⓐ Ⓑ Ⓒ Ⓓ Ⓔ	57. Ⓐ Ⓑ Ⓒ Ⓓ Ⓔ Ⓕ Ⓖ Ⓗ	83. Ⓐ Ⓑ Ⓒ Ⓓ Ⓔ
6. Ⓐ Ⓑ Ⓒ Ⓓ Ⓔ	32. Ⓐ Ⓑ Ⓒ Ⓓ Ⓔ	58. Ⓐ Ⓑ Ⓒ Ⓓ Ⓔ Ⓕ Ⓖ Ⓗ	84. Ⓐ Ⓑ Ⓒ Ⓓ Ⓔ
7. Ⓐ Ⓑ Ⓒ Ⓓ Ⓔ	33. Ⓐ Ⓑ Ⓒ Ⓓ Ⓔ	59. Ⓐ Ⓑ Ⓒ Ⓓ Ⓔ Ⓕ Ⓖ Ⓗ	85. Ⓐ Ⓑ Ⓒ Ⓓ Ⓔ
8. Ⓐ Ⓑ Ⓒ Ⓓ Ⓔ	34. Ⓐ Ⓑ Ⓒ Ⓓ Ⓔ	60. Ⓐ Ⓑ Ⓒ Ⓓ Ⓔ Ⓕ Ⓖ Ⓗ	86. Ⓐ Ⓑ Ⓒ Ⓓ Ⓔ
9. Ⓐ Ⓑ Ⓒ Ⓓ Ⓔ	35. Ⓐ Ⓑ Ⓒ Ⓓ Ⓔ	61. Ⓐ Ⓑ Ⓒ Ⓓ Ⓔ Ⓕ Ⓖ Ⓗ	87. Ⓐ Ⓑ Ⓒ Ⓓ Ⓔ
10. Ⓐ Ⓑ Ⓒ Ⓓ Ⓔ	36. Ⓐ Ⓑ Ⓒ Ⓓ Ⓔ	62. Ⓐ Ⓑ Ⓒ Ⓓ Ⓔ Ⓕ Ⓖ Ⓗ	88. Ⓐ Ⓑ Ⓒ Ⓓ Ⓔ
11. Ⓐ Ⓑ Ⓒ Ⓓ Ⓔ	37. Ⓐ Ⓑ Ⓒ Ⓓ Ⓔ	63. Ⓐ Ⓑ Ⓒ Ⓓ Ⓔ Ⓕ Ⓖ Ⓗ	89. Ⓐ Ⓑ Ⓒ Ⓓ Ⓔ
12. Ⓐ Ⓑ Ⓒ Ⓓ Ⓔ	38. Ⓐ Ⓑ Ⓒ Ⓓ Ⓔ	64. Ⓐ Ⓑ Ⓒ Ⓓ Ⓔ Ⓕ Ⓖ Ⓗ	90. Ⓐ Ⓑ Ⓒ Ⓓ Ⓔ
13. Ⓐ Ⓑ Ⓒ Ⓓ Ⓔ	39. Ⓐ Ⓑ Ⓒ Ⓓ Ⓔ	65. Ⓐ Ⓑ Ⓒ Ⓓ Ⓔ	91. Ⓐ Ⓑ Ⓒ Ⓓ Ⓔ
14. Ⓐ Ⓑ Ⓒ Ⓓ Ⓔ	40. Ⓐ Ⓑ Ⓒ Ⓓ Ⓔ	66. Ⓐ Ⓑ Ⓒ Ⓓ Ⓔ	92. Ⓐ Ⓑ Ⓒ Ⓓ Ⓔ
15. Ⓐ Ⓑ Ⓒ Ⓓ Ⓔ	41. Ⓐ Ⓑ Ⓒ Ⓓ Ⓔ	67. Ⓐ Ⓑ Ⓒ Ⓓ Ⓔ	93. Ⓐ Ⓑ Ⓒ Ⓓ Ⓔ
16. Ⓐ Ⓑ Ⓒ Ⓓ Ⓔ	42. Ⓐ Ⓑ Ⓒ Ⓓ Ⓔ	68. Ⓐ Ⓑ Ⓒ Ⓓ Ⓔ Ⓕ	94. Ⓐ Ⓑ Ⓒ Ⓓ Ⓔ
17. Ⓐ Ⓑ Ⓒ Ⓓ Ⓔ	43. Ⓐ Ⓑ Ⓒ Ⓓ Ⓔ	69. Ⓐ Ⓑ Ⓒ Ⓓ Ⓔ Ⓕ	95. Ⓐ Ⓑ Ⓒ Ⓓ Ⓔ
18. Ⓐ Ⓑ Ⓒ Ⓓ Ⓔ	44. Ⓐ Ⓑ Ⓒ Ⓓ Ⓔ	70. Ⓐ Ⓑ Ⓒ Ⓓ Ⓔ Ⓕ	96. Ⓐ Ⓑ Ⓒ Ⓓ Ⓔ
19. Ⓐ Ⓑ Ⓒ Ⓓ Ⓔ	45. Ⓐ Ⓑ Ⓒ Ⓓ Ⓔ	71. Ⓐ Ⓑ Ⓒ Ⓓ Ⓔ Ⓕ	97. Ⓐ Ⓑ Ⓒ Ⓓ Ⓔ
20. Ⓐ Ⓑ Ⓒ Ⓓ Ⓔ	46. Ⓐ Ⓑ Ⓒ Ⓓ Ⓔ	72. Ⓐ Ⓑ Ⓒ Ⓓ Ⓔ Ⓕ	98. Ⓐ Ⓑ Ⓒ Ⓓ Ⓔ
21. Ⓐ Ⓑ Ⓒ Ⓓ Ⓔ	47. Ⓐ Ⓑ Ⓒ Ⓓ Ⓔ	73. Ⓐ Ⓑ Ⓒ Ⓓ Ⓔ Ⓕ	99. Ⓐ Ⓑ Ⓒ Ⓓ Ⓔ
22. Ⓐ Ⓑ Ⓒ Ⓓ Ⓔ	48. Ⓐ Ⓑ Ⓒ Ⓓ Ⓔ	74. Ⓐ Ⓑ Ⓒ Ⓓ Ⓔ	100. Ⓐ Ⓑ Ⓒ Ⓓ Ⓔ
23. Ⓐ Ⓑ Ⓒ Ⓓ Ⓔ	49. Ⓐ Ⓑ Ⓒ Ⓓ Ⓔ	75. Ⓐ Ⓑ Ⓒ Ⓓ Ⓔ	101. Ⓐ Ⓑ Ⓒ Ⓓ Ⓔ
24. Ⓐ Ⓑ Ⓒ Ⓓ Ⓔ	50. Ⓐ Ⓑ Ⓒ Ⓓ Ⓔ	76. Ⓐ Ⓑ Ⓒ Ⓓ Ⓔ	102. Ⓐ Ⓑ Ⓒ Ⓓ Ⓔ
25. Ⓐ Ⓑ Ⓒ Ⓓ Ⓔ	51. Ⓐ Ⓑ Ⓒ Ⓓ Ⓔ	77. Ⓐ Ⓑ Ⓒ Ⓓ Ⓔ	103. Ⓐ Ⓑ Ⓒ Ⓓ Ⓔ
26. Ⓐ Ⓑ Ⓒ Ⓓ Ⓔ	52. Ⓐ Ⓑ Ⓒ Ⓓ Ⓔ	78. Ⓐ Ⓑ Ⓒ Ⓓ Ⓔ	104. Ⓐ Ⓑ Ⓒ Ⓓ Ⓔ

105. Ⓐ Ⓑ Ⓒ Ⓓ Ⓔ
106. Ⓐ Ⓑ Ⓒ Ⓓ Ⓔ
107. Ⓐ Ⓑ Ⓒ Ⓓ Ⓔ
108. Ⓐ Ⓑ Ⓒ Ⓓ Ⓔ
109. Ⓐ Ⓑ Ⓒ Ⓓ Ⓔ
110. Ⓐ Ⓑ Ⓒ Ⓓ Ⓔ
111. Ⓐ Ⓑ Ⓒ Ⓓ Ⓔ
112. Ⓐ Ⓑ Ⓒ Ⓓ Ⓔ
113. Ⓐ Ⓑ Ⓒ Ⓓ Ⓔ
114. Ⓐ Ⓑ Ⓒ Ⓓ Ⓔ
115. Ⓐ Ⓑ Ⓒ Ⓓ Ⓔ
116. Ⓐ Ⓑ Ⓒ Ⓓ Ⓔ
117. Ⓐ Ⓑ Ⓒ Ⓓ Ⓔ
118. Ⓐ Ⓑ Ⓒ Ⓓ Ⓔ
119. Ⓐ Ⓑ Ⓒ Ⓓ Ⓔ
120. Ⓐ Ⓑ Ⓒ Ⓓ Ⓔ
121. Ⓐ Ⓑ Ⓒ Ⓓ Ⓔ
122. Ⓐ Ⓑ Ⓒ Ⓓ Ⓔ
123. Ⓐ Ⓑ Ⓒ Ⓓ Ⓔ
124. Ⓐ Ⓑ Ⓒ Ⓓ Ⓔ
125. Ⓐ Ⓑ Ⓒ Ⓓ Ⓔ
126. Ⓐ Ⓑ Ⓒ Ⓓ Ⓔ
127. Ⓐ Ⓑ Ⓒ Ⓓ Ⓔ
128. Ⓐ Ⓑ Ⓒ Ⓓ Ⓔ
129. Ⓐ Ⓑ Ⓒ Ⓓ Ⓔ
130. Ⓐ Ⓑ Ⓒ Ⓓ Ⓔ
131. Ⓐ Ⓑ Ⓒ Ⓓ Ⓔ
132. Ⓐ Ⓑ Ⓒ Ⓓ Ⓔ
133. Ⓐ Ⓑ Ⓒ Ⓓ Ⓔ
134. Ⓐ Ⓑ Ⓒ Ⓓ Ⓔ
135. Ⓐ Ⓑ Ⓒ Ⓓ Ⓔ
136. Ⓐ Ⓑ Ⓒ Ⓓ Ⓔ
137. Ⓐ Ⓑ Ⓒ Ⓓ Ⓔ
138. Ⓐ Ⓑ Ⓒ Ⓓ Ⓔ
139. Ⓐ Ⓑ Ⓒ Ⓓ Ⓔ
140. Ⓐ Ⓑ Ⓒ Ⓓ Ⓔ
141. Ⓐ Ⓑ Ⓒ Ⓓ Ⓔ
142. Ⓐ Ⓑ Ⓒ Ⓓ Ⓔ
143. Ⓐ Ⓑ Ⓒ Ⓓ Ⓔ
144. Ⓐ Ⓑ Ⓒ Ⓓ Ⓔ
145. Ⓐ Ⓑ Ⓒ Ⓓ Ⓔ
146. Ⓐ Ⓑ Ⓒ Ⓓ Ⓔ
147. Ⓐ Ⓑ Ⓒ Ⓓ Ⓔ
148. Ⓐ Ⓑ Ⓒ Ⓓ Ⓔ
149. Ⓐ Ⓑ Ⓒ Ⓓ Ⓔ
150. Ⓐ Ⓑ Ⓒ Ⓓ Ⓔ
151. Ⓐ Ⓑ Ⓒ Ⓓ Ⓔ
152. Ⓐ Ⓑ Ⓒ Ⓓ Ⓔ
153. Ⓐ Ⓑ Ⓒ Ⓓ Ⓔ

154. Ⓐ Ⓑ Ⓒ Ⓓ Ⓔ
155. Ⓐ Ⓑ Ⓒ Ⓓ Ⓔ
156. Ⓐ Ⓑ Ⓒ Ⓓ Ⓔ
157. Ⓐ Ⓑ Ⓒ Ⓓ Ⓔ
158. Ⓐ Ⓑ Ⓒ Ⓓ Ⓔ
159. Ⓐ Ⓑ Ⓒ Ⓓ Ⓔ
160. Ⓐ Ⓑ Ⓒ Ⓓ Ⓔ
161. Ⓐ Ⓑ Ⓒ Ⓓ Ⓔ
162. Ⓐ Ⓑ Ⓒ Ⓓ Ⓔ
163. Ⓐ Ⓑ Ⓒ Ⓓ Ⓔ
164. Ⓐ Ⓑ Ⓒ Ⓓ Ⓔ
165. Ⓐ Ⓑ Ⓒ Ⓓ Ⓔ
166. Ⓐ Ⓑ Ⓒ Ⓓ Ⓔ
167. Ⓐ Ⓑ Ⓒ Ⓓ Ⓔ Ⓕ
168. Ⓐ Ⓑ Ⓒ Ⓓ Ⓔ Ⓕ
169. Ⓐ Ⓑ Ⓒ Ⓓ Ⓔ Ⓕ
170. Ⓐ Ⓑ Ⓒ Ⓓ Ⓔ Ⓕ
171. Ⓐ Ⓑ Ⓒ Ⓓ Ⓔ Ⓕ
172. Ⓐ Ⓑ Ⓒ Ⓓ Ⓔ Ⓕ
173. Ⓐ Ⓑ Ⓒ Ⓓ Ⓔ
174. Ⓐ Ⓑ Ⓒ Ⓓ Ⓔ
175. Ⓐ Ⓑ Ⓒ Ⓓ Ⓔ
176. Ⓐ Ⓑ Ⓒ Ⓓ Ⓔ
177. Ⓐ Ⓑ Ⓒ Ⓓ Ⓔ
178. Ⓐ Ⓑ Ⓒ Ⓓ Ⓔ
179. Ⓐ Ⓑ Ⓒ Ⓓ Ⓔ
180. Ⓐ Ⓑ Ⓒ Ⓓ Ⓔ
181. Ⓐ Ⓑ Ⓒ Ⓓ Ⓔ
182. Ⓐ Ⓑ Ⓒ Ⓓ Ⓔ
183. Ⓐ Ⓑ Ⓒ Ⓓ Ⓔ
184. Ⓐ Ⓑ Ⓒ Ⓓ Ⓔ
185. Ⓐ Ⓑ Ⓒ Ⓓ Ⓔ
186. Ⓐ Ⓑ Ⓒ Ⓓ Ⓔ
187. Ⓐ Ⓑ Ⓒ Ⓓ Ⓔ
188. Ⓐ Ⓑ Ⓒ Ⓓ Ⓔ
189. Ⓐ Ⓑ Ⓒ Ⓓ Ⓔ
190. Ⓐ Ⓑ Ⓒ Ⓓ Ⓔ
191. Ⓐ Ⓑ Ⓒ Ⓓ Ⓔ Ⓕ Ⓖ Ⓗ Ⓘ Ⓙ
192. Ⓐ Ⓑ Ⓒ Ⓓ Ⓔ Ⓕ Ⓖ Ⓗ Ⓘ Ⓙ
193. Ⓐ Ⓑ Ⓒ Ⓓ Ⓔ Ⓕ Ⓖ Ⓗ Ⓘ Ⓙ
194. Ⓐ Ⓑ Ⓒ Ⓓ Ⓔ Ⓕ Ⓖ Ⓗ Ⓘ Ⓙ
195. Ⓐ Ⓑ Ⓒ Ⓓ Ⓔ Ⓕ Ⓖ Ⓗ Ⓘ Ⓙ
196. Ⓐ Ⓑ Ⓒ Ⓓ Ⓔ Ⓕ Ⓖ Ⓗ Ⓘ Ⓙ
197. Ⓐ Ⓑ Ⓒ Ⓓ Ⓔ Ⓕ Ⓖ Ⓗ Ⓘ Ⓙ
198. Ⓐ Ⓑ Ⓒ Ⓓ Ⓔ Ⓕ Ⓖ Ⓗ Ⓘ Ⓙ
199. Ⓐ Ⓑ Ⓒ Ⓓ Ⓔ Ⓕ Ⓖ Ⓗ Ⓘ Ⓙ
200. Ⓐ Ⓑ Ⓒ Ⓓ Ⓔ Ⓕ Ⓖ Ⓗ Ⓘ Ⓙ
201. Ⓐ Ⓑ Ⓒ Ⓓ Ⓔ
202. Ⓐ Ⓑ Ⓒ Ⓓ Ⓔ

203. Ⓐ Ⓑ Ⓒ Ⓓ Ⓔ
204. Ⓐ Ⓑ Ⓒ Ⓓ Ⓔ
205. Ⓐ Ⓑ Ⓒ Ⓓ Ⓔ
206. Ⓐ Ⓑ Ⓒ Ⓓ Ⓔ
207. Ⓐ Ⓑ Ⓒ Ⓓ Ⓔ
208. Ⓐ Ⓑ Ⓒ Ⓓ Ⓔ
209. Ⓐ Ⓑ Ⓒ Ⓓ Ⓔ
210. Ⓐ Ⓑ Ⓒ Ⓓ Ⓔ
211. Ⓐ Ⓑ Ⓒ Ⓓ Ⓔ
212. Ⓐ Ⓑ Ⓒ Ⓓ Ⓔ
213. Ⓐ Ⓑ Ⓒ Ⓓ Ⓔ
214. Ⓐ Ⓑ Ⓒ Ⓓ Ⓔ
215. Ⓐ Ⓑ Ⓒ Ⓓ Ⓔ
216. Ⓐ Ⓑ Ⓒ Ⓓ Ⓔ
217. Ⓐ Ⓑ Ⓒ Ⓓ Ⓔ
218. Ⓐ Ⓑ Ⓒ Ⓓ Ⓔ
219. Ⓐ Ⓑ Ⓒ Ⓓ Ⓔ
220. Ⓐ Ⓑ Ⓒ Ⓓ Ⓔ
221. Ⓐ Ⓑ Ⓒ Ⓓ Ⓔ
222. Ⓐ Ⓑ Ⓒ Ⓓ Ⓔ
223. Ⓐ Ⓑ Ⓒ Ⓓ Ⓔ
224. Ⓐ Ⓑ Ⓒ Ⓓ Ⓔ
225. Ⓐ Ⓑ Ⓒ Ⓓ Ⓔ
226. Ⓐ Ⓑ Ⓒ Ⓓ Ⓔ
227. Ⓐ Ⓑ Ⓒ Ⓓ Ⓔ
228. Ⓐ Ⓑ Ⓒ Ⓓ Ⓔ
229. Ⓐ Ⓑ Ⓒ Ⓓ Ⓔ
230. Ⓐ Ⓑ Ⓒ Ⓓ Ⓔ
231. Ⓐ Ⓑ Ⓒ Ⓓ Ⓔ
232. Ⓐ Ⓑ Ⓒ Ⓓ Ⓔ
233. Ⓐ Ⓑ Ⓒ Ⓓ Ⓔ
234. Ⓐ Ⓑ Ⓒ Ⓓ Ⓔ
235. Ⓐ Ⓑ Ⓒ Ⓓ Ⓔ
236. Ⓐ Ⓑ Ⓒ Ⓓ Ⓔ
237. Ⓐ Ⓑ Ⓒ Ⓓ Ⓔ
238. Ⓐ Ⓑ Ⓒ Ⓓ Ⓔ
239. Ⓐ Ⓑ Ⓒ Ⓓ Ⓔ
240. Ⓐ Ⓑ Ⓒ Ⓓ Ⓔ
241. Ⓐ Ⓑ Ⓒ Ⓓ Ⓔ Ⓕ Ⓖ
242. Ⓐ Ⓑ Ⓒ Ⓓ Ⓔ Ⓕ Ⓖ
243. Ⓐ Ⓑ Ⓒ Ⓓ Ⓔ Ⓕ Ⓖ
244. Ⓐ Ⓑ Ⓒ Ⓓ Ⓔ Ⓕ Ⓖ
245. Ⓐ Ⓑ Ⓒ Ⓓ Ⓔ Ⓕ Ⓖ
246. Ⓐ Ⓑ Ⓒ Ⓓ Ⓔ Ⓕ Ⓖ
247. Ⓐ Ⓑ Ⓒ Ⓓ Ⓔ Ⓕ Ⓖ
248. Ⓐ Ⓑ Ⓒ Ⓓ Ⓔ
249. Ⓐ Ⓑ Ⓒ Ⓓ Ⓔ
250. Ⓐ Ⓑ Ⓒ Ⓓ Ⓔ
251. Ⓐ Ⓑ Ⓒ Ⓓ Ⓔ

252. Ⓐ Ⓑ Ⓒ Ⓓ Ⓔ
253. Ⓐ Ⓑ Ⓒ Ⓓ Ⓔ
254. Ⓐ Ⓑ Ⓒ Ⓓ Ⓔ
255. Ⓐ Ⓑ Ⓒ Ⓓ Ⓔ
256. Ⓐ Ⓑ Ⓒ Ⓓ Ⓔ
257. Ⓐ Ⓑ Ⓒ Ⓓ Ⓔ
258. Ⓐ Ⓑ Ⓒ Ⓓ Ⓔ
259. Ⓐ Ⓑ Ⓒ Ⓓ Ⓔ
260. Ⓐ Ⓑ Ⓒ Ⓓ Ⓔ
261. Ⓐ Ⓑ Ⓒ Ⓓ Ⓔ
262. Ⓐ Ⓑ Ⓒ Ⓓ Ⓔ
263. Ⓐ Ⓑ Ⓒ Ⓓ Ⓔ
264. Ⓐ Ⓑ Ⓒ Ⓓ Ⓔ
265. Ⓐ Ⓑ Ⓒ Ⓓ Ⓔ
266. Ⓐ Ⓑ Ⓒ Ⓓ Ⓔ
267. Ⓐ Ⓑ Ⓒ Ⓓ Ⓔ
268. Ⓐ Ⓑ Ⓒ Ⓓ Ⓔ
269. Ⓐ Ⓑ Ⓒ Ⓓ Ⓔ
270. Ⓐ Ⓑ Ⓒ Ⓓ Ⓔ
271. Ⓐ Ⓑ Ⓒ Ⓓ Ⓔ
272. Ⓐ Ⓑ Ⓒ Ⓓ Ⓔ
273. Ⓐ Ⓑ Ⓒ Ⓓ Ⓔ
274. Ⓐ Ⓑ Ⓒ Ⓓ Ⓔ
275. Ⓐ Ⓑ Ⓒ Ⓓ Ⓔ
276. Ⓐ Ⓑ Ⓒ Ⓓ Ⓔ
277. Ⓐ Ⓑ Ⓒ Ⓓ Ⓔ
278. Ⓐ Ⓑ Ⓒ Ⓓ Ⓔ
279. Ⓐ Ⓑ Ⓒ Ⓓ Ⓔ
280. Ⓐ Ⓑ Ⓒ Ⓓ Ⓔ
281. Ⓐ Ⓑ Ⓒ Ⓓ Ⓔ
282. Ⓐ Ⓑ Ⓒ Ⓓ Ⓔ
283. Ⓐ Ⓑ Ⓒ Ⓓ Ⓔ
284. Ⓐ Ⓑ Ⓒ Ⓓ Ⓔ
285. Ⓐ Ⓑ Ⓒ Ⓓ Ⓔ
286. Ⓐ Ⓑ Ⓒ Ⓓ Ⓔ
287. Ⓐ Ⓑ Ⓒ Ⓓ Ⓔ
288. Ⓐ Ⓑ Ⓒ Ⓓ Ⓔ
289. Ⓐ Ⓑ Ⓒ Ⓓ Ⓔ
290. Ⓐ Ⓑ Ⓒ Ⓓ Ⓔ
291. Ⓐ Ⓑ Ⓒ Ⓓ Ⓔ
292. Ⓐ Ⓑ Ⓒ Ⓓ Ⓔ
293. Ⓐ Ⓑ Ⓒ Ⓓ Ⓔ
294. Ⓐ Ⓑ Ⓒ Ⓓ Ⓔ
295. Ⓐ Ⓑ Ⓒ Ⓓ Ⓔ
296. Ⓐ Ⓑ Ⓒ Ⓓ Ⓔ
297. Ⓐ Ⓑ Ⓒ Ⓓ Ⓔ
298. Ⓐ Ⓑ Ⓒ Ⓓ Ⓔ
299. Ⓐ Ⓑ Ⓒ Ⓓ Ⓔ
300. Ⓐ Ⓑ Ⓒ Ⓓ Ⓔ

Answer Sheet for Comprehensive Practice Exam

Name _____ Date _____
    Last   First   Middle

Directions:

1. Using pencil, fill in only one circle representing your answer for each question.
2. Keeping your marks inside the circle, blacken the circle completely.
3. Completely erase any answer you wish to change, and make no stray marks.

Correct: Ⓐ ● Ⓒ Ⓓ Ⓔ Ⓕ Ⓖ Ⓗ Ⓘ Ⓙ   Wrong: Ⓧ ⓐ ○ Ⓓ Ⓔ Ⓕ Ⓖ Ⓗ Ⓘ Ⓙ

1. Ⓐ Ⓑ Ⓒ Ⓓ Ⓔ	27. Ⓐ Ⓑ Ⓒ Ⓓ Ⓔ	53. Ⓐ Ⓑ Ⓒ Ⓓ Ⓔ	79. Ⓐ Ⓑ Ⓒ Ⓓ Ⓔ
2. Ⓐ Ⓑ Ⓒ Ⓓ Ⓔ	28. Ⓐ Ⓑ Ⓒ Ⓓ Ⓔ	54. Ⓐ Ⓑ Ⓒ Ⓓ Ⓔ	80. Ⓐ Ⓑ Ⓒ Ⓓ Ⓔ
3. Ⓐ Ⓑ Ⓒ Ⓓ Ⓔ	29. Ⓐ Ⓑ Ⓒ Ⓓ Ⓔ	55. Ⓐ Ⓑ Ⓒ Ⓓ Ⓔ	81. Ⓐ Ⓑ Ⓒ Ⓓ Ⓔ
4. Ⓐ Ⓑ Ⓒ Ⓓ Ⓔ	30. Ⓐ Ⓑ Ⓒ Ⓓ Ⓔ	56. Ⓐ Ⓑ Ⓒ Ⓓ Ⓔ	82. Ⓐ Ⓑ Ⓒ Ⓓ Ⓔ
5. Ⓐ Ⓑ Ⓒ Ⓓ Ⓔ	31. Ⓐ Ⓑ Ⓒ Ⓓ Ⓔ	57. Ⓐ Ⓑ Ⓒ Ⓓ Ⓔ Ⓕ Ⓖ Ⓗ	83. Ⓐ Ⓑ Ⓒ Ⓓ Ⓔ
6. Ⓐ Ⓑ Ⓒ Ⓓ Ⓔ	32. Ⓐ Ⓑ Ⓒ Ⓓ Ⓔ	58. Ⓐ Ⓑ Ⓒ Ⓓ Ⓔ Ⓕ Ⓖ Ⓗ	84. Ⓐ Ⓑ Ⓒ Ⓓ Ⓔ
7. Ⓐ Ⓑ Ⓒ Ⓓ Ⓔ	33. Ⓐ Ⓑ Ⓒ Ⓓ Ⓔ	59. Ⓐ Ⓑ Ⓒ Ⓓ Ⓔ Ⓕ Ⓖ Ⓗ	85. Ⓐ Ⓑ Ⓒ Ⓓ Ⓔ
8. Ⓐ Ⓑ Ⓒ Ⓓ Ⓔ	34. Ⓐ Ⓑ Ⓒ Ⓓ Ⓔ	60. Ⓐ Ⓑ Ⓒ Ⓓ Ⓔ Ⓕ Ⓖ Ⓗ	86. Ⓐ Ⓑ Ⓒ Ⓓ Ⓔ
9. Ⓐ Ⓑ Ⓒ Ⓓ Ⓔ	35. Ⓐ Ⓑ Ⓒ Ⓓ Ⓔ	61. Ⓐ Ⓑ Ⓒ Ⓓ Ⓔ Ⓕ Ⓖ Ⓗ	87. Ⓐ Ⓑ Ⓒ Ⓓ Ⓔ
10. Ⓐ Ⓑ Ⓒ Ⓓ Ⓔ	36. Ⓐ Ⓑ Ⓒ Ⓓ Ⓔ	62. Ⓐ Ⓑ Ⓒ Ⓓ Ⓔ Ⓕ Ⓖ Ⓗ	88. Ⓐ Ⓑ Ⓒ Ⓓ Ⓔ
11. Ⓐ Ⓑ Ⓒ Ⓓ Ⓔ	37. Ⓐ Ⓑ Ⓒ Ⓓ Ⓔ	63. Ⓐ Ⓑ Ⓒ Ⓓ Ⓔ Ⓕ Ⓖ Ⓗ	89. Ⓐ Ⓑ Ⓒ Ⓓ Ⓔ
12. Ⓐ Ⓑ Ⓒ Ⓓ Ⓔ	38. Ⓐ Ⓑ Ⓒ Ⓓ Ⓔ	64. Ⓐ Ⓑ Ⓒ Ⓓ Ⓔ Ⓕ Ⓖ Ⓗ	90. Ⓐ Ⓑ Ⓒ Ⓓ Ⓔ
13. Ⓐ Ⓑ Ⓒ Ⓓ Ⓔ	39. Ⓐ Ⓑ Ⓒ Ⓓ Ⓔ	65. Ⓐ Ⓑ Ⓒ Ⓓ Ⓔ	91. Ⓐ Ⓑ Ⓒ Ⓓ Ⓔ
14. Ⓐ Ⓑ Ⓒ Ⓓ Ⓔ	40. Ⓐ Ⓑ Ⓒ Ⓓ Ⓔ	66. Ⓐ Ⓑ Ⓒ Ⓓ Ⓔ	92. Ⓐ Ⓑ Ⓒ Ⓓ Ⓔ
15. Ⓐ Ⓑ Ⓒ Ⓓ Ⓔ	41. Ⓐ Ⓑ Ⓒ Ⓓ Ⓔ	67. Ⓐ Ⓑ Ⓒ Ⓓ Ⓔ	93. Ⓐ Ⓑ Ⓒ Ⓓ Ⓔ
16. Ⓐ Ⓑ Ⓒ Ⓓ Ⓔ	42. Ⓐ Ⓑ Ⓒ Ⓓ Ⓔ	68. Ⓐ Ⓑ Ⓒ Ⓓ Ⓔ Ⓕ	94. Ⓐ Ⓑ Ⓒ Ⓓ Ⓔ
17. Ⓐ Ⓑ Ⓒ Ⓓ Ⓔ	43. Ⓐ Ⓑ Ⓒ Ⓓ Ⓔ	69. Ⓐ Ⓑ Ⓒ Ⓓ Ⓔ Ⓕ	95. Ⓐ Ⓑ Ⓒ Ⓓ Ⓔ
18. Ⓐ Ⓑ Ⓒ Ⓓ Ⓔ	44. Ⓐ Ⓑ Ⓒ Ⓓ Ⓔ	70. Ⓐ Ⓑ Ⓒ Ⓓ Ⓔ Ⓕ	96. Ⓐ Ⓑ Ⓒ Ⓓ Ⓔ
19. Ⓐ Ⓑ Ⓒ Ⓓ Ⓔ	45. Ⓐ Ⓑ Ⓒ Ⓓ Ⓔ	71. Ⓐ Ⓑ Ⓒ Ⓓ Ⓔ Ⓕ	97. Ⓐ Ⓑ Ⓒ Ⓓ Ⓔ
20. Ⓐ Ⓑ Ⓒ Ⓓ Ⓔ	46. Ⓐ Ⓑ Ⓒ Ⓓ Ⓔ	72. Ⓐ Ⓑ Ⓒ Ⓓ Ⓔ Ⓕ	98. Ⓐ Ⓑ Ⓒ Ⓓ Ⓔ
21. Ⓐ Ⓑ Ⓒ Ⓓ Ⓔ	47. Ⓐ Ⓑ Ⓒ Ⓓ Ⓔ	73. Ⓐ Ⓑ Ⓒ Ⓓ Ⓔ Ⓕ	99. Ⓐ Ⓑ Ⓒ Ⓓ Ⓔ
22. Ⓐ Ⓑ Ⓒ Ⓓ Ⓔ	48. Ⓐ Ⓑ Ⓒ Ⓓ Ⓔ	74. Ⓐ Ⓑ Ⓒ Ⓓ Ⓔ	100. Ⓐ Ⓑ Ⓒ Ⓓ Ⓔ
23. Ⓐ Ⓑ Ⓒ Ⓓ Ⓔ	49. Ⓐ Ⓑ Ⓒ Ⓓ Ⓔ	75. Ⓐ Ⓑ Ⓒ Ⓓ Ⓔ	101. Ⓐ Ⓑ Ⓒ Ⓓ Ⓔ
24. Ⓐ Ⓑ Ⓒ Ⓓ Ⓔ	50. Ⓐ Ⓑ Ⓒ Ⓓ Ⓔ	76. Ⓐ Ⓑ Ⓒ Ⓓ Ⓔ	102. Ⓐ Ⓑ Ⓒ Ⓓ Ⓔ
25. Ⓐ Ⓑ Ⓒ Ⓓ Ⓔ	51. Ⓐ Ⓑ Ⓒ Ⓓ Ⓔ	77. Ⓐ Ⓑ Ⓒ Ⓓ Ⓔ	103. Ⓐ Ⓑ Ⓒ Ⓓ Ⓔ
26. Ⓐ Ⓑ Ⓒ Ⓓ Ⓔ	52. Ⓐ Ⓑ Ⓒ Ⓓ Ⓔ	78. Ⓐ Ⓑ Ⓒ Ⓓ Ⓔ	104. Ⓐ Ⓑ Ⓒ Ⓓ Ⓔ

105. Ⓐ Ⓑ Ⓒ Ⓓ Ⓔ	154. Ⓐ Ⓑ Ⓒ Ⓓ Ⓔ	203. Ⓐ Ⓑ Ⓒ Ⓓ Ⓔ	252. Ⓐ Ⓑ Ⓒ Ⓓ Ⓔ
106. Ⓐ Ⓑ Ⓒ Ⓓ Ⓔ	155. Ⓐ Ⓑ Ⓒ Ⓓ Ⓔ	204. Ⓐ Ⓑ Ⓒ Ⓓ Ⓔ	253. Ⓐ Ⓑ Ⓒ Ⓓ Ⓔ
107. Ⓐ Ⓑ Ⓒ Ⓓ Ⓔ	156. Ⓐ Ⓑ Ⓒ Ⓓ Ⓔ	205. Ⓐ Ⓑ Ⓒ Ⓓ Ⓔ	254. Ⓐ Ⓑ Ⓒ Ⓓ Ⓔ
108. Ⓐ Ⓑ Ⓒ Ⓓ Ⓔ	157. Ⓐ Ⓑ Ⓒ Ⓓ Ⓔ	206. Ⓐ Ⓑ Ⓒ Ⓓ Ⓔ	255. Ⓐ Ⓑ Ⓒ Ⓓ Ⓔ
109. Ⓐ Ⓑ Ⓒ Ⓓ Ⓔ	158. Ⓐ Ⓑ Ⓒ Ⓓ Ⓔ	207. Ⓐ Ⓑ Ⓒ Ⓓ Ⓔ	256. Ⓐ Ⓑ Ⓒ Ⓓ Ⓔ
110. Ⓐ Ⓑ Ⓒ Ⓓ Ⓔ	159. Ⓐ Ⓑ Ⓒ Ⓓ Ⓔ	208. Ⓐ Ⓑ Ⓒ Ⓓ Ⓔ	257. Ⓐ Ⓑ Ⓒ Ⓓ Ⓔ
111. Ⓐ Ⓑ Ⓒ Ⓓ Ⓔ	160. Ⓐ Ⓑ Ⓒ Ⓓ Ⓔ	209. Ⓐ Ⓑ Ⓒ Ⓓ Ⓔ	258. Ⓐ Ⓑ Ⓒ Ⓓ Ⓔ
112. Ⓐ Ⓑ Ⓒ Ⓓ Ⓔ	161. Ⓐ Ⓑ Ⓒ Ⓓ Ⓔ	210. Ⓐ Ⓑ Ⓒ Ⓓ Ⓔ	259. Ⓐ Ⓑ Ⓒ Ⓓ Ⓔ
113. Ⓐ Ⓑ Ⓒ Ⓓ Ⓔ	162. Ⓐ Ⓑ Ⓒ Ⓓ Ⓔ	211. Ⓐ Ⓑ Ⓒ Ⓓ Ⓔ	260. Ⓐ Ⓑ Ⓒ Ⓓ Ⓔ
114. Ⓐ Ⓑ Ⓒ Ⓓ Ⓔ	163. Ⓐ Ⓑ Ⓒ Ⓓ Ⓔ	212. Ⓐ Ⓑ Ⓒ Ⓓ Ⓔ	261. Ⓐ Ⓑ Ⓒ Ⓓ Ⓔ
115. Ⓐ Ⓑ Ⓒ Ⓓ Ⓔ	164. Ⓐ Ⓑ Ⓒ Ⓓ Ⓔ	213. Ⓐ Ⓑ Ⓒ Ⓓ Ⓔ	262. Ⓐ Ⓑ Ⓒ Ⓓ Ⓔ
116. Ⓐ Ⓑ Ⓒ Ⓓ Ⓔ	165. Ⓐ Ⓑ Ⓒ Ⓓ Ⓔ	214. Ⓐ Ⓑ Ⓒ Ⓓ Ⓔ	263. Ⓐ Ⓑ Ⓒ Ⓓ Ⓔ
117. Ⓐ Ⓑ Ⓒ Ⓓ Ⓔ	166. Ⓐ Ⓑ Ⓒ Ⓓ Ⓔ	215. Ⓐ Ⓑ Ⓒ Ⓓ Ⓔ	264. Ⓐ Ⓑ Ⓒ Ⓓ Ⓔ
118. Ⓐ Ⓑ Ⓒ Ⓓ Ⓔ	167. Ⓐ Ⓑ Ⓒ Ⓓ Ⓔ Ⓕ	216. Ⓐ Ⓑ Ⓒ Ⓓ Ⓔ	265. Ⓐ Ⓑ Ⓒ Ⓓ Ⓔ
119. Ⓐ Ⓑ Ⓒ Ⓓ Ⓔ	168. Ⓐ Ⓑ Ⓒ Ⓓ Ⓔ Ⓕ	217. Ⓐ Ⓑ Ⓒ Ⓓ Ⓔ	266. Ⓐ Ⓑ Ⓒ Ⓓ Ⓔ
120. Ⓐ Ⓑ Ⓒ Ⓓ Ⓔ	169. Ⓐ Ⓑ Ⓒ Ⓓ Ⓔ Ⓕ	218. Ⓐ Ⓑ Ⓒ Ⓓ Ⓔ	267. Ⓐ Ⓑ Ⓒ Ⓓ Ⓔ
121. Ⓐ Ⓑ Ⓒ Ⓓ Ⓔ	170. Ⓐ Ⓑ Ⓒ Ⓓ Ⓔ Ⓕ	219. Ⓐ Ⓑ Ⓒ Ⓓ Ⓔ	268. Ⓐ Ⓑ Ⓒ Ⓓ Ⓔ
122. Ⓐ Ⓑ Ⓒ Ⓓ Ⓔ	171. Ⓐ Ⓑ Ⓒ Ⓓ Ⓔ Ⓕ	220. Ⓐ Ⓑ Ⓒ Ⓓ Ⓔ	269. Ⓐ Ⓑ Ⓒ Ⓓ Ⓔ
123. Ⓐ Ⓑ Ⓒ Ⓓ Ⓔ	172. Ⓐ Ⓑ Ⓒ Ⓓ Ⓔ Ⓕ	221. Ⓐ Ⓑ Ⓒ Ⓓ Ⓔ	270. Ⓐ Ⓑ Ⓒ Ⓓ Ⓔ
124. Ⓐ Ⓑ Ⓒ Ⓓ Ⓔ	173. Ⓐ Ⓑ Ⓒ Ⓓ Ⓔ	222. Ⓐ Ⓑ Ⓒ Ⓓ Ⓔ	271. Ⓐ Ⓑ Ⓒ Ⓓ Ⓔ
125. Ⓐ Ⓑ Ⓒ Ⓓ Ⓔ	174. Ⓐ Ⓑ Ⓒ Ⓓ Ⓔ	223. Ⓐ Ⓑ Ⓒ Ⓓ Ⓔ	272. Ⓐ Ⓑ Ⓒ Ⓓ Ⓔ
126. Ⓐ Ⓑ Ⓒ Ⓓ Ⓔ	175. Ⓐ Ⓑ Ⓒ Ⓓ Ⓔ	224. Ⓐ Ⓑ Ⓒ Ⓓ Ⓔ	273. Ⓐ Ⓑ Ⓒ Ⓓ Ⓔ
127. Ⓐ Ⓑ Ⓒ Ⓓ Ⓔ	176. Ⓐ Ⓑ Ⓒ Ⓓ Ⓔ	225. Ⓐ Ⓑ Ⓒ Ⓓ Ⓔ	274. Ⓐ Ⓑ Ⓒ Ⓓ Ⓔ
128. Ⓐ Ⓑ Ⓒ Ⓓ Ⓔ	177. Ⓐ Ⓑ Ⓒ Ⓓ Ⓔ	226. Ⓐ Ⓑ Ⓒ Ⓓ Ⓔ	275. Ⓐ Ⓑ Ⓒ Ⓓ Ⓔ
129. Ⓐ Ⓑ Ⓒ Ⓓ Ⓔ	178. Ⓐ Ⓑ Ⓒ Ⓓ Ⓔ	227. Ⓐ Ⓑ Ⓒ Ⓓ Ⓔ	276. Ⓐ Ⓑ Ⓒ Ⓓ Ⓔ
130. Ⓐ Ⓑ Ⓒ Ⓓ Ⓔ	179. Ⓐ Ⓑ Ⓒ Ⓓ Ⓔ	228. Ⓐ Ⓑ Ⓒ Ⓓ Ⓔ	277. Ⓐ Ⓑ Ⓒ Ⓓ Ⓔ
131. Ⓐ Ⓑ Ⓒ Ⓓ Ⓔ	180. Ⓐ Ⓑ Ⓒ Ⓓ Ⓔ	229. Ⓐ Ⓑ Ⓒ Ⓓ Ⓔ	278. Ⓐ Ⓑ Ⓒ Ⓓ Ⓔ
132. Ⓐ Ⓑ Ⓒ Ⓓ Ⓔ	181. Ⓐ Ⓑ Ⓒ Ⓓ Ⓔ	230. Ⓐ Ⓑ Ⓒ Ⓓ Ⓔ	279. Ⓐ Ⓑ Ⓒ Ⓓ Ⓔ
133. Ⓐ Ⓑ Ⓒ Ⓓ Ⓔ	182. Ⓐ Ⓑ Ⓒ Ⓓ Ⓔ	231. Ⓐ Ⓑ Ⓒ Ⓓ Ⓔ	280. Ⓐ Ⓑ Ⓒ Ⓓ Ⓔ
134. Ⓐ Ⓑ Ⓒ Ⓓ Ⓔ	183. Ⓐ Ⓑ Ⓒ Ⓓ Ⓔ	232. Ⓐ Ⓑ Ⓒ Ⓓ Ⓔ	281. Ⓐ Ⓑ Ⓒ Ⓓ Ⓔ
135. Ⓐ Ⓑ Ⓒ Ⓓ Ⓔ	184. Ⓐ Ⓑ Ⓒ Ⓓ Ⓔ	233. Ⓐ Ⓑ Ⓒ Ⓓ Ⓔ	282. Ⓐ Ⓑ Ⓒ Ⓓ Ⓔ
136. Ⓐ Ⓑ Ⓒ Ⓓ Ⓔ	185. Ⓐ Ⓑ Ⓒ Ⓓ Ⓔ	234. Ⓐ Ⓑ Ⓒ Ⓓ Ⓔ	283. Ⓐ Ⓑ Ⓒ Ⓓ Ⓔ
137. Ⓐ Ⓑ Ⓒ Ⓓ Ⓔ	186. Ⓐ Ⓑ Ⓒ Ⓓ Ⓔ	235. Ⓐ Ⓑ Ⓒ Ⓓ Ⓔ	284. Ⓐ Ⓑ Ⓒ Ⓓ Ⓔ
138. Ⓐ Ⓑ Ⓒ Ⓓ Ⓔ	187. Ⓐ Ⓑ Ⓒ Ⓓ Ⓔ	236. Ⓐ Ⓑ Ⓒ Ⓓ Ⓔ	285. Ⓐ Ⓑ Ⓒ Ⓓ Ⓔ
139. Ⓐ Ⓑ Ⓒ Ⓓ Ⓔ	188. Ⓐ Ⓑ Ⓒ Ⓓ Ⓔ	237. Ⓐ Ⓑ Ⓒ Ⓓ Ⓔ	286. Ⓐ Ⓑ Ⓒ Ⓓ Ⓔ
140. Ⓐ Ⓑ Ⓒ Ⓓ Ⓔ	189. Ⓐ Ⓑ Ⓒ Ⓓ Ⓔ	238. Ⓐ Ⓑ Ⓒ Ⓓ Ⓔ	287. Ⓐ Ⓑ Ⓒ Ⓓ Ⓔ
141. Ⓐ Ⓑ Ⓒ Ⓓ Ⓔ	190. Ⓐ Ⓑ Ⓒ Ⓓ Ⓔ	239. Ⓐ Ⓑ Ⓒ Ⓓ Ⓔ	288. Ⓐ Ⓑ Ⓒ Ⓓ Ⓔ
142. Ⓐ Ⓑ Ⓒ Ⓓ Ⓔ	191. Ⓐ Ⓑ Ⓒ Ⓓ Ⓔ Ⓕ Ⓖ Ⓗ Ⓘ Ⓙ	240. Ⓐ Ⓑ Ⓒ Ⓓ Ⓔ	289. Ⓐ Ⓑ Ⓒ Ⓓ Ⓔ
143. Ⓐ Ⓑ Ⓒ Ⓓ Ⓔ	192. Ⓐ Ⓑ Ⓒ Ⓓ Ⓔ Ⓕ Ⓖ Ⓗ Ⓘ Ⓙ	241. Ⓐ Ⓑ Ⓒ Ⓓ Ⓔ Ⓕ Ⓖ	290. Ⓐ Ⓑ Ⓒ Ⓓ Ⓔ
144. Ⓐ Ⓑ Ⓒ Ⓓ Ⓔ	193. Ⓐ Ⓑ Ⓒ Ⓓ Ⓔ Ⓕ Ⓖ Ⓗ Ⓘ Ⓙ	242. Ⓐ Ⓑ Ⓒ Ⓓ Ⓔ Ⓕ Ⓖ	291. Ⓐ Ⓑ Ⓒ Ⓓ Ⓔ
145. Ⓐ Ⓑ Ⓒ Ⓓ Ⓔ	194. Ⓐ Ⓑ Ⓒ Ⓓ Ⓔ Ⓕ Ⓖ Ⓗ Ⓘ Ⓙ	243. Ⓐ Ⓑ Ⓒ Ⓓ Ⓔ Ⓕ Ⓖ	292. Ⓐ Ⓑ Ⓒ Ⓓ Ⓔ
146. Ⓐ Ⓑ Ⓒ Ⓓ Ⓔ	195. Ⓐ Ⓑ Ⓒ Ⓓ Ⓔ Ⓕ Ⓖ Ⓗ Ⓘ Ⓙ	244. Ⓐ Ⓑ Ⓒ Ⓓ Ⓔ Ⓕ Ⓖ	293. Ⓐ Ⓑ Ⓒ Ⓓ Ⓔ
147. Ⓐ Ⓑ Ⓒ Ⓓ Ⓔ	196. Ⓐ Ⓑ Ⓒ Ⓓ Ⓔ Ⓕ Ⓖ Ⓗ Ⓘ Ⓙ	245. Ⓐ Ⓑ Ⓒ Ⓓ Ⓔ Ⓕ Ⓖ	294. Ⓐ Ⓑ Ⓒ Ⓓ Ⓔ
148. Ⓐ Ⓑ Ⓒ Ⓓ Ⓔ	197. Ⓐ Ⓑ Ⓒ Ⓓ Ⓔ Ⓕ Ⓖ Ⓗ Ⓘ Ⓙ	246. Ⓐ Ⓑ Ⓒ Ⓓ Ⓔ Ⓕ Ⓖ	295. Ⓐ Ⓑ Ⓒ Ⓓ Ⓔ
149. Ⓐ Ⓑ Ⓒ Ⓓ Ⓔ	198. Ⓐ Ⓑ Ⓒ Ⓓ Ⓔ Ⓕ Ⓖ Ⓗ Ⓘ Ⓙ	247. Ⓐ Ⓑ Ⓒ Ⓓ Ⓔ Ⓕ Ⓖ	296. Ⓐ Ⓑ Ⓒ Ⓓ Ⓔ
150. Ⓐ Ⓑ Ⓒ Ⓓ Ⓔ	199. Ⓐ Ⓑ Ⓒ Ⓓ Ⓔ Ⓕ Ⓖ Ⓗ Ⓘ Ⓙ	248. Ⓐ Ⓑ Ⓒ Ⓓ Ⓔ	297. Ⓐ Ⓑ Ⓒ Ⓓ Ⓔ
151. Ⓐ Ⓑ Ⓒ Ⓓ Ⓔ	200. Ⓐ Ⓑ Ⓒ Ⓓ Ⓔ Ⓕ Ⓖ Ⓗ Ⓘ Ⓙ	249. Ⓐ Ⓑ Ⓒ Ⓓ Ⓔ	298. Ⓐ Ⓑ Ⓒ Ⓓ Ⓔ
152. Ⓐ Ⓑ Ⓒ Ⓓ Ⓔ	201. Ⓐ Ⓑ Ⓒ Ⓓ Ⓔ	250. Ⓐ Ⓑ Ⓒ Ⓓ Ⓔ	299. Ⓐ Ⓑ Ⓒ Ⓓ Ⓔ
153. Ⓐ Ⓑ Ⓒ Ⓓ Ⓔ	202. Ⓐ Ⓑ Ⓒ Ⓓ Ⓔ	251. Ⓐ Ⓑ Ⓒ Ⓓ Ⓔ	300. Ⓐ Ⓑ Ⓒ Ⓓ Ⓔ

Answer Sheet for Comprehensive Practice Exam

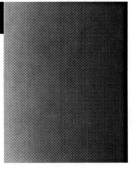

Name _____ Date _____

       Last   First   Middle

Directions:

1. Using pencil, fill in only one circle representing your answer for each question.
2. Keeping your marks inside the circle, blacken the circle completely.
3. Completely erase any answer you wish to change, and make no stray marks.

Correct: Ⓐ ● Ⓒ Ⓓ Ⓔ Ⓕ Ⓖ Ⓗ Ⓘ Ⓙ   Wrong: Ⓧ ⊜ ○ ⊘ ⊘ Ⓕ Ⓖ Ⓗ Ⓘ Ⓙ

1. Ⓐ Ⓑ Ⓒ Ⓓ Ⓔ
2. Ⓐ Ⓑ Ⓒ Ⓓ Ⓔ
3. Ⓐ Ⓑ Ⓒ Ⓓ Ⓔ
4. Ⓐ Ⓑ Ⓒ Ⓓ Ⓔ
5. Ⓐ Ⓑ Ⓒ Ⓓ Ⓔ
6. Ⓐ Ⓑ Ⓒ Ⓓ Ⓔ
7. Ⓐ Ⓑ Ⓒ Ⓓ Ⓔ
8. Ⓐ Ⓑ Ⓒ Ⓓ Ⓔ
9. Ⓐ Ⓑ Ⓒ Ⓓ Ⓔ
10. Ⓐ Ⓑ Ⓒ Ⓓ Ⓔ
11. Ⓐ Ⓑ Ⓒ Ⓓ Ⓔ
12. Ⓐ Ⓑ Ⓒ Ⓓ Ⓔ
13. Ⓐ Ⓑ Ⓒ Ⓓ Ⓔ
14. Ⓐ Ⓑ Ⓒ Ⓓ Ⓔ
15. Ⓐ Ⓑ Ⓒ Ⓓ Ⓔ
16. Ⓐ Ⓑ Ⓒ Ⓓ Ⓔ
17. Ⓐ Ⓑ Ⓒ Ⓓ Ⓔ
18. Ⓐ Ⓑ Ⓒ Ⓓ Ⓔ
19. Ⓐ Ⓑ Ⓒ Ⓓ Ⓔ
20. Ⓐ Ⓑ Ⓒ Ⓓ Ⓔ
21. Ⓐ Ⓑ Ⓒ Ⓓ Ⓔ
22. Ⓐ Ⓑ Ⓒ Ⓓ Ⓔ
23. Ⓐ Ⓑ Ⓒ Ⓓ Ⓔ
24. Ⓐ Ⓑ Ⓒ Ⓓ Ⓔ
25. Ⓐ Ⓑ Ⓒ Ⓓ Ⓔ
26. Ⓐ Ⓑ Ⓒ Ⓓ Ⓔ

27. Ⓐ Ⓑ Ⓒ Ⓓ Ⓔ
28. Ⓐ Ⓑ Ⓒ Ⓓ Ⓔ
29. Ⓐ Ⓑ Ⓒ Ⓓ Ⓔ
30. Ⓐ Ⓑ Ⓒ Ⓓ Ⓔ
31. Ⓐ Ⓑ Ⓒ Ⓓ Ⓔ
32. Ⓐ Ⓑ Ⓒ Ⓓ Ⓔ
33. Ⓐ Ⓑ Ⓒ Ⓓ Ⓔ
34. Ⓐ Ⓑ Ⓒ Ⓓ Ⓔ
35. Ⓐ Ⓑ Ⓒ Ⓓ Ⓔ
36. Ⓐ Ⓑ Ⓒ Ⓓ Ⓔ
37. Ⓐ Ⓑ Ⓒ Ⓓ Ⓔ
38. Ⓐ Ⓑ Ⓒ Ⓓ Ⓔ
39. Ⓐ Ⓑ Ⓒ Ⓓ Ⓔ
40. Ⓐ Ⓑ Ⓒ Ⓓ Ⓔ
41. Ⓐ Ⓑ Ⓒ Ⓓ Ⓔ
42. Ⓐ Ⓑ Ⓒ Ⓓ Ⓔ
43. Ⓐ Ⓑ Ⓒ Ⓓ Ⓔ
44. Ⓐ Ⓑ Ⓒ Ⓓ Ⓔ
45. Ⓐ Ⓑ Ⓒ Ⓓ Ⓔ
46. Ⓐ Ⓑ Ⓒ Ⓓ Ⓔ
47. Ⓐ Ⓑ Ⓒ Ⓓ Ⓔ
48. Ⓐ Ⓑ Ⓒ Ⓓ Ⓔ
49. Ⓐ Ⓑ Ⓒ Ⓓ Ⓔ
50. Ⓐ Ⓑ Ⓒ Ⓓ Ⓔ
51. Ⓐ Ⓑ Ⓒ Ⓓ Ⓔ
52. Ⓐ Ⓑ Ⓒ Ⓓ Ⓔ

53. Ⓐ Ⓑ Ⓒ Ⓓ Ⓔ
54. Ⓐ Ⓑ Ⓒ Ⓓ Ⓔ
55. Ⓐ Ⓑ Ⓒ Ⓓ Ⓔ
56. Ⓐ Ⓑ Ⓒ Ⓓ Ⓔ
57. Ⓐ Ⓑ Ⓒ Ⓓ Ⓔ Ⓕ Ⓖ Ⓗ
58. Ⓐ Ⓑ Ⓒ Ⓓ Ⓔ Ⓕ Ⓖ Ⓗ
59. Ⓐ Ⓑ Ⓒ Ⓓ Ⓔ Ⓕ Ⓖ Ⓗ
60. Ⓐ Ⓑ Ⓒ Ⓓ Ⓔ Ⓕ Ⓖ Ⓗ
61. Ⓐ Ⓑ Ⓒ Ⓓ Ⓔ Ⓕ Ⓖ Ⓗ
62. Ⓐ Ⓑ Ⓒ Ⓓ Ⓔ Ⓕ Ⓖ Ⓗ
63. Ⓐ Ⓑ Ⓒ Ⓓ Ⓔ Ⓕ Ⓖ Ⓗ
64. Ⓐ Ⓑ Ⓒ Ⓓ Ⓔ Ⓕ Ⓖ Ⓗ
65. Ⓐ Ⓑ Ⓒ Ⓓ Ⓔ
66. Ⓐ Ⓑ Ⓒ Ⓓ Ⓔ
67. Ⓐ Ⓑ Ⓒ Ⓓ Ⓔ
68. Ⓐ Ⓑ Ⓒ Ⓓ Ⓔ Ⓕ
69. Ⓐ Ⓑ Ⓒ Ⓓ Ⓔ Ⓕ
70. Ⓐ Ⓑ Ⓒ Ⓓ Ⓔ Ⓕ
71. Ⓐ Ⓑ Ⓒ Ⓓ Ⓔ Ⓕ
72. Ⓐ Ⓑ Ⓒ Ⓓ Ⓔ Ⓕ
73. Ⓐ Ⓑ Ⓒ Ⓓ Ⓔ Ⓕ
74. Ⓐ Ⓑ Ⓒ Ⓓ Ⓔ
75. Ⓐ Ⓑ Ⓒ Ⓓ Ⓔ
76. Ⓐ Ⓑ Ⓒ Ⓓ Ⓔ
77. Ⓐ Ⓑ Ⓒ Ⓓ Ⓔ
78. Ⓐ Ⓑ Ⓒ Ⓓ Ⓔ

79. Ⓐ Ⓑ Ⓒ Ⓓ Ⓔ
80. Ⓐ Ⓑ Ⓒ Ⓓ Ⓔ
81. Ⓐ Ⓑ Ⓒ Ⓓ Ⓔ
82. Ⓐ Ⓑ Ⓒ Ⓓ Ⓔ
83. Ⓐ Ⓑ Ⓒ Ⓓ Ⓔ
84. Ⓐ Ⓑ Ⓒ Ⓓ Ⓔ
85. Ⓐ Ⓑ Ⓒ Ⓓ Ⓔ
86. Ⓐ Ⓑ Ⓒ Ⓓ Ⓔ
87. Ⓐ Ⓑ Ⓒ Ⓓ Ⓔ
88. Ⓐ Ⓑ Ⓒ Ⓓ Ⓔ
89. Ⓐ Ⓑ Ⓒ Ⓓ Ⓔ
90. Ⓐ Ⓑ Ⓒ Ⓓ Ⓔ
91. Ⓐ Ⓑ Ⓒ Ⓓ Ⓔ
92. Ⓐ Ⓑ Ⓒ Ⓓ Ⓔ
93. Ⓐ Ⓑ Ⓒ Ⓓ Ⓔ
94. Ⓐ Ⓑ Ⓒ Ⓓ Ⓔ
95. Ⓐ Ⓑ Ⓒ Ⓓ Ⓔ
96. Ⓐ Ⓑ Ⓒ Ⓓ Ⓔ
97. Ⓐ Ⓑ Ⓒ Ⓓ Ⓔ
98. Ⓐ Ⓑ Ⓒ Ⓓ Ⓔ
99. Ⓐ Ⓑ Ⓒ Ⓓ Ⓔ
100. Ⓐ Ⓑ Ⓒ Ⓓ Ⓔ
101. Ⓐ Ⓑ Ⓒ Ⓓ Ⓔ
102. Ⓐ Ⓑ Ⓒ Ⓓ Ⓔ
103. Ⓐ Ⓑ Ⓒ Ⓓ Ⓔ
104. Ⓐ Ⓑ Ⓒ Ⓓ Ⓔ

105. Ⓐ Ⓑ Ⓒ Ⓓ Ⓔ
106. Ⓐ Ⓑ Ⓒ Ⓓ Ⓔ
107. Ⓐ Ⓑ Ⓒ Ⓓ Ⓔ
108. Ⓐ Ⓑ Ⓒ Ⓓ Ⓔ
109. Ⓐ Ⓑ Ⓒ Ⓓ Ⓔ
110. Ⓐ Ⓑ Ⓒ Ⓓ Ⓔ
111. Ⓐ Ⓑ Ⓒ Ⓓ Ⓔ
112. Ⓐ Ⓑ Ⓒ Ⓓ Ⓔ
113. Ⓐ Ⓑ Ⓒ Ⓓ Ⓔ
114. Ⓐ Ⓑ Ⓒ Ⓓ Ⓔ
115. Ⓐ Ⓑ Ⓒ Ⓓ Ⓔ
116. Ⓐ Ⓑ Ⓒ Ⓓ Ⓔ
117. Ⓐ Ⓑ Ⓒ Ⓓ Ⓔ
118. Ⓐ Ⓑ Ⓒ Ⓓ Ⓔ
119. Ⓐ Ⓑ Ⓒ Ⓓ Ⓔ
120. Ⓐ Ⓑ Ⓒ Ⓓ Ⓔ
121. Ⓐ Ⓑ Ⓒ Ⓓ Ⓔ
122. Ⓐ Ⓑ Ⓒ Ⓓ Ⓔ
123. Ⓐ Ⓑ Ⓒ Ⓓ Ⓔ
124. Ⓐ Ⓑ Ⓒ Ⓓ Ⓔ
125. Ⓐ Ⓑ Ⓒ Ⓓ Ⓔ
126. Ⓐ Ⓑ Ⓒ Ⓓ Ⓔ
127. Ⓐ Ⓑ Ⓒ Ⓓ Ⓔ
128. Ⓐ Ⓑ Ⓒ Ⓓ Ⓔ
129. Ⓐ Ⓑ Ⓒ Ⓓ Ⓔ
130. Ⓐ Ⓑ Ⓒ Ⓓ Ⓔ
131. Ⓐ Ⓑ Ⓒ Ⓓ Ⓔ
132. Ⓐ Ⓑ Ⓒ Ⓓ Ⓔ
133. Ⓐ Ⓑ Ⓒ Ⓓ Ⓔ
134. Ⓐ Ⓑ Ⓒ Ⓓ Ⓔ
135. Ⓐ Ⓑ Ⓒ Ⓓ Ⓔ
136. Ⓐ Ⓑ Ⓒ Ⓓ Ⓔ
137. Ⓐ Ⓑ Ⓒ Ⓓ Ⓔ
138. Ⓐ Ⓑ Ⓒ Ⓓ Ⓔ
139. Ⓐ Ⓑ Ⓒ Ⓓ Ⓔ
140. Ⓐ Ⓑ Ⓒ Ⓓ Ⓔ
141. Ⓐ Ⓑ Ⓒ Ⓓ Ⓔ
142. Ⓐ Ⓑ Ⓒ Ⓓ Ⓔ
143. Ⓐ Ⓑ Ⓒ Ⓓ Ⓔ
144. Ⓐ Ⓑ Ⓒ Ⓓ Ⓔ
145. Ⓐ Ⓑ Ⓒ Ⓓ Ⓔ
146. Ⓐ Ⓑ Ⓒ Ⓓ Ⓔ
147. Ⓐ Ⓑ Ⓒ Ⓓ Ⓔ
148. Ⓐ Ⓑ Ⓒ Ⓓ Ⓔ
149. Ⓐ Ⓑ Ⓒ Ⓓ Ⓔ
150. Ⓐ Ⓑ Ⓒ Ⓓ Ⓔ
151. Ⓐ Ⓑ Ⓒ Ⓓ Ⓔ
152. Ⓐ Ⓑ Ⓒ Ⓓ Ⓔ
153. Ⓐ Ⓑ Ⓒ Ⓓ Ⓔ

154. Ⓐ Ⓑ Ⓒ Ⓓ Ⓔ
155. Ⓐ Ⓑ Ⓒ Ⓓ Ⓔ
156. Ⓐ Ⓑ Ⓒ Ⓓ Ⓔ
157. Ⓐ Ⓑ Ⓒ Ⓓ Ⓔ
158. Ⓐ Ⓑ Ⓒ Ⓓ Ⓔ
159. Ⓐ Ⓑ Ⓒ Ⓓ Ⓔ
160. Ⓐ Ⓑ Ⓒ Ⓓ Ⓔ
161. Ⓐ Ⓑ Ⓒ Ⓓ Ⓔ
162. Ⓐ Ⓑ Ⓒ Ⓓ Ⓔ
163. Ⓐ Ⓑ Ⓒ Ⓓ Ⓔ
164. Ⓐ Ⓑ Ⓒ Ⓓ Ⓔ
165. Ⓐ Ⓑ Ⓒ Ⓓ Ⓔ
166. Ⓐ Ⓑ Ⓒ Ⓓ Ⓔ
167. Ⓐ Ⓑ Ⓒ Ⓓ Ⓔ Ⓕ
168. Ⓐ Ⓑ Ⓒ Ⓓ Ⓔ Ⓕ
169. Ⓐ Ⓑ Ⓒ Ⓓ Ⓔ Ⓕ
170. Ⓐ Ⓑ Ⓒ Ⓓ Ⓔ Ⓕ
171. Ⓐ Ⓑ Ⓒ Ⓓ Ⓔ Ⓕ
172. Ⓐ Ⓑ Ⓒ Ⓓ Ⓔ Ⓕ
173. Ⓐ Ⓑ Ⓒ Ⓓ Ⓔ
174. Ⓐ Ⓑ Ⓒ Ⓓ Ⓔ
175. Ⓐ Ⓑ Ⓒ Ⓓ Ⓔ
176. Ⓐ Ⓑ Ⓒ Ⓓ Ⓔ
177. Ⓐ Ⓑ Ⓒ Ⓓ Ⓔ
178. Ⓐ Ⓑ Ⓒ Ⓓ Ⓔ
179. Ⓐ Ⓑ Ⓒ Ⓓ Ⓔ
180. Ⓐ Ⓑ Ⓒ Ⓓ Ⓔ
181. Ⓐ Ⓑ Ⓒ Ⓓ Ⓔ
182. Ⓐ Ⓑ Ⓒ Ⓓ Ⓔ
183. Ⓐ Ⓑ Ⓒ Ⓓ Ⓔ
184. Ⓐ Ⓑ Ⓒ Ⓓ Ⓔ
185. Ⓐ Ⓑ Ⓒ Ⓓ Ⓔ
186. Ⓐ Ⓑ Ⓒ Ⓓ Ⓔ
187. Ⓐ Ⓑ Ⓒ Ⓓ Ⓔ
188. Ⓐ Ⓑ Ⓒ Ⓓ Ⓔ
189. Ⓐ Ⓑ Ⓒ Ⓓ Ⓔ
190. Ⓐ Ⓑ Ⓒ Ⓓ Ⓔ
191. Ⓐ Ⓑ Ⓒ Ⓓ Ⓔ Ⓕ Ⓖ Ⓗ Ⓘ Ⓙ
192. Ⓐ Ⓑ Ⓒ Ⓓ Ⓔ Ⓕ Ⓖ Ⓗ Ⓘ Ⓙ
193. Ⓐ Ⓑ Ⓒ Ⓓ Ⓔ Ⓕ Ⓖ Ⓗ Ⓘ Ⓙ
194. Ⓐ Ⓑ Ⓒ Ⓓ Ⓔ Ⓕ Ⓖ Ⓗ Ⓘ Ⓙ
195. Ⓐ Ⓑ Ⓒ Ⓓ Ⓔ Ⓕ Ⓖ Ⓗ Ⓘ Ⓙ
196. Ⓐ Ⓑ Ⓒ Ⓓ Ⓔ Ⓕ Ⓖ Ⓗ Ⓘ Ⓙ
197. Ⓐ Ⓑ Ⓒ Ⓓ Ⓔ Ⓕ Ⓖ Ⓗ Ⓘ Ⓙ
198. Ⓐ Ⓑ Ⓒ Ⓓ Ⓔ Ⓕ Ⓖ Ⓗ Ⓘ Ⓙ
199. Ⓐ Ⓑ Ⓒ Ⓓ Ⓔ Ⓕ Ⓖ Ⓗ Ⓘ Ⓙ
200. Ⓐ Ⓑ Ⓒ Ⓓ Ⓔ Ⓕ Ⓖ Ⓗ Ⓘ Ⓙ
201. Ⓐ Ⓑ Ⓒ Ⓓ Ⓔ
202. Ⓐ Ⓑ Ⓒ Ⓓ Ⓔ

203. Ⓐ Ⓑ Ⓒ Ⓓ Ⓔ
204. Ⓐ Ⓑ Ⓒ Ⓓ Ⓔ
205. Ⓐ Ⓑ Ⓒ Ⓓ Ⓔ
206. Ⓐ Ⓑ Ⓒ Ⓓ Ⓔ
207. Ⓐ Ⓑ Ⓒ Ⓓ Ⓔ
208. Ⓐ Ⓑ Ⓒ Ⓓ Ⓔ
209. Ⓐ Ⓑ Ⓒ Ⓓ Ⓔ
210. Ⓐ Ⓑ Ⓒ Ⓓ Ⓔ
211. Ⓐ Ⓑ Ⓒ Ⓓ Ⓔ
212. Ⓐ Ⓑ Ⓒ Ⓓ Ⓔ
213. Ⓐ Ⓑ Ⓒ Ⓓ Ⓔ
214. Ⓐ Ⓑ Ⓒ Ⓓ Ⓔ
215. Ⓐ Ⓑ Ⓒ Ⓓ Ⓔ
216. Ⓐ Ⓑ Ⓒ Ⓓ Ⓔ
217. Ⓐ Ⓑ Ⓒ Ⓓ Ⓔ
218. Ⓐ Ⓑ Ⓒ Ⓓ Ⓔ
219. Ⓐ Ⓑ Ⓒ Ⓓ Ⓔ
220. Ⓐ Ⓑ Ⓒ Ⓓ Ⓔ
221. Ⓐ Ⓑ Ⓒ Ⓓ Ⓔ
222. Ⓐ Ⓑ Ⓒ Ⓓ Ⓔ
223. Ⓐ Ⓑ Ⓒ Ⓓ Ⓔ
224. Ⓐ Ⓑ Ⓒ Ⓓ Ⓔ
225. Ⓐ Ⓑ Ⓒ Ⓓ Ⓔ
226. Ⓐ Ⓑ Ⓒ Ⓓ Ⓔ
227. Ⓐ Ⓑ Ⓒ Ⓓ Ⓔ
228. Ⓐ Ⓑ Ⓒ Ⓓ Ⓔ
229. Ⓐ Ⓑ Ⓒ Ⓓ Ⓔ
230. Ⓐ Ⓑ Ⓒ Ⓓ Ⓔ
231. Ⓐ Ⓑ Ⓒ Ⓓ Ⓔ
232. Ⓐ Ⓑ Ⓒ Ⓓ Ⓔ
233. Ⓐ Ⓑ Ⓒ Ⓓ Ⓔ
234. Ⓐ Ⓑ Ⓒ Ⓓ Ⓔ
235. Ⓐ Ⓑ Ⓒ Ⓓ Ⓔ
236. Ⓐ Ⓑ Ⓒ Ⓓ Ⓔ
237. Ⓐ Ⓑ Ⓒ Ⓓ Ⓔ
238. Ⓐ Ⓑ Ⓒ Ⓓ Ⓔ
239. Ⓐ Ⓑ Ⓒ Ⓓ Ⓔ
240. Ⓐ Ⓑ Ⓒ Ⓓ Ⓔ
241. Ⓐ Ⓑ Ⓒ Ⓓ Ⓔ Ⓕ Ⓖ
242. Ⓐ Ⓑ Ⓒ Ⓓ Ⓔ Ⓕ Ⓖ
243. Ⓐ Ⓑ Ⓒ Ⓓ Ⓔ Ⓕ Ⓖ
244. Ⓐ Ⓑ Ⓒ Ⓓ Ⓔ Ⓕ Ⓖ
245. Ⓐ Ⓑ Ⓒ Ⓓ Ⓔ Ⓕ Ⓖ
246. Ⓐ Ⓑ Ⓒ Ⓓ Ⓔ Ⓕ Ⓖ
247. Ⓐ Ⓑ Ⓒ Ⓓ Ⓔ Ⓕ Ⓖ
248. Ⓐ Ⓑ Ⓒ Ⓓ Ⓔ
249. Ⓐ Ⓑ Ⓒ Ⓓ Ⓔ
250. Ⓐ Ⓑ Ⓒ Ⓓ Ⓔ
251. Ⓐ Ⓑ Ⓒ Ⓓ Ⓔ

252. Ⓐ Ⓑ Ⓒ Ⓓ Ⓔ
253. Ⓐ Ⓑ Ⓒ Ⓓ Ⓔ
254. Ⓐ Ⓑ Ⓒ Ⓓ Ⓔ
255. Ⓐ Ⓑ Ⓒ Ⓓ Ⓔ
256. Ⓐ Ⓑ Ⓒ Ⓓ Ⓔ
257. Ⓐ Ⓑ Ⓒ Ⓓ Ⓔ
258. Ⓐ Ⓑ Ⓒ Ⓓ Ⓔ
259. Ⓐ Ⓑ Ⓒ Ⓓ Ⓔ
260. Ⓐ Ⓑ Ⓒ Ⓓ Ⓔ
261. Ⓐ Ⓑ Ⓒ Ⓓ Ⓔ
262. Ⓐ Ⓑ Ⓒ Ⓓ Ⓔ
263. Ⓐ Ⓑ Ⓒ Ⓓ Ⓔ
264. Ⓐ Ⓑ Ⓒ Ⓓ Ⓔ
265. Ⓐ Ⓑ Ⓒ Ⓓ Ⓔ
266. Ⓐ Ⓑ Ⓒ Ⓓ Ⓔ
267. Ⓐ Ⓑ Ⓒ Ⓓ Ⓔ
268. Ⓐ Ⓑ Ⓒ Ⓓ Ⓔ
269. Ⓐ Ⓑ Ⓒ Ⓓ Ⓔ
270. Ⓐ Ⓑ Ⓒ Ⓓ Ⓔ
271. Ⓐ Ⓑ Ⓒ Ⓓ Ⓔ
272. Ⓐ Ⓑ Ⓒ Ⓓ Ⓔ
273. Ⓐ Ⓑ Ⓒ Ⓓ Ⓔ
274. Ⓐ Ⓑ Ⓒ Ⓓ Ⓔ
275. Ⓐ Ⓑ Ⓒ Ⓓ Ⓔ
276. Ⓐ Ⓑ Ⓒ Ⓓ Ⓔ
277. Ⓐ Ⓑ Ⓒ Ⓓ Ⓔ
278. Ⓐ Ⓑ Ⓒ Ⓓ Ⓔ
279. Ⓐ Ⓑ Ⓒ Ⓓ Ⓔ
280. Ⓐ Ⓑ Ⓒ Ⓓ Ⓔ
281. Ⓐ Ⓑ Ⓒ Ⓓ Ⓔ
282. Ⓐ Ⓑ Ⓒ Ⓓ Ⓔ
283. Ⓐ Ⓑ Ⓒ Ⓓ Ⓔ
284. Ⓐ Ⓑ Ⓒ Ⓓ Ⓔ
285. Ⓐ Ⓑ Ⓒ Ⓓ Ⓔ
286. Ⓐ Ⓑ Ⓒ Ⓓ Ⓔ
287. Ⓐ Ⓑ Ⓒ Ⓓ Ⓔ
288. Ⓐ Ⓑ Ⓒ Ⓓ Ⓔ
289. Ⓐ Ⓑ Ⓒ Ⓓ Ⓔ
290. Ⓐ Ⓑ Ⓒ Ⓓ Ⓔ
291. Ⓐ Ⓑ Ⓒ Ⓓ Ⓔ
292. Ⓐ Ⓑ Ⓒ Ⓓ Ⓔ
293. Ⓐ Ⓑ Ⓒ Ⓓ Ⓔ
294. Ⓐ Ⓑ Ⓒ Ⓓ Ⓔ
295. Ⓐ Ⓑ Ⓒ Ⓓ Ⓔ
296. Ⓐ Ⓑ Ⓒ Ⓓ Ⓔ
297. Ⓐ Ⓑ Ⓒ Ⓓ Ⓔ
298. Ⓐ Ⓑ Ⓒ Ⓓ Ⓔ
299. Ⓐ Ⓑ Ⓒ Ⓓ Ⓔ
300. Ⓐ Ⓑ Ⓒ Ⓓ Ⓔ

Answer Sheet for Comprehensive Practice Exam

Name _____ Date _____
               Last   First   Middle

Directions:

1. Using pencil, fill in only one circle representing your answer for each question.
2. Keeping your marks inside the circle, blacken the circle completely.
3. Completely erase any answer you wish to change, and make no stray marks.

Correct: Ⓐ ● Ⓒ Ⓓ Ⓔ Ⓕ Ⓖ Ⓗ Ⓘ Ⓙ   Wrong: ⊗ ⊜ ○ ☑ ⊘ Ⓕ Ⓖ Ⓗ Ⓘ Ⓙ

1. Ⓐ Ⓑ Ⓒ Ⓓ Ⓔ	27. Ⓐ Ⓑ Ⓒ Ⓓ Ⓔ	53. Ⓐ Ⓑ Ⓒ Ⓓ Ⓔ	79. Ⓐ Ⓑ Ⓒ Ⓓ Ⓔ
2. Ⓐ Ⓑ Ⓒ Ⓓ Ⓔ	28. Ⓐ Ⓑ Ⓒ Ⓓ Ⓔ	54. Ⓐ Ⓑ Ⓒ Ⓓ Ⓔ	80. Ⓐ Ⓑ Ⓒ Ⓓ Ⓔ
3. Ⓐ Ⓑ Ⓒ Ⓓ Ⓔ	29. Ⓐ Ⓑ Ⓒ Ⓓ Ⓔ	55. Ⓐ Ⓑ Ⓒ Ⓓ Ⓔ	81. Ⓐ Ⓑ Ⓒ Ⓓ Ⓔ
4. Ⓐ Ⓑ Ⓒ Ⓓ Ⓔ	30. Ⓐ Ⓑ Ⓒ Ⓓ Ⓔ	56. Ⓐ Ⓑ Ⓒ Ⓓ Ⓔ	82. Ⓐ Ⓑ Ⓒ Ⓓ Ⓔ
5. Ⓐ Ⓑ Ⓒ Ⓓ Ⓔ	31. Ⓐ Ⓑ Ⓒ Ⓓ Ⓔ	57. Ⓐ Ⓑ Ⓒ Ⓓ Ⓔ Ⓕ Ⓖ Ⓗ	83. Ⓐ Ⓑ Ⓒ Ⓓ Ⓔ
6. Ⓐ Ⓑ Ⓒ Ⓓ Ⓔ	32. Ⓐ Ⓑ Ⓒ Ⓓ Ⓔ	58. Ⓐ Ⓑ Ⓒ Ⓓ Ⓔ Ⓕ Ⓖ Ⓗ	84. Ⓐ Ⓑ Ⓒ Ⓓ Ⓔ
7. Ⓐ Ⓑ Ⓒ Ⓓ Ⓔ	33. Ⓐ Ⓑ Ⓒ Ⓓ Ⓔ	59. Ⓐ Ⓑ Ⓒ Ⓓ Ⓔ Ⓕ Ⓖ Ⓗ	85. Ⓐ Ⓑ Ⓒ Ⓓ Ⓔ
8. Ⓐ Ⓑ Ⓒ Ⓓ Ⓔ	34. Ⓐ Ⓑ Ⓒ Ⓓ Ⓔ	60. Ⓐ Ⓑ Ⓒ Ⓓ Ⓔ Ⓕ Ⓖ Ⓗ	86. Ⓐ Ⓑ Ⓒ Ⓓ Ⓔ
9. Ⓐ Ⓑ Ⓒ Ⓓ Ⓔ	35. Ⓐ Ⓑ Ⓒ Ⓓ Ⓔ	61. Ⓐ Ⓑ Ⓒ Ⓓ Ⓔ Ⓕ Ⓖ Ⓗ	87. Ⓐ Ⓑ Ⓒ Ⓓ Ⓔ
10. Ⓐ Ⓑ Ⓒ Ⓓ Ⓔ	36. Ⓐ Ⓑ Ⓒ Ⓓ Ⓔ	62. Ⓐ Ⓑ Ⓒ Ⓓ Ⓔ Ⓕ Ⓖ Ⓗ	88. Ⓐ Ⓑ Ⓒ Ⓓ Ⓔ
11. Ⓐ Ⓑ Ⓒ Ⓓ Ⓔ	37. Ⓐ Ⓑ Ⓒ Ⓓ Ⓔ	63. Ⓐ Ⓑ Ⓒ Ⓓ Ⓔ Ⓕ Ⓖ Ⓗ	89. Ⓐ Ⓑ Ⓒ Ⓓ Ⓔ
12. Ⓐ Ⓑ Ⓒ Ⓓ Ⓔ	38. Ⓐ Ⓑ Ⓒ Ⓓ Ⓔ	64. Ⓐ Ⓑ Ⓒ Ⓓ Ⓔ Ⓕ Ⓖ Ⓗ	90. Ⓐ Ⓑ Ⓒ Ⓓ Ⓔ
13. Ⓐ Ⓑ Ⓒ Ⓓ Ⓔ	39. Ⓐ Ⓑ Ⓒ Ⓓ Ⓔ	65. Ⓐ Ⓑ Ⓒ Ⓓ Ⓔ	91. Ⓐ Ⓑ Ⓒ Ⓓ Ⓔ
14. Ⓐ Ⓑ Ⓒ Ⓓ Ⓔ	40. Ⓐ Ⓑ Ⓒ Ⓓ Ⓔ	66. Ⓐ Ⓑ Ⓒ Ⓓ Ⓔ	92. Ⓐ Ⓑ Ⓒ Ⓓ Ⓔ
15. Ⓐ Ⓑ Ⓒ Ⓓ Ⓔ	41. Ⓐ Ⓑ Ⓒ Ⓓ Ⓔ	67. Ⓐ Ⓑ Ⓒ Ⓓ Ⓔ	93. Ⓐ Ⓑ Ⓒ Ⓓ Ⓔ
16. Ⓐ Ⓑ Ⓒ Ⓓ Ⓔ	42. Ⓐ Ⓑ Ⓒ Ⓓ Ⓔ	68. Ⓐ Ⓑ Ⓒ Ⓓ Ⓔ Ⓕ	94. Ⓐ Ⓑ Ⓒ Ⓓ Ⓔ
17. Ⓐ Ⓑ Ⓒ Ⓓ Ⓔ	43. Ⓐ Ⓑ Ⓒ Ⓓ Ⓔ	69. Ⓐ Ⓑ Ⓒ Ⓓ Ⓔ Ⓕ	95. Ⓐ Ⓑ Ⓒ Ⓓ Ⓔ
18. Ⓐ Ⓑ Ⓒ Ⓓ Ⓔ	44. Ⓐ Ⓑ Ⓒ Ⓓ Ⓔ	70. Ⓐ Ⓑ Ⓒ Ⓓ Ⓔ Ⓕ	96. Ⓐ Ⓑ Ⓒ Ⓓ Ⓔ
19. Ⓐ Ⓑ Ⓒ Ⓓ Ⓔ	45. Ⓐ Ⓑ Ⓒ Ⓓ Ⓔ	71. Ⓐ Ⓑ Ⓒ Ⓓ Ⓔ Ⓕ	97. Ⓐ Ⓑ Ⓒ Ⓓ Ⓔ
20. Ⓐ Ⓑ Ⓒ Ⓓ Ⓔ	46. Ⓐ Ⓑ Ⓒ Ⓓ Ⓔ	72. Ⓐ Ⓑ Ⓒ Ⓓ Ⓔ Ⓕ	98. Ⓐ Ⓑ Ⓒ Ⓓ Ⓔ
21. Ⓐ Ⓑ Ⓒ Ⓓ Ⓔ	47. Ⓐ Ⓑ Ⓒ Ⓓ Ⓔ	73. Ⓐ Ⓑ Ⓒ Ⓓ Ⓔ Ⓕ	99. Ⓐ Ⓑ Ⓒ Ⓓ Ⓔ
22. Ⓐ Ⓑ Ⓒ Ⓓ Ⓔ	48. Ⓐ Ⓑ Ⓒ Ⓓ Ⓔ	74. Ⓐ Ⓑ Ⓒ Ⓓ Ⓔ	100. Ⓐ Ⓑ Ⓒ Ⓓ Ⓔ
23. Ⓐ Ⓑ Ⓒ Ⓓ Ⓔ	49. Ⓐ Ⓑ Ⓒ Ⓓ Ⓔ	75. Ⓐ Ⓑ Ⓒ Ⓓ Ⓔ	101. Ⓐ Ⓑ Ⓒ Ⓓ Ⓔ
24. Ⓐ Ⓑ Ⓒ Ⓓ Ⓔ	50. Ⓐ Ⓑ Ⓒ Ⓓ Ⓔ	76. Ⓐ Ⓑ Ⓒ Ⓓ Ⓔ	102. Ⓐ Ⓑ Ⓒ Ⓓ Ⓔ
25. Ⓐ Ⓑ Ⓒ Ⓓ Ⓔ	51. Ⓐ Ⓑ Ⓒ Ⓓ Ⓔ	77. Ⓐ Ⓑ Ⓒ Ⓓ Ⓔ	103. Ⓐ Ⓑ Ⓒ Ⓓ Ⓔ
26. Ⓐ Ⓑ Ⓒ Ⓓ Ⓔ	52. Ⓐ Ⓑ Ⓒ Ⓓ Ⓔ	78. Ⓐ Ⓑ Ⓒ Ⓓ Ⓔ	104. Ⓐ Ⓑ Ⓒ Ⓓ Ⓔ

105. Ⓐ Ⓑ Ⓒ Ⓓ Ⓔ	154. Ⓐ Ⓑ Ⓒ Ⓓ Ⓔ	203. Ⓐ Ⓑ Ⓒ Ⓓ Ⓔ	252. Ⓐ Ⓑ Ⓒ Ⓓ Ⓔ
106. Ⓐ Ⓑ Ⓒ Ⓓ Ⓔ	155. Ⓐ Ⓑ Ⓒ Ⓓ Ⓔ	204. Ⓐ Ⓑ Ⓒ Ⓓ Ⓔ	253. Ⓐ Ⓑ Ⓒ Ⓓ Ⓔ
107. Ⓐ Ⓑ Ⓒ Ⓓ Ⓔ	156. Ⓐ Ⓑ Ⓒ Ⓓ Ⓔ	205. Ⓐ Ⓑ Ⓒ Ⓓ Ⓔ	254. Ⓐ Ⓑ Ⓒ Ⓓ Ⓔ
108. Ⓐ Ⓑ Ⓒ Ⓓ Ⓔ	157. Ⓐ Ⓑ Ⓒ Ⓓ Ⓔ	206. Ⓐ Ⓑ Ⓒ Ⓓ Ⓔ	255. Ⓐ Ⓑ Ⓒ Ⓓ Ⓔ
109. Ⓐ Ⓑ Ⓒ Ⓓ Ⓔ	158. Ⓐ Ⓑ Ⓒ Ⓓ Ⓔ	207. Ⓐ Ⓑ Ⓒ Ⓓ Ⓔ	256. Ⓐ Ⓑ Ⓒ Ⓓ Ⓔ
110. Ⓐ Ⓑ Ⓒ Ⓓ Ⓔ	159. Ⓐ Ⓑ Ⓒ Ⓓ Ⓔ	208. Ⓐ Ⓑ Ⓒ Ⓓ Ⓔ	257. Ⓐ Ⓑ Ⓒ Ⓓ Ⓔ
111. Ⓐ Ⓑ Ⓒ Ⓓ Ⓔ	160. Ⓐ Ⓑ Ⓒ Ⓓ Ⓔ	209. Ⓐ Ⓑ Ⓒ Ⓓ Ⓔ	258. Ⓐ Ⓑ Ⓒ Ⓓ Ⓔ
112. Ⓐ Ⓑ Ⓒ Ⓓ Ⓔ	161. Ⓐ Ⓑ Ⓒ Ⓓ Ⓔ	210. Ⓐ Ⓑ Ⓒ Ⓓ Ⓔ	259. Ⓐ Ⓑ Ⓒ Ⓓ Ⓔ
113. Ⓐ Ⓑ Ⓒ Ⓓ Ⓔ	162. Ⓐ Ⓑ Ⓒ Ⓓ Ⓔ	211. Ⓐ Ⓑ Ⓒ Ⓓ Ⓔ	260. Ⓐ Ⓑ Ⓒ Ⓓ Ⓔ
114. Ⓐ Ⓑ Ⓒ Ⓓ Ⓔ	163. Ⓐ Ⓑ Ⓒ Ⓓ Ⓔ	212. Ⓐ Ⓑ Ⓒ Ⓓ Ⓔ	261. Ⓐ Ⓑ Ⓒ Ⓓ Ⓔ
115. Ⓐ Ⓑ Ⓒ Ⓓ Ⓔ	164. Ⓐ Ⓑ Ⓒ Ⓓ Ⓔ	213. Ⓐ Ⓑ Ⓒ Ⓓ Ⓔ	262. Ⓐ Ⓑ Ⓒ Ⓓ Ⓔ
116. Ⓐ Ⓑ Ⓒ Ⓓ Ⓔ	165. Ⓐ Ⓑ Ⓒ Ⓓ Ⓔ	214. Ⓐ Ⓑ Ⓒ Ⓓ Ⓔ	263. Ⓐ Ⓑ Ⓒ Ⓓ Ⓔ
117. Ⓐ Ⓑ Ⓒ Ⓓ Ⓔ	166. Ⓐ Ⓑ Ⓒ Ⓓ Ⓔ	215. Ⓐ Ⓑ Ⓒ Ⓓ Ⓔ	264. Ⓐ Ⓑ Ⓒ Ⓓ Ⓔ
118. Ⓐ Ⓑ Ⓒ Ⓓ Ⓔ	167. Ⓐ Ⓑ Ⓒ Ⓓ Ⓔ Ⓕ	216. Ⓐ Ⓑ Ⓒ Ⓓ Ⓔ	265. Ⓐ Ⓑ Ⓒ Ⓓ Ⓔ
119. Ⓐ Ⓑ Ⓒ Ⓓ Ⓔ	168. Ⓐ Ⓑ Ⓒ Ⓓ Ⓔ Ⓕ	217. Ⓐ Ⓑ Ⓒ Ⓓ Ⓔ	266. Ⓐ Ⓑ Ⓒ Ⓓ Ⓔ
120. Ⓐ Ⓑ Ⓒ Ⓓ Ⓔ	169. Ⓐ Ⓑ Ⓒ Ⓓ Ⓔ Ⓕ	218. Ⓐ Ⓑ Ⓒ Ⓓ Ⓔ	267. Ⓐ Ⓑ Ⓒ Ⓓ Ⓔ
121. Ⓐ Ⓑ Ⓒ Ⓓ Ⓔ	170. Ⓐ Ⓑ Ⓒ Ⓓ Ⓔ Ⓕ	219. Ⓐ Ⓑ Ⓒ Ⓓ Ⓔ	268. Ⓐ Ⓑ Ⓒ Ⓓ Ⓔ
122. Ⓐ Ⓑ Ⓒ Ⓓ Ⓔ	171. Ⓐ Ⓑ Ⓒ Ⓓ Ⓔ Ⓕ	220. Ⓐ Ⓑ Ⓒ Ⓓ Ⓔ	269. Ⓐ Ⓑ Ⓒ Ⓓ Ⓔ
123. Ⓐ Ⓑ Ⓒ Ⓓ Ⓔ	172. Ⓐ Ⓑ Ⓒ Ⓓ Ⓔ Ⓕ	221. Ⓐ Ⓑ Ⓒ Ⓓ Ⓔ	270. Ⓐ Ⓑ Ⓒ Ⓓ Ⓔ
124. Ⓐ Ⓑ Ⓒ Ⓓ Ⓔ	173. Ⓐ Ⓑ Ⓒ Ⓓ Ⓔ	222. Ⓐ Ⓑ Ⓒ Ⓓ Ⓔ	271. Ⓐ Ⓑ Ⓒ Ⓓ Ⓔ
125. Ⓐ Ⓑ Ⓒ Ⓓ Ⓔ	174. Ⓐ Ⓑ Ⓒ Ⓓ Ⓔ	223. Ⓐ Ⓑ Ⓒ Ⓓ Ⓔ	272. Ⓐ Ⓑ Ⓒ Ⓓ Ⓔ
126. Ⓐ Ⓑ Ⓒ Ⓓ Ⓔ	175. Ⓐ Ⓑ Ⓒ Ⓓ Ⓔ	224. Ⓐ Ⓑ Ⓒ Ⓓ Ⓔ	273. Ⓐ Ⓑ Ⓒ Ⓓ Ⓔ
127. Ⓐ Ⓑ Ⓒ Ⓓ Ⓔ	176. Ⓐ Ⓑ Ⓒ Ⓓ Ⓔ	225. Ⓐ Ⓑ Ⓒ Ⓓ Ⓔ	274. Ⓐ Ⓑ Ⓒ Ⓓ Ⓔ
128. Ⓐ Ⓑ Ⓒ Ⓓ Ⓔ	177. Ⓐ Ⓑ Ⓒ Ⓓ Ⓔ	226. Ⓐ Ⓑ Ⓒ Ⓓ Ⓔ	275. Ⓐ Ⓑ Ⓒ Ⓓ Ⓔ
129. Ⓐ Ⓑ Ⓒ Ⓓ Ⓔ	178. Ⓐ Ⓑ Ⓒ Ⓓ Ⓔ	227. Ⓐ Ⓑ Ⓒ Ⓓ Ⓔ	276. Ⓐ Ⓑ Ⓒ Ⓓ Ⓔ
130. Ⓐ Ⓑ Ⓒ Ⓓ Ⓔ	179. Ⓐ Ⓑ Ⓒ Ⓓ Ⓔ	228. Ⓐ Ⓑ Ⓒ Ⓓ Ⓔ	277. Ⓐ Ⓑ Ⓒ Ⓓ Ⓔ
131. Ⓐ Ⓑ Ⓒ Ⓓ Ⓔ	180. Ⓐ Ⓑ Ⓒ Ⓓ Ⓔ	229. Ⓐ Ⓑ Ⓒ Ⓓ Ⓔ	278. Ⓐ Ⓑ Ⓒ Ⓓ Ⓔ
132. Ⓐ Ⓑ Ⓒ Ⓓ Ⓔ	181. Ⓐ Ⓑ Ⓒ Ⓓ Ⓔ	230. Ⓐ Ⓑ Ⓒ Ⓓ Ⓔ	279. Ⓐ Ⓑ Ⓒ Ⓓ Ⓔ
133. Ⓐ Ⓑ Ⓒ Ⓓ Ⓔ	182. Ⓐ Ⓑ Ⓒ Ⓓ Ⓔ	231. Ⓐ Ⓑ Ⓒ Ⓓ Ⓔ	280. Ⓐ Ⓑ Ⓒ Ⓓ Ⓔ
134. Ⓐ Ⓑ Ⓒ Ⓓ Ⓔ	183. Ⓐ Ⓑ Ⓒ Ⓓ Ⓔ	232. Ⓐ Ⓑ Ⓒ Ⓓ Ⓔ	281. Ⓐ Ⓑ Ⓒ Ⓓ Ⓔ
135. Ⓐ Ⓑ Ⓒ Ⓓ Ⓔ	184. Ⓐ Ⓑ Ⓒ Ⓓ Ⓔ	233. Ⓐ Ⓑ Ⓒ Ⓓ Ⓔ	282. Ⓐ Ⓑ Ⓒ Ⓓ Ⓔ
136. Ⓐ Ⓑ Ⓒ Ⓓ Ⓔ	185. Ⓐ Ⓑ Ⓒ Ⓓ Ⓔ	234. Ⓐ Ⓑ Ⓒ Ⓓ Ⓔ	283. Ⓐ Ⓑ Ⓒ Ⓓ Ⓔ
137. Ⓐ Ⓑ Ⓒ Ⓓ Ⓔ	186. Ⓐ Ⓑ Ⓒ Ⓓ Ⓔ	235. Ⓐ Ⓑ Ⓒ Ⓓ Ⓔ	284. Ⓐ Ⓑ Ⓒ Ⓓ Ⓔ
138. Ⓐ Ⓑ Ⓒ Ⓓ Ⓔ	187. Ⓐ Ⓑ Ⓒ Ⓓ Ⓔ	236. Ⓐ Ⓑ Ⓒ Ⓓ Ⓔ	285. Ⓐ Ⓑ Ⓒ Ⓓ Ⓔ
139. Ⓐ Ⓑ Ⓒ Ⓓ Ⓔ	188. Ⓐ Ⓑ Ⓒ Ⓓ Ⓔ	237. Ⓐ Ⓑ Ⓒ Ⓓ Ⓔ	286. Ⓐ Ⓑ Ⓒ Ⓓ Ⓔ
140. Ⓐ Ⓑ Ⓒ Ⓓ Ⓔ	189. Ⓐ Ⓑ Ⓒ Ⓓ Ⓔ	238. Ⓐ Ⓑ Ⓒ Ⓓ Ⓔ	287. Ⓐ Ⓑ Ⓒ Ⓓ Ⓔ
141. Ⓐ Ⓑ Ⓒ Ⓓ Ⓔ	190. Ⓐ Ⓑ Ⓒ Ⓓ Ⓔ	239. Ⓐ Ⓑ Ⓒ Ⓓ Ⓔ	288. Ⓐ Ⓑ Ⓒ Ⓓ Ⓔ
142. Ⓐ Ⓑ Ⓒ Ⓓ Ⓔ	191. Ⓐ Ⓑ Ⓒ Ⓓ Ⓔ Ⓕ Ⓖ Ⓗ Ⓘ Ⓙ	240. Ⓐ Ⓑ Ⓒ Ⓓ Ⓔ	289. Ⓐ Ⓑ Ⓒ Ⓓ Ⓔ
143. Ⓐ Ⓑ Ⓒ Ⓓ Ⓔ	192. Ⓐ Ⓑ Ⓒ Ⓓ Ⓔ Ⓕ Ⓖ Ⓗ Ⓘ Ⓙ	241. Ⓐ Ⓑ Ⓒ Ⓓ Ⓔ Ⓕ Ⓖ	290. Ⓐ Ⓑ Ⓒ Ⓓ Ⓔ
144. Ⓐ Ⓑ Ⓒ Ⓓ Ⓔ	193. Ⓐ Ⓑ Ⓒ Ⓓ Ⓔ Ⓕ Ⓖ Ⓗ Ⓘ Ⓙ	242. Ⓐ Ⓑ Ⓒ Ⓓ Ⓔ Ⓕ Ⓖ	291. Ⓐ Ⓑ Ⓒ Ⓓ Ⓔ
145. Ⓐ Ⓑ Ⓒ Ⓓ Ⓔ	194. Ⓐ Ⓑ Ⓒ Ⓓ Ⓔ Ⓕ Ⓖ Ⓗ Ⓘ Ⓙ	243. Ⓐ Ⓑ Ⓒ Ⓓ Ⓔ Ⓕ Ⓖ	292. Ⓐ Ⓑ Ⓒ Ⓓ Ⓔ
146. Ⓐ Ⓑ Ⓒ Ⓓ Ⓔ	195. Ⓐ Ⓑ Ⓒ Ⓓ Ⓔ Ⓕ Ⓖ Ⓗ Ⓘ Ⓙ	244. Ⓐ Ⓑ Ⓒ Ⓓ Ⓔ Ⓕ Ⓖ	293. Ⓐ Ⓑ Ⓒ Ⓓ Ⓔ
147. Ⓐ Ⓑ Ⓒ Ⓓ Ⓔ	196. Ⓐ Ⓑ Ⓒ Ⓓ Ⓔ Ⓕ Ⓖ Ⓗ Ⓘ Ⓙ	245. Ⓐ Ⓑ Ⓒ Ⓓ Ⓔ Ⓕ Ⓖ	294. Ⓐ Ⓑ Ⓒ Ⓓ Ⓔ
148. Ⓐ Ⓑ Ⓒ Ⓓ Ⓔ	197. Ⓐ Ⓑ Ⓒ Ⓓ Ⓔ Ⓕ Ⓖ Ⓗ Ⓘ Ⓙ	246. Ⓐ Ⓑ Ⓒ Ⓓ Ⓔ Ⓕ Ⓖ	295. Ⓐ Ⓑ Ⓒ Ⓓ Ⓔ
149. Ⓐ Ⓑ Ⓒ Ⓓ Ⓔ	198. Ⓐ Ⓑ Ⓒ Ⓓ Ⓔ Ⓕ Ⓖ Ⓗ Ⓘ Ⓙ	247. Ⓐ Ⓑ Ⓒ Ⓓ Ⓔ Ⓕ Ⓖ	296. Ⓐ Ⓑ Ⓒ Ⓓ Ⓔ
150. Ⓐ Ⓑ Ⓒ Ⓓ Ⓔ	199. Ⓐ Ⓑ Ⓒ Ⓓ Ⓔ Ⓕ Ⓖ Ⓗ Ⓘ Ⓙ	248. Ⓐ Ⓑ Ⓒ Ⓓ Ⓔ	297. Ⓐ Ⓑ Ⓒ Ⓓ Ⓔ
151. Ⓐ Ⓑ Ⓒ Ⓓ Ⓔ	200. Ⓐ Ⓑ Ⓒ Ⓓ Ⓔ Ⓕ Ⓖ Ⓗ Ⓘ Ⓙ	249. Ⓐ Ⓑ Ⓒ Ⓓ Ⓔ	298. Ⓐ Ⓑ Ⓒ Ⓓ Ⓔ
152. Ⓐ Ⓑ Ⓒ Ⓓ Ⓔ	201. Ⓐ Ⓑ Ⓒ Ⓓ Ⓔ	250. Ⓐ Ⓑ Ⓒ Ⓓ Ⓔ	299. Ⓐ Ⓑ Ⓒ Ⓓ Ⓔ
153. Ⓐ Ⓑ Ⓒ Ⓓ Ⓔ	202. Ⓐ Ⓑ Ⓒ Ⓓ Ⓔ	251. Ⓐ Ⓑ Ⓒ Ⓓ Ⓔ	300. Ⓐ Ⓑ Ⓒ Ⓓ Ⓔ

Answers to Comprehensive Practice Exam

1. B	31. A	61. F	91. B	121. B	151. B	181. A	211. A	241. G	271. C
2. C	32. B	62. H	92. B	122. B	152. B	182. C	212. D	242. F	272. A
3. D	33. A	63. A	93. A	123. B	153. C	183. B	213. B	243. E	273. B
4. B	34. C	64. B	94. A	124. A	154. A	184. C	214. C	244. A	274. B
5. B	35. C	65. A	95. A	125. C	155. B	185. B	215. A	245. C	275. C
6. D	36. C	66. B	96. B	126. B	156. B	186. D	216. C	246. D	276. B
7. B	37. A	67. C	97. B	127. A	157. B	187. A	217. B	247. B	277. B
8. D	38. B	68. C	98. B	128. E	158. B	188. B	218. D	248. C	278. C
9. D	39. B	69. B	99. D	129. D	159. A	189. A	219. B	249. A	279. A
10. B	40. A	70. E	100. A	130. C	160. B	190. D	220. B	250. C	280. B
11. C	41. E	71. D	101. A	131. B	161. C	191. D	221. C	251. B	281. D
12. C	42. D	72. F	102. B	132. A	162. B	192. J	222. B	252. A	282. D
13. B	43. C	73. A	103. B	133. B	163. B	193. E	223. C	253. D	283. D
14. B	44. B	74. B	104. A	134. B	164. C	194. A	224. C	254. B	284. D
15. A	45. B	75. D	105. C	135. D	165. C	195. F	225. A	255. C	285. C
16. C	46. A	76. C	106. A	136. B	166. B	196. C	226. B	256. B	286. C
17. A	47. B	77. A	107. A	137. B	167. C	197. H	227. D	257. C	287. A
18. D	48. A	78. A	108. D	138. C	168. E	198. I	228. A	258. B	288. C
19. B	49. B	79. B	109. D	139. B	169. D	199. B	229. E	259. B	289. B
20. B	50. C	80. A	110. B	140. A	170. B	200. G	230. B	260. C	290. D
21. B	51. A	81. C	111. C	141. C	171. A	201. C	231. B	261. B	291. A
22. B	52. D	82. B	112. C	142. B	172. F	202. B	232. B	262. A	292. A
23. A	53. C	83. D	113. C	143. D	173. A	203. E	233. C	263. D	293. A
24. C	54. A	84. A	114. B	144. C	174. A	204. B	234. A	264. B	294. B
25. C	55. C	85. C	115. A	145. B	175. A	205. A	235. B	265. C	295. C
26. A	56. B	86. D	116. A	146. B	176. A	206. C	236. C	266. C	296. A
27. A	57. E	87. C	117. C	147. B	177. C	207. D	237. C	267. A	297. B
28. B	58. D	88. B	118. D	148. A	178. B	208. D	238. A	268. B	298. B
29. B	59. C	89. A	119. D	149. D	179. A	209. B	239. A	269. C	299. B
30. B	60. G	90. A	120. A	150. B	180. A	210. B	240. D	270. B	300. B

Glossary

abandonment discontinuation of care after treatment has started but prior to completion

abscess localized accumulation of infection in an area formed by the degeneration of soft tissue or bone

abutment a tooth or implant used as retention for a fixed or removable prosthesis

acid attack the action of bacterial waste products on the surfaces of the teeth

acquired pellicle a colorless film composed of sugar molecules, which is constantly being produced in the mouth

act of commission an "act" that a reasonable and prudent professional would perform

act of omission an "act" that a reasonable and prudent professional would not perform

ALARA in radiography, an acronym standing for "as low as reasonably achievable."

alginate an irreversible hydrocolloid impression material

allergy a reaction by the body to a specific allergen

alveolar process the projection of the maxilla and mandible that encompasses and supports the teeth. Also called the alveolar ridge

alveolitis an infection, which is related to the loss or disturbance of the blood clot, following the extraction of a tooth. Also called "dry socket."

amalgam a combination of metals, one of the constituents of which is mercury

analgesics medications that relieve pain without causing excessive drowsiness

anaphylactic shock a sudden allergic reaction

anaphylaxis a severe allergic reaction resulting in rash, difficulty breathing, and sometimes death

anesthesia medications to produce the temporary loss of feeling, sensation, and sometimes consciousness

anesthesiologist medical doctor who is trained to administer local and general anesthetics

anesthetic medications that are designed to produce the temporary loss of feeling or sensation, either generally or locally

angle's classification of malocclusion a system of classifying malocclusion set up by orthodontist Edward Hartley Angle (1855–1930)

anode the positive ion of an x-ray

antagonistic teeth that occlude one another in the dental arch

anterior teeth the central and lateral incisors and the cuspids in the maxillary and mandibular arches

antibodies a substance that is produced by the body in the presence of an antigen

antibiotics medications given to combat infections of a bacterial nature

antigen a cellular protein that causes antibody formation by the body

antiseptic a preparation used topically to minimize surface microbes

apex the tip of the root of the tooth

apicoectomy the surgical removal of the apex of the tooth

attachment apparatus tissues that include the cementum, alveolar process, and the periodontal ligament. These tissues work together to support the tooth in its proper position in the arch

avulsed torn away with force

barbiturates sedatives that produce a hypnotic or calming effect

behavior modification techniques   techniques used in pediatric dentistry to control the behavior of the child during treatment

behavior management   managing the pediatric dental patient who is experiencing discomfort or anxiety through various methods such as the show-and-tell method or with antianxiety medications

bioburden   any visible disposable waste such as bloody gauze, saliva-soaked cotton rolls, tissue, or bone that is generated during operative procedures

biohazard   infectious waste generated by dental treatment

biological monitoring   the testing and monitoring of a sterilizing device, using specialized testing strips, for effectiveness

biopsy   the removal of a tissue for evaluation

bisecting angle technique   a technique in the exposure of radiographs in which the central beam bisects the right angle that is formed by the long axis of the tooth and the film packet

bite registration   using impression material to capture the relationship of the maxillary and mandibular bite

bitewing radiographs   intraoral films that show the anatomic crown and a portion of the root of the maxillary and mandibular teeth when in centric occlusion

bloodborne   any disease that can be transmitted through contact with blood or body fluids that are contaminated with blood, saliva, or other bodily fluids

blood pressure   the pressure exerted on the arterial walls by the blood

Board of Dental Examiners   the state agency that is responsible for administration of examinations for licensure and enforces the statutes and rules as they apply to the practice of dentistry within that state

bracket   in orthodontics, a small device that attaches to the facial aspect of the teeth and holds an arch wire in place

brand name   a drug whose name is protected by trademark

bridge   a fixed prosthesis that consists of a pontic (replacement tooth) attached to abutments to replace one or more missing teeth called the abutment

broach, barbed   an endodontic instrument with sharp projections that is used to remove large amounts of pulpal tissue

buccal   relating to the cheek

buccal tube   a tube to hold an arch wire in place; located on the buccal aspect of the mandibular molar band

bur, friction grip   a bur used in a high-speed contra-angle handpiece that has a smooth shank

bur, latch type   a bur used in a slow-speed latch-type contra-angle that has a notch at the end of the bur

burnisher   a hand instrument that is used to smooth and seal the margin of a restoration

calculus   a deposit of organic mineralized substances that adheres to tooth structures

capitation   an insurance plan under which the dentist has contracted to provide all or most of his dental services to the insurance plan subscribers. Payment is issued to the dentist on a per-capita basis

cardiac arrest   the complete cessation of the heart

caries   dental decay

carver   a hand instrument used to shape the occlusal or interproximal surfaces of a restoration

cast crown   full coverage crown manufactured by using a metal shell and adhering porcelain or gold to the outside

catalyst   a material that when introduced to a base begins a chemical reaction

cathode   a negative electrode from which electrons are emitted

cavity   a lesion or hole resulting from dental decay

cavity liner   the material placed over the pulpal area of the preparation to soothe irritated or sensitive pulp. Used to stimulate secondary dentin

cavity varnish   applied under amalgam to seal dentin tubules and prevent thermal sensitivity. Is not compatible with composite resin restorative material

cementoenamel junction   the junction of the enamel of the crown and the cementum of the root at the cervix (neck) of the tooth

cementum   the substance that covers the root surface of the tooth

Centers for Disease Control   a federal agency that tracks, monitors, and investigates infectious diseases

centric occlusion   when the jaws are closed in a position that produces stable contact between the mandible and maxilla

cephalometric   an extraoral radiograph used to study the dentofacial bones and tissues of the face and jaws

chemical injury   damage of tissue such as skin, eye, mouth, or other mucous membrane or non-intact skin resulting from a liquid or a dry chemical exposure incident

child abuse   any negligent or criminal act against a child

chisel   a hand instrument used to remove undermined enamel during the cavity preparation stage

classifications of motion   motions divided into classes to identify the body movements of the dental health-care worker

clinical examination   a patient examination limited to the examination of extraoral structures

clock positions   an imaginary clock placed over the patient's face with the patient's face being in the center. The dental team members take positions at various times so that they may be positioned to access the patient easily

collimation   narrowing the main beam of radiation by reducing radiation outside the main beam

communication   a technique by which thoughts or ideas are conveyed between two or more people

composite   plastic tooth-colored filling material

composite resin restoration   a restoration which contains a tooth colored plastic material. Usually used for anterior restoration because of their esthetic purposes. This plastic material is comprised of acrylic resin monomers and approximately 70% inorganic filler such as glass, quartz, or silicate. Composite resin restorations can be light-cured or self-cured

conscious sedation   a level of consciousness that permits the patient to respond to commands and maintain an airway without assistance

consumables   supply items that are "used up," for example, restorative materials or radiography film

coordination of benefits   a method of combining benefits that are paid by more than one insurance plan

co-payment   the beneficiary's share of the fees after the plan has paid the dentist

core buildup   material comprised of plastics or amalgam and used to increase retention for a tooth missing large amounts of natural structure

coronal polishing   a procedure in which plaque and extrinsic stains are removed from the coronal portion of the teeth using an abrasive and a prophy angle and cup or brush

CPR   acronym for cardiopulmonary resuscitation which is the delivery of life support by artificial means

cranial bones   eight bones that make up the hard protective covering which houses the brain

cranial nerves   twelve pairs of nerves that serve both sensory and motor functions of the body. They are generally named for the area that they serve

critical instruments   instruments that penetrate bone and soft tissue that must be sterilized after each patient use

cross-bite   malocclusion in which the buccal surfaces of the maxillary teeth are situated labially to the mandibular teeth

cross-contamination   the spread of pathogenic organisms by contact with contaminated items such as drawer handles, instruments, or hard surfaces

crown, cast   a cast restoration that covers the entire anatomic crown of the tooth

curettage   scraping or cleaning of necrotic material with a curette

curette   a periodontal hand instrument with sharp cutting edges and a rounded toe

cuspid   an anterior tooth with a long thick root. Also known as a canine

debridement   the removal of debris by either mechanical or chemical means

deciduous teeth   the first set of dentition comprised of twenty teeth, also referred to as deciduous, baby, or milk teeth

deductible   a sum of money that must be paid by the patient before any benefits are paid to the dentist

dental claim forms   standardized forms containing itemized dental treatment which are submitted to an insurance carrier for payment

dental dam   a thin piece of latex used with a clamp and frame to prevent moisture and saliva from entering the oral cavity during operative procedures

dental history   a comprehensive report of all dental treatment that has been performed on a patient

dental implants   artificial teeth that have been attached to anchors that have been surgically implanted into the alveolar ridge

dental insurance   a contract for the patient provided by an outside source whereby a premium is paid by the insured and compensation is provided by the insurance company for dental treatment

Dental Practice Act   a written law as it applies to dentistry. Each state has a dental practice act that contains the legal restrictions on the dental health-care worker and the practice of dentistry in that state

dentin   the material forming the bulk of the tooth just below the enamel

dentition   the teeth as they appear in the dental arch

denture   a prosthesis to replace missing teeth within the same arch. May be complete (full) or partial

dependents   the spouse and children who are covered by the insured

diabetic emergency   the result of an inadequate insulin supply that can lead to unconsciousness, coma, and eventually death unless treated

diastolic pressure   the blood pressure during the relaxation phase of the heart

disclosing solution   a coloring agent applied to the teeth that causes the staining of the components of plaque

disinfectant   an agent used to kill pathogenic microorganisms

distal   away from the midline

distocclusion   when the mandibular teeth occlude distally to their normal relationship to the maxillary teeth

Drug Enforcement Agency   the branch of the federal government that tracks, investigates, and monitors any activity relating to the legal or illegal selling, dispensing, or use of controlled substances

dry socket   see alveolitis

dual coverage   coverage for a patient under more than one insurance plan

due care   a legal term meaning just, proper, and sufficient care for the patient

elastomeric impression material   rubber base impression material used for permanent prosthetic impressions

electron   a negatively charged atomic particle with very low mass

elevator   surgical instrument used to elevate the tooth out of the alveolar socket

enamel   the hard tissue that covers the anatomic crown of the tooth

endodontic explorer   endodontic instrument used to locate canals during endodontic therapy

endodontic file   small hand instrument used to debride and shape the root canal during root canal therapy

endogenous stain   a stain that occurs on the inside of a tooth

Environmental Protection Agency   a division of the federal government that monitors and regulates environmental concerns such as water, air, and pollution

epilepsy   a disorder characterized by sudden attacks of unconsciousness and may or may not accompany convulsions

ethics   a set of standards as it relates to actions that are right and wrong when practicing dentistry

exfoliation   the normal shedding of primary teeth

exfoliative cytology   a type of biopsy that involves the mechanical scraping of cells from the area of concern for closer inspection under a microscope

exodontics   the practice of removing teeth from the oral cavity as performed by a dentist

external marketing   marketing that centers around attracting new patients to the practice. Newspaper advertisements, coupons, and commercials are examples of external marketing

extraction   the removal of teeth by surgical means

extraoral factors   considerations during the examination that relate to any factors outside the mouth such as musculature, mental state, and so on

extrinsic stain   a stain that occurs on the outside of the tooth and can be removed by polishing with an abrasive and rubber cup or brush

facial   pertaining to the buccal or labial surfaces

facial bones   fourteen bones that make up the shape of the face

festooning   the shaping of material or tissue to simulate normal tissue appearance

filtration in radiography, the filtering of less desirable x-rays during the exposure process using an aluminum filter

first aid the rendering of primary care to an injured victim until a trained professional arrives on the scene or the victim is transported to a medical facility

fixed appliances any appliances that are attached to the teeth

fixed bridge a fixed prosthesis replacing two or more teeth

fixed overhead business expenses that occur on a regular basis such as rent on the building or salaries to the employees

flap surgery any surgical procedure that requires the laying of a flap. For example; root planing, osseous surgery, or coronal repositioning of gingival tissue

fluorides, systemic fluorides ingested into the body. They can be found in water, food, or supplements

fluorides, topical fluorides applied directly onto the teeth. They can be applied by rinses, fluoridated toothpaste, and topical fluoride applications

fluorosis mottled appearance of the enamel caused by excessive fluoride intake

framework the metal skeleton portion of the removable partial denture

frenum a fold of tissue that attaches the cheeks and lips to the alveolar process

frontal sinuses hollow air-filled cavities located above the forehead and within the frontal bone which produces mucus, provides resonance when speaking, and lightens the weight of the skull

fulcrum placement of the fingers that stabilizes the wrist during the use of dental instruments

full denture a removable prosthesis that replaces an entire arch with teeth and tissues

gag reflex protective mechanism located in the posterior part of the mouth that prevents the aspiration of foreign objects

Gates-Glidden burs endodontic drills that enlarge the root canal during endodontic therapy

generic a drug that is not protected by a trademark

germicide a solution that can kill all microorganisms except spores

gingiva the tissue that surrounds a tooth

gingiva, attached the tissue that extends from the gingival margin to the alveolar mucosa

gingiva, free the part of the gingiva that surrounds the tooth in a collarlike fashion

gingival curettage the removal of necrotic tissue within the periodontal pocket

gingival retraction retraction of gingival tissue to gain access to the entire anatomical crown

gingivectomy the surgical removal of gingival tissue

gingivitis inflammation of the gingiva characterized by red, inflamed, bleeding, gingival tissue

gingivoplasty a surgical procedure to correct gingival abnormalities

glass ionomer cement permanent cement containing fluoride and having the ability to chemically bond to tooth structures

graft the complete removal of tissue from one region of the mouth which is placed in another region of the mouth to reinforce an area which has been damaged by disease or trauma

gutta-percha an inert rubber type of filling material used in endodontic treatment

hand-cutting instruments instruments used to remove undermined enamel and shape cavity preparations

hand instruments instruments used under the direction of the operator, as opposed to a motor driven handpiece

handpiece a motor driven instrument which can hold rotary devices such as burs and other attachments used in the delivery of dental treatment. Handpieces can come in several different types; slow-speed, high-speed, contra-angle, sonic, surgical, and laser

hazard communication a plan of action for handling any hazardous chemicals or materials in the dental office

hemisection separating a tooth in two halves at the furcation

hemostats scissorlike instruments used to hold or grasp objects during dental procedures

high-speed handpiece a handpiece which rotates and reaches speeds of up to 450,000 rpm. This handpiece is used primarily for removing enamel or other tooth structures

high volume evacuator tip a tip that fits onto the evacuator hose and is used to remove saliva and debris from the oral cavity

hoe   a dental hand instrument used in restorative dentistry. It has an angled end and is used to shape the cavity preparation

hydrocolloid impression material   a reversible or irreversible impression material used in the fabrication of fixed and removable prosthetics

incident report   a report filed when an accident occurs in the dental office

incisal   relating to the biting edge of an anterior tooth

infiltration   technique of placing anesthetic solution directly into the area that surrounds the tooth

inlay   a cast restoration designed to restore one, two, or three surfaces of the prepared tooth

insured   the person who has the insurance policy in his or her name

interproximal   between the proximal surfaces of adjacent teeth

intraoral examination   a clinical examination that includes inspection of teeth, intraoral tissues, and other structures of the oral cavity

intraoral factors   considerations during the examination that relate to the structures within the oral cavity

intrinsic stain   a stain that occurs within tooth structures

inventory and supplies   itemized materials that are ordered, tracked, and used by the dental office in the course of delivering dental treatment

irrigating solution   solution used to irrigate within the root canals or around the gingival tissues

jurisprudence   the law as it applies to dentistry

kilovoltage   measured as 1000 volts of electricity. Determines the quality or penetrating power of x-rays that are emitted

labial   relating to the lip

labioversion   the excessive protrusion of the maxillary anterior teeth over the lips

lawsuit   a legal action filed by a plaintiff alleging wrongdoing

Lentulo spiral   a small instrument that fits into the slow-speed handpiece and is used to deliver cement into the root canal during the obturation process

lingual   relating to the tongue

linguoversion   when the teeth are in their functional bite, the anterior teeth are positioned behind the mandibular incisors

lining mucosa   a thin tissue that lines the inside of the cheeks, vestibule, lips, and soft palate

litigation   when a lawsuit is presented to a court of law for ruling

local anesthesia   the temporary loss of feeling in a specific area

malocclusion   an abnormal bite

malpractice   the failure to use due care and judgment when treating a patient

masticatory mucosa   a tough keratinized tissue that covers the hard palate and gingiva. It is able to withstand chewing forces and regular oral hygiene maintenance

maxillary sinuses   hollow air-filled cavities located within the maxilla. These are the largest of the paranasal sinuses

maximum permissible dose   a term that describes the amount of exposure of radiation that the dental health-care worker can be safely exposed to without suffering from damaging effects

medical history   a detailed report of the patient's medical background

mesioclusion   a malocclusion in which the body of the mandible is in mesial relationship to the maxilla. This condition gives the appearance of the mandible protruding over the maxilla

midline   an imaginary line that divides the body into two halves

milliampere   a measurement equal to one-thousandth of an ampere. Milliamperage determines the quantity (amount) of x-rays that are emitted

mobility test   manually testing the degree of movement of a tooth within its socket. The higher degree of movement indicates injury or trauma from disease or other means

molar   a posterior tooth with a broad occlusal chewing surface

narcotic   a drug that is used as an analgesic and may cause physiological or psychological dependence

necrotic   dead or dying

needle holders   an instrument that resembles locking hemostats and is used to manipulate the needle during the suturing procedure

negligence   failure to practice due care when treating a patient

neutroclusion   when the jaws are at rest, the relationship of the maxilla and mandible are in a normal mesiodistal relationship

nib   the working end of a dental hand instrument

nitrous oxide   a combination of two gases, nitrogen and oxygen, that when used together produces a mild sedative effect

noncritical instruments   instruments that do not come into contact with blood or saliva. They can be cleaned with antimicrobial soap after each use

nonverbal cues   the act of sending messages to others with facial gestures, body movements, and attitudes which can reflect the overall feeling of an individual

non-vital   dead or not alive as in pulpal tissues

obturation   the process of filling the root canal

occlusal   relating to the chewing surfaces of the posterior teeth

occlusion   the relationship of the chewing surface of all teeth

onlay   a cast restoration designed to restore the occlusal and some proximal surfaces of a posterior tooth

open bite   a malocclusion where the anterior teeth do not occlude in any functional position

opposing model   a reproduction of the area opposite the area being treated

orthodontic radiography   a series of radiographic surveys (full series, cephalometric, or panelipse), which are used in the planning phase and ongoing treatment of the orthodontic patient

orthognathic surgery   surgery performed to restore the normal relationship of the jaws and supporting structures

osseous surgery   surgical procedures involving the alveolar bone

overbite   the vertical protrusion of upper teeth over the lowers

overcrowding   malpositioned teeth in the dental arch, which can cause an increase in caries formation or difficulty with mastication

overjet   horizontal protrusion of upper teeth over the lowers

palate, hard   the anterior part of the roof of the mouth, which has the hard bony underlying layer

palate, soft   the part of the palate that is posterior to the hard palate

palliative   providing immediate relief

palm grasp   a technique to grasp the instrument in the palm of the hand as in passing surgical forceps or using a dental dam clamp forceps

panoramic radiograph   an extraoral radiograph that produces an x-ray of the entire dentition along with the supporting tissues and the lower portion of the facial structures

paper points   single-use items made of paper used to dry the inside of the canals during endodontic therapy

papoose board   a device used to restrain a child's upper torso during dental treatment

paralleling technique   the technique consisting of placing the film packet parallel to the longitudinal axis of the tooth and directing the central ray perpendicular to the tooth and the film packet

partial denture   a prosthetic unit containing artificial teeth supported on a framework with acrylic and metal attachments

patient management   the methods of managing a patient to alleviate fear, anxiety, or discomfort. The goal of patient management is to maintain a positive setting while delivering quality dental treatment in a non-threatening atmosphere

pediatric dentist   a dentist who specializes in the preventive care and delivery of treatment to the dental patient from infancy into adolescence

pediatric dental office design   the specialized "open concept" design of the dental office to accommodate the younger patient by offering a non-threatening environment which includes entertainment and reading material appropriate for the pediatric dental patient

pedodontist   a dentist who specializes in the diseases and treatment of the primary dentition

Peeso reamer   a long shanked bur used in endodontic treatment to enlarge the canal

pen grasp   an instrument-holding technique that enables the operator to hold the instrument like a pen so that the little finger and third finger can act as a fulcrum

percussion test   an examination technique that involves short tapping actions on the teeth to reveal sensitivity of the tooth

periapical   surrounding the apex of the root of the tooth

periapical abscess   localized infection around the root or apex of a tooth

periapical radiograph   an intraoral film that shows the entire tooth and surrounding structures

periodontal abscess   localized infection in and around the tissues of the tooth

periodontal dressing a dressing that is used for the protection of a periodontal surgical site during the first part of healing

periodontal ligament the tissues that support and affix the tooth in its socket

periodontal pocket a formation in the sulcular space between the gingiva and alveolar bone. Healthy periodontal pockets are 1–3 millimeters

periodontal probe a device used to measure the periodontal pocket depth

periosteal elevator a surgical instrument used to unattach or reflect soft tissue from the alveolar bone

personal protective equipment (PPE) gloves, masks, goggles, gowns, and face shields used to protect the health-care worker from a potential exposure to bloodborne pathogens

pharmacology the study of drugs as they relate to medicinal uses

pin retention a small pinlike metallic device used under a restoration to aid in the prevention of the displacement of that restoration

plaque a buildup of bacteria, cellular debris, and bacterial products

polycarboxylate cement a permanent cement used as a luting agent for crown and bridge

pontic an artificial tooth that replaces one or more teeth

position indicator device (PID) in radiography, a lead extension attached to the tubehead. It guides the primary beam at the target

post a stainless steel device fitted into the root canal of an endodontically treated tooth. This device improves the retention of any fixed prosthetic device that is placed over it

post build up used when a tooth has been endodontically treated. A post is cemented into the canal of the treated tooth and a build up material is added to the coronal portion. This adds a larger area of retention and strength to the tooth prior to the placement of a permanent restoration

posterior toward the back of the oral cavity

posterior teeth teeth comprising the maxillary and mandibular premolars and molars

premedication medications taken prior to any treatment. This would include any antibiotics or antianxieties

prescription any written order for medication to be dispensed by the pharmacist

preventive dentistry delivery of dental care that is centered on delivering care to avoid the occurrence of dental problems. This would include radiographs, regular prophylaxis, and examinations

primary radiation the main beam of radiation emitted from the x-ray unit

prophylaxis, dental a procedure performed by either a licensed dentist or a dental hygienist in which there is complete removal of calculus, debris, stains, and plaque from the teeth

prosthesis a replacement for a missing tooth or teeth and tissues as in a denture or partial

protrusion the condition of being pushed forward

pulp the vital portion of the tooth

pulpectomy the complete removal of the pulp from a tooth

pulpitis inflammation of the dental pulp

pulpotomy the partial removal of the dental pulp usually from the coronal portion

pulp vitality testing diagnostic testing to determine whether the pulp of a tooth is vital (alive) or non-vital (dead)

pulse number of beats produced by the expansion and relaxation of the arterial vessels of the body

pumice ground volcanic ash used to polish natural teeth and some fixed and removable prostheses

rad a basic unit of measurement of ionizing radiation. It is expressed as Gray (Gy)

radiation safety precautions to protect the operator and patient from unnecessary exposure to radiation

radiograph an image projected onto a piece of dental film using the generation of ionizing radiation targeted at the film packet and tooth or teeth to be exposed

recall systems various systems established in the dental office to bring patients back into the practice for routine cleanings, adjustments, and general maintenance appointments. Considered an important part of preventive dentistry

recession loss of part or all of the attached gingiva over the root portion of a tooth

release of information form the patient's written consent to release information regarding dental care and related conditions

rem a basic measurement of ionizing radiation. It is expressed as Sievert (Sv)

removable appliance an appliance that is designed to be seated and removed by the patient

retraction, gingival   a procedure in which temporary tissue displacement is used to widen the gingival sulcus before taking an impression

retrusion   a position of the mandible as far posterior as possible from the centric position, as related to the maxilla

rongeur   a surgical instrument used to nip or remove bone fragments

root amputation   the surgical removal of the root of a tooth

root canal therapy   the removal of the pulpal tissues within the coronal and root portions of the tooth. An inert material is then placed inside the pulp canals and chamber to restore the bulk of the tooth

root planing   the removal of plaque and subgingival calculus from the roots of the teeth

rubber points   points which have been incorporated with a polishing agent and are used to polish metallic restorations

rubber stops   small stops used on endodontic files to note the length of the canal during instrumentation. These stops prevent the accidental perforation of the canal

rugae   a series of folds in the tissue found on the roof of the mouth

saliva ejector   also referred to as "slow speed" evacuator. A thin, single-use attachment connected to its own suction device, used to evacuate saliva from the oral cavity

scaling   the removal of plaque and calculus from the crown and root surfaces of the teeth with the use of curettes and scalers

scalpel   a surgical blade used to create an incision

sealant   resin material used to seal pits and fissures to protect against caries

sedative   a drug administered to diminish excitability and create a calming effect

semicritical instruments   instruments which do not penetrate soft tissue or bone. These instruments require sterilization after each use

shaft   the stem of an instrument designed to provide leverage during use

sharps   characterized as biohazard waste and consisting of orthodontic wires, needles, blades, and broken instruments

sharps management   the method of disposing or handling of any item that is considered to be sharps waste. For example, some of these items would include used needles, blades, endodontic files and broaches, and orthodontic wires

single-ended instrument   hand instrument that has only one working end

single-use instrument   instrument designed to be used only once and then discarded

space maintainer   appliance used after the loss of a primary tooth to maintain the space in the arch until the permanent tooth erupts

sphygmomanometer   a manual blood pressure cuff

spreaders   an endodontic instrument used to manipulate gutta-percha into the canal

State Board of Dental Examiners   the administrative body within its own state that regulates and supervises the practice of dentistry

state Dental Practice Act   the law as it is written that contains the legal restrictions for the dentist and the dental health-care worker in their own state

sterilization   the eradication of all pathogenic organisms

stethoscope   a device used to listen to the heartbeat

stippling   a texture that resembles an orange peel and is reminiscent of healthy gingival tissue

stones   attachments used to polish amalgam, gold, and natural tooth surfaces

stops   small, round, sterile pieces of rubber or plastic that are placed on endodontic instruments to mark the working length

subgingival calculus   hardened deposits found beneath the margin of the gingiva

sulcular fluid   fluid found within the sulcus of the tooth

supragingival calculus   hardened deposits found above the margin of the gingiva

surgical aspirating tip   a specialized suction tip used during surgical procedures. It is smaller in diameter than a standard HVE tip and is used in a wiping motion to keep the surgical field clear of blood and saliva

surgical curette   a surgical instrument used to remove necrotic material from the alveolar socket following an extraction

surgical dressing   see periodontal dressing

surgical stent   a clear acrylic retainer used in the interim for healing and splinting purposes following oral or periodontal surgery

surgical suction tip   a suction tip designed to be used in a wiping or sweeping motion to remove blood and saliva during oral surgery procedures. Surgical suction tips are much smaller in diameter than those used in restorative dentistry

suture   a ligature placed to close an incision

svedopter   a slow-speed saliva ejector that has a curled working end to aid in tissue retraction as well as elimination of saliva from the area of treatment

syncope   fainting

synergistic   when two drugs work together to produce a heightened effect

systolic pressure   the pressure of the blood on the arterial walls, which designates the contraction of the heart muscle

target   the tungsten block which is embedded in the face of the anode. This tungsten block is bombarded by electrons from the cathode which is located in an x-ray tube

temperature   the degree of hot or coldness. The normal temperature for a healthy human is 98.6°F.

three-way syringe   a device equipped with a water and air delivery system. Used to dry and irrigate the oral cavity. Can be used either as air or water or a combination mist

tissue forceps   a surgical instrument that resembles cotton pliers. It is used to reflect tissue away from the surgical area

tofflemire   a matrix retainer and band setup used to replace the missing wall of a tooth while the restoration is being placed

topical anesthetic   a topical ointment used on the oral mucosa to create a temporary diminished feeling

transillumination test   the process of passing a light through the coronal portion of the tooth to detect fractures

treatment plan   a written or discussed plan for delivering treatment presented to the patient prior to the start of the actual treatment

tubehead   the part of the x-ray unit where ionizing radiation is generated

ultrasonic scaling   the use of an ultrasonic scaler to remove calculus from the tooth structures

ultrasonic handpiece   handpieces which remove heavy deposits from tooth surfaces by producing a high-frequency electrical current which mechanically vibrates the deposits from the tooth structures

unit   one part of a whole

universal numbering system   a universally accepted method for identifying teeth by the numbers 1–32 for permanent teeth and the letters A–T for primary teeth

universal precautions   a set of precautions designed to prevent transmission of bloodborne pathogens in a health-care setting

vasoconstrictor   a substance that causes blood vessels to narrow and constrict

vitality   the degree to which a tooth is alive

vitalometer   an electrical device used to register the vitality of the tooth

vital signs   a combination of blood pressure, temperature, respiration, and pulse to establish a baseline for overall patient health

written consent   when a detailed explanation of the diagnosis, prescribed treatment and treatment outcome have been presented to the patient, and a statement outlining the entire planned treatment is signed by the patient before treatment is rendered

working end   the end of the dental instrument designed to perform a task

working length   in endodontic therapy, it is the length of the canal that is established for debriding

x-ray   invisible, penetrable waves of electromagnetic energy, which travel at the speed of light and are used in exposing dental radiographs

zinc phosphate cement   a dental cement used to cement inlays, onlays, and crowns. Composed of zinc oxide and magnesium oxide in a phosphoric acid and water suspension

Appendix A
Index of Abbreviations

Following are examples of abbreviations commonly used in dentistry.

A	amp	d.d.	Let it be given to	lat	lateral
@	at	DO	disto-occlusal	Lt	left
aa	of each	DOB	date of birth		
abs	abscess	Dx	diagnosis	M	mesial
a.c.	before meals			mand	mandibular
a.d.	alternating days	endo	endodontics	max	maxillary
adj.	adjustment	exam	examination	mm	millimeter
anes	anesthetic	Ext	extraction	MO	mesio-occlusal
ant	anterior			MOD	mesio-occlusal-distal
		ff	following		
B	buccal	FGC	full gold crown	norm	normal
BCC	basal cell carcinoma	FH	family history		
BF	bone fragment	FLD	full lower denture	occ	occlusal
bib	drink	FMX	full mouth x-ray	o.d.	every day
b.i.d.	twice a day	frag	fragment	OH	oral hygiene
BP	blood pressure	FUD	full upper denture	OHI	oral hygiene instruction
BS	blood sugar	Fx	fracture	o.m.	every morning
BWX	bitewing x-ray			o.n.	every night
Bx	biopsy	ging	gingiva		
				pano	panorex
C	centigrade or 100	H	hour	PFM	porcelain fused to metal
c	with	h.d.	at hour of bedtime	PLD	partial lower denture
Ca	carcinoma	hr	hour	PO	postoperative
caps	capsules	h.s.	hour of sleep	p.o.	by mouth
cav	cavity	Hx	history	prep	preparation
CC	chief complaint			p.r.n.	as required for
comp	composite	I or Inc	incisal	prog	prognosis
cur	curettage	imp	impression	pt	patient
crn	crown			PUD	partial upper denture
		L	lingual	Px	prophylaxis
D	distal	lab	laboratory		

q	every		surg	surgery
q.d.	every day		Sx	symptom
q.h.	every hour			
q.2h	every two hours		tab	tablet
q4-6h	every four to six hours		temp	temporary
q.i.d.	four times a day		t.i.d.	three times a day
			TLC	tender loving care
RCT	root canal therapy		TMJ	temporomandibular joint
Rt	right		Tx	treatment
Rx	prescription			
			ZOE	zinc oxide eugenol
s	without			
sig	take thou (directions for use)			
stat	immediately			

Appendix B
Resources

The following are publications that can be used as study sources for the Dental Assisting National Board Examination.

Bird, D., A. Ehrlich, and H. Torres. *Essentials of Dental Assisting.* 2nd ed. Philadelphia: W. B. Saunders, 1996.

1999 Candidate Guide for the Dental Assisting National Board, Inc.

Chasteen, J. E., and C. Miyaski-Ching. *Chasteen's Essentials of Clinical Dental Assisting.* 5th ed. St. Louis: C.V. Mosby, 1996.

Dofka, C. M. *Competency Skills for the Dental Assistant.* Albany, N.Y.: Delmar, 1996.

Ehrlich, A. *Nutrition and Dental Health.* 2nd ed. Albany, N.Y.: Delmar, 1994.

Ehrlich, A., D. Robinson, and H. Torres. *Modern Dental Assisting.* 6th ed. Philadelphia: W.B. Saunders, 1999.

Fehrenbach, J.F., and S.W. Herring. *Illustrated Anatomy of the Head and Neck.* 2nd ed. Philadelphia: W.B. Saunders, 1996.

Finkbeiner, B.L., and C.S. Johnson. *Comprehensive Dental Assisting.* St. Louis: C.V. Mosby, 1995.

Giaquinto, C., and R. Albano. *Dental Assisting Test Preparation.* Upper Saddle River, N.J.: Brady/Prentice Hall, 1996.

Little, J., D. Falace, C. Miller, and N. Rhodus. *Dental Management of the Medically Compromised Patient.* 5th ed. St. Louis: C. V. Mosby, 1997.

Malamed, S. F. *Handbook of Medical Emergencies in the Dental Office.* 4th ed. St. Louis: C.V. Mosby, 1993.

Phinney, D. J., and J. H. Halstead. *Delmar's Dental Assisting: A Comprehensive Approach.* Albany, N.Y.: Delmar, 2000.

Phillips, R. W., and B. D. Moore. *Elements of Dental Materials for Dental Hygienists and Dental Assistants.* 5th ed. Philadelphia: W.B. Saunders, 1994.

Sonis, S. T. *Dental Secrets: Questions You Will Be Asked on Rounds, in the Clinic, on Oral Exams, on Board Examinations.* 2nd ed. Philadelphia: Hanley and Belfus, 1999.

Zwemer, T.J. *Boucher's Clinical Dental Terminology: Glossary of Accepted Terms in All Disciplines of Dentistry.* 4th ed. St. Louis: C.V. Mosby, 1993.

Appendix C
Pathways

The following are pathways that will lead to qualification for the Dental Assisting National Board Examination.

Pathway I
Graduation from a dental assisting or dental hygiene program that is accredited by the American Dental Association.

And
Current cardiopulmonary resuscitation (CPR) certification with the American Heart Association or American Red Cross.

Pathway II
High school graduation or equivalent.

And
Two (2) years of full-time employment experience (3,500 hours) and a written recommendation by your dentist/employer.

And
Current cardiopulmonary resuscitation (CPR) certification with the American Heart Association or the American Red Cross.

Pathway III
Status as a current or previous DANB CDA or graduation from a DDS or DMD program accredited by the American Dental Association.

And
Current cardiopulmonary resuscitation (CPR) certification with the American Heart Association or American Red Cross.

Pathway IV
High school graduation or equivalent.

And
A minimum of four (4) years part-time work experience (at least 3,500 hours accumulated over a 48-month period) as a dental assistant verified by dentist-employer.

And
Current cardiopulmonary resuscitation (CPR) certification with the American Heart Association or American Red Cross.

Appendix D
Additional Certifications

The following are additional certification offered by the Dental Assisting National Board.

Radiation Health and Safety Examination (RHS)
100 questions regarding radiation health
and safety

Infection Control Examination (ICE)
100 questions regarding infection control in
the dental field

Certified Orthodontic Assistant Examination
(COA)
The exam includes:
Infection control—100 questions
Orthodontic assisting—210 questions

Certified Oral and Maxillofacial Surgery
Assistant Examination (COMSA)
The exam includes:
Infection control—100 questions
Oral and maxillofacial surgery—220 questions

Certified Dental Practice Management (CDPMA)
The exam includes:
275 questions regarding dental practice
management

Each component has its own pathways
for entrance.
Contact DANB at (800) FOR-DANB for details.

Appendix E
Internet Access

The following provide Internet access for information related to dentistry.

American Dental Assistants Association
http://home.fuse.net/kspradlin/adaainfo.htm

American Dental Association
http://www.ada.org

Centers for Disease Control
http://www.cdc.gov

Dental Assisting National Board
http://www.dentalassisting.com

Occupational Safety and Health Administration
http://www.osha.gov

Bibliography

The following sources were used in compiling the review materials contained in this manual.

Bird, D., A. Ehrlich, D. Robinson, and H. Torres. *Modern Dental Assisting.* 6th ed. Philadelphia: W.B. Saunders, 1999.

California Board of Dental Examiners Infection Control Handbook. Centers for Disease Control Recommendations, July 1994.

1999 Candidate Guide for the Dental Assisting National Board, Inc.

Dofka, C.M. *Competency Skills for the Dental Assistant.* Albany, N.Y.: Delmar, 1996.

Ehrlich, A. *Nutrition and Dental Health.* 2nd ed. Albany, N.Y.: Delmar, 1994.

Fehrenbach, J.F., and S.W. Herring. *Illustrated Anatomy of the Head and Neck.* Philadelphia: W. B. Saunders, 1996.

Finkbeiner B. L. and C. G. Johnson. *Comprehensive Review of Clinical Dental Assisting.* St. Louis: C.V. Mosby, 1995.

Frommer, H.H. *Radiology for Dental Auxiliaries.* 6th ed. St. Louis: C. V. Mosby, 1995.

Malamed, S. F. *Handbook of Medical Emergencies in the Dental Office.* 4th ed. St. Louis: C.V. Mosby, 1993.

Miller, C. H., and C. Palenik. *Infection Control and Management of Hazardous Materials for the Dental Health Team.* 2nd ed. St. Louis: C.V. Mosby, 1998.

Olson, S. *Dental Radiography Laboratory Manual.* Philadelphia: W.B. Saunders, 1995.

Zwemer, T. J. *Boucher's Clinical Dental Terminology.* 4th ed. A glossary of accepted terms in all disciplines of dentistry. St. Louis: C.V. Mosby, 1993.